SORORITY OF SURVIVAL

SORORITY OF SURVIVAL

Katherine A. Newman

Kroshka Books
Commack, New York
1998

Editorial Production: Susan Boriotti
Office Manager: Annette Hellinger
Graphics: Frank Grucci and John M. T'lustachowski
Information Editor: Tatiana Shohov
Book Production: Donna Dennis, Patrick Devin, Christine Mathosian and Tammy Sauter
Circulation: Maryanne Schmidt
Marketing/Sales: Cathy DeGregory

Library of Congress Cataloging-in-Publication Data

Newman, Katherine A.
    Sorority of Survival: Memoirs of a Multiple / Katherine A. Newman.
        p. cm.
    ISBN 1-56072-346-7
    1. Multiple personality—Patients—Miscellanea. 2. Multiple personality—Patients—Biography. 3. Newman, Katherine A.—Mental health.
    I. Title.
RC569.5.M8N49   1996
616.85'236'0092—dc20   96-25582
                                          CIP

Copyright © 1998 by   Katherine A. Newman
                    Nova Science Publishers, Inc.
                    6080 Jericho Turnpike, Suite 207
                    Commack, New York 11725
                    Tele. 516-499-3103 Fax 516-499-3146
                    e-mail: Novascil@aol.com, Novascience@earthlink.net
                    Web Site: http://www.nexusworld.com/nova

Printed in the United States of America

This book is dedicated to Dr. Gregory A. Wilets, who learned of the secret and diligently worked with my case through the roughest years of my life. It is also dedicated to Dr. Loraine Martin, who later became my therapist and would not let anything slide by. She furnished me the opportunity to do some of my best work toward recovery. Also, to my young niece Stephanie, who, in eleven short years, has taught many about love. From her I have learned about courage and the importance of hope and to fight for life. Finally, to the Group, the Sorority, without whose continual support and cooperation, this book could never have happened.

C ONTENTS

PREFACE

I've always felt that truth is the best medicine, and what a better way to get at the truth than directly from the horse's mouth — or mind? That's why I have decided to put my true identity(ies) on the line and present you with my story.

Life as a multiple personality is not a simple life. It can be both heaven and hell at the same time. To say the least, one's life is interesting and unpredictable.

More is being learned about multiple personalities all the time. A valuable source to the public and practitioners would be a biographical sketch of a multiple's own personalities. Things can become lost and muddied through an intermediary.

I and my Group, or Sorority, have all agreed to tell everything; no matter how good or bad the truth is. Some of the truths I have been searching for may come forward. My physicians feel something of this nature will be helpful to my therapy, but may also give other multiples some needed hope.

Katherine and Francie are two of my known alters. They will help me write about my life in general, as they are the most competent at this sort of thing. Katherine is the writer of the Group, and Francie is the Group historian.

Michele M. Newman

PROLOGUE

Michele Marie Newman is a 40 year old white female living in Denver, Colorado. She was born in Sheridan, Wyoming and spent most of her childhood there. She has now lived in Denver for the past eighteen years.

Her personalities began at a very early age. At first they were just make-believe friends. But, in time, they became separate identities; real people. She calls them her Group, or Sorority. Michele has been aware of them since their beginning, but never let anyone know about this Group until 1984. Each personality evolved out of a necessity to survive a situation which Michele, alone, could not deal with or manage on her own.

Michele is an intelligent woman who has been through a lot and experienced a lot in her lifetime. Most multiples have a high level of intelligence — it takes some smarts to create separate identities to face situations on an appropriate basis. Unlike most multiples, she did not experience traumatic physical abuse. Her abuse was emotional rather than physical. There was an occurrence of incest in her history, though.

In addition to multiple personalities, Michele has been diagnosed as having manic-depression (bipolar illness) and pseudo-seizures. This has placed additional complications on her treatment. Like most multiples, she has had her series of various psychological diagnoses and treatments until the truth finally came out.

With Francie's help, I will try to convey to you what Michele's life has been like from as early as we can remember and have documentation for, through the present day. This portion will be written in the first person, as though things were happening and being done by Michele, as they are from her memories. I will put these memories into words for her. This will be less confusing. Then, at the end of Michele's story, each Group member will give an accounting of their life and the roles they had in Michele's life thus far. We will tell when we were born and the lives we live and have lived. The autobiographical sketches of each Group member will be written by that member with my writing just a brief introduction as to where that member falls within the Group. Where one is available, a photo will accompany that biographical sketch.

This story will be broken into parts. Each part represents a move and a different physical environment Michele has been exposed to. Things changed with these moves and so did some of the Group members. Some were strengthened. New ones evolved.

Katherine A. Newman

INTRODUCTION

What's it like to be classified as having multiple personalities? I've found it to be love, chaos and friendship all rolled together. Despite conflicts, misunderstandings and confusion, my alters have been a close-knit family I can rely on. Sisters (and brothers), like in a sorority. They are there when you need them, and sometimes when you don't.

I never thought of my alters as separate identities, though that's what they are. They started as friends and companions; someone to be there in a time of need. I remember spending more time growing up with my Group than my own brother and sister. In fact, I remember very little time being spent with my sister.

Just about every Group member got their beginning to make it possible for me to face the day to day situations life brought. Some were companions in my introverted loneliness. Others took talents and skills I had and developed them into specialties. I have sisters who give me wisdom and organization and the abilities to do things that are beyond my moral standards. I have one to work as a check and balance within the system. There's even some to pull me back to the simpler times of a child. Together, the earlier members helped me make it through childhood and life with an alcoholic parent.

My alters did not start out with names; however, when the names were told to me, there was little uncertainty behind them. I assume everyone in the Group has always had a name, but until my secret sorority was identified and found out, there was no real need for names. I always communicated with them on their basis of talent, skill or otherwise. When you talk with family members one on one, you don't use their real names in the conversation. That's how it was for me.

My Group has generally had a sense of cohesiveness to it, except for two periods of time. Between 1968 and 1972, and 1980 to 1989. Things are fairly stable now and a sense of cooperation has been present. I attribute this to my being less influenced by stress and pressure and to the present regimen of medication I am on.

It was agreed upon, from the start, that no matter who was present, that member would always answer to 'Michele.' It's what you might call a secret pact to keep a secret a secret. It was important to me that no one knew about the others. I had this horrible fear of losing any one of my sisters and brothers whom I'd grown to love and care about deeply. They have been the only true, lifelong friends and family I've had. Losing any one of them, no matter how good or bad their past, would be devastating. It would be like losing my real brother or sister, or worse, like it was when I lost my real father.

I have been in counseling or psychotherapy off and on since 1971. Only after a Group reunion in 1984, during a vacation, was it decided to let someone in on my secret sorority. It was not going to be an obvious disclosure, however. Something had been going wrong in the Group for some time and we seemed to be pulling apart into separate directions from one another. It was decided that Dr. Wilets, our therapist at the time, would be the one to learn about this secret. Everyone seemed to trust him and he had a genuine concern over our wellbeing. He had been confused about my behavior and if my therapy was going to progress, he would need to know what was really going on.

Among the many doctors and therapists I had seen, I had been labeled from depressed to suicidal to psychotic to schizophrenic to severely depressed to neurotic to manic-depressive. Numerous long-term hospitalizations occurred as a result. I felt it was time to lay it all on the line and find out once and for all just how crazy I really was.

I knew I had mood swings — some severe, but never really considered myself as having multiple personalities in terms of a diagnosis. I didn't think my behavior fell into the realm of what little I knew about the illness. I was confused. Dr. Wilets knew of this illness before my own family. Only when it was certain that this was the correct diagnosis, did I fill my family in on the secret. They do have a little better understanding of my behavior, but I feel they are still in disbelief and denial of it.

This illness has created a lot of problems for me workwise and financially. If I hadn't been given the opportunity to take an early retirement option with my employer in 1985, I would have certainly been fired from my position. My absences due to hospitalizations were excessive. I got into such financial trouble by Group members doing their own thing, that in January of 1986, I was informed that my only option would be to file bankruptcy. The filing finally took place in June. It took six months to get organized enough to get all the paperwork together and to the attorney.

Other problems include knowing or remembering what may have been said or done by one of the Group members. Early on, I did not have strong co-consciousness with my alters. I might have said something to or promised someone something and have no memory of it. This began happening a lot at work and was one thing that got me into trouble. This happened more on a social basis, though. Someone would see me and talk to me as if we were the best of friends, and I'd swear I didn't know them nor had never met them. There sometimes may have been a puzzling familiarity to them but that would be all. Blanking out periods of time also happens a lot and goes hand in hand with what I've just explained. I'd forget about going places or doing things on vacations or trips, or even during the course of a normal day. I left Dr. Wilets' office one night, not exactly myself. I went somewhere between 6:30 p.m. and midnight and put about 70 miles on my truck. I'm still not certain of where all I went that night.

Some of my alters have developed certain physical ailments. For three years, I had been diagnosed as having complex partial seizures/temporal lobe seizures, or epilepsy with all the symptoms. Now I'm told they were, in reality, pseudo-seizures. Not all the alters have them. I've also been diagnosed as having functional bowel syndrome at various times. On occasion, I have blood in my stools. I was hospitalized for having bloody diarrhea. When tests were done on me, everything came back normal. It was a pure mystery. I did have witnesses at the hospital when I was admitted that it was real. At times I have been found to have mitral valve prolapse — a type of low grade heart murmur. It is not always heard when I have examinations.

I'm told that research has found that some personalities not only have different characteristics, but may very possibly have certain physiological ailments others don't have. I've been witnessed and monitored having a grand mal seizure and abnormal EEG's, then turn around and have seizures with normal EEG's, or vice versa. I find this to be one of the most difficult parts of my illness to deal with. I'm often finding myself not calling a doctor when something seems to be wrong, for fear that once I'm seen, they find nothing.

Dr. Frank W. Putnam, Jr., whom I saw at the National Institute of Health in Bethesda, Maryland, told me that some multiples grow out of this illness once they feel safe in their existence. It is thought to be a phase, generally more common to women in their late twenties and early thirties. Others with MPD have their personalities fused and integrated back into one, the host. Then, others decide to continue to coexist with a better understanding and communication within the internal family. I love and depend on my alters too much to fuse them together. I will be content if I can live the rest of my life with my alters present in a cooperative cohabitation of my body and mind.

Now that you have had some background on who I am, it is time to tell you my life's story. It has been complex but very exciting. I would not have traded it were I have it all to do over again, because it has made me the strong person I am today. You don't learn to value life until you have almost lost it.

THE DIAGNOSIS

I can't believe it has been just over 10 years since my secret got out. I have made such progress in coming to grips with who belongs to this body and what we are all about. The decision has been made against integration. I need everyone in the Group, so I have agreed to a coop setting for use of my body. So far things seem to be working quite well.

It was the first of June 1984 and I had just returned from an eleven day trip to Montana and the Pacific Northwest. I drove to Billings, Montana from Denver to attend a regional meeting for a professional organization I belonged to. At the conclusion of the meeting, I continued my trip to Anacortes, Washington, the Olympic Peninsula and on to Oregon where I spent some time with some close friends from my college days. From there I went down the California coast before heading due east to Reno, Nevada. I came home by way of Salt Lake City. I took this trip entirely alone — so I thought.

Shortly after my return, I had an appointment with my psychiatrist, Dr. Greg Wilets. I had been seeing him for about three years for an extreme case of chronic depression which had worsened in the previous few years. I was so excited to tell him of my trip and all the beautiful scenery I had encountered along the way. It had been an exhausting trip, but somehow I seemed to have been rejuvenated by it and almost felt like a kid again.

About two-thirds of the way through my session, Dr. Wilets stopped me for some clarification. It seems that I had been using "we" throughout the conversation as if someone had gone with me. I drew a long pause. I wasn't aware of what I had been doing. I didn't know just how to answer him. Then I realized what had happened. A lifetime secret had finally leaked out. Something I didn't consciously want or plan to happen. I had some explaining to do and wasn't quite sure how to do it.

Dr. Wilets sat back and took a deep breath. Something he had considered before but was not sure of had surfaced. He proceeded to explain to me that he now believed that I was suffering from Multiple Personality Disorder. He briefly described the basics of the illness and remarked how, if indeed I was a multiple, many questions regarding my therapy and hospitalizations were about to clear up. It was time for my session to end but he did not want to leave this hanging in the air. We set another appointment for a few days later.

I had the difficult task of trying to explain to him that I had a group of friends who had been present a good deal of the time throughout my life. All my life I had been very introverted and lonely. To accommodate this loneliness I developed a menagerie of friends. I call them my Group or Sorority. To me they were make believe and just voices to keep me company. Many times I thought it was just my conscience talking to me. I told him that I sensed their presence on my trip. In fact, the trip turned out to be not only a vacation, but a reunion rolled into one.

I had lost track of these friends though they were always with me. They had been with me, all right, but doing things without my knowledge. I had lapses of memory and found myself in situations I normally would not be caught dead engaging in.

At my next session we tried to piece things together and put them in perspective. The Group finally became comfortable enough with someone who I felt I could trust and would care about me. It was about time. I had been seeing Dr. Wilets quite regularly for a considerable amount of time. I had been through a number of hospitalizations, including shock treatments, a whole regiment of drug therapies, and some major self-destructive incidents. Through all of this he was always there for me to see that I would make it through in one piece. He suggested that I try to get in touch with all my inner selves and draw some kind of organization chart.

I struggled for the next several days trying to get "in touch" with my so-called other personalities. I went through some of my old medical papers and came across a drawing that I had done earlier, before this diagnosis, that identified different aspects of voices that had made themselves known to me. I think Dr. Wilets had remembered this drawing before me and that was why he was so quick to come up with this new MPD diagnosis. These different parts of me were really identified only by what they were known to my system as. They were nameless and only had labels.

I had drawn a picture of a child standing on a table with descriptive over its head, balloons and parts of the body identified. At the top of the drawing was Self-Annihilation, followed by the Big Guy, Pain, Destructiveness, Ms. Sexy, Hate/Anger, and Depression. The balloons I was holding were labeled: Writing, Photographic, Art/Design, and Vocal. Then there was my body. My head was called Shelley. My arms were Talent and Perfectionist. Michele was the upper torso. I had a belt labeled Mania and legs as Tomboy and The Kid. The table I was standing on was identified as Mom.

Up until this major breakthrough, Dr. Wilets had been treating me primarily for Bipolar Depression and Self-destructive behavior. He was baffled by some of the strange mood swings I would encounter and behavior that was quite unlike the Michele he knew. Much of this was seen during hospitalizations for severe episodes of depression.

My therapy was about to take off in a new direction. Over the course of my next several sessions, the emphasis changed from my problem of depression to trying to explain and understand the "we" that I kept referring to. From these sessions we would hopefully get some answers to problems and questions he had developed concerning me as a patient. We would try to learn about the trauma in my childhood that caused me to split and continue to split to maintain a level of bearable existence. I had some memories, but nothing seemed quite as traumatic as that experienced by most known multiples. Certainly there were memories that were held by some alters that were kept from me as a safeguard.

My sessions intensified and were more frequent. Early in my new therapy those alters who did decide to show themselves came forth slowly and with nameless identities. It wasn't long before a very vocal and destructive alter showed herself. This one was quick to give herself a name. She identified herself as Chrissy. Not until several years later would we learn she was using the name of another alter as a front. Her true name was unknown until a near fatal incident in 1989. She became very adamant about her suicidal feelings. She was not at all interested in going into the hospital. This concerned Dr. Wilets deeply. He was dealing with new individuals he was not familiar with, so he thought.

He received a panic call from me about midday the day after this session. I was sounding real depressed and desperate. He suggested I come in for an emergency session that afternoon. I agreed because I was not in control of my feelings. I was becoming overwhelmed with these new senses and awareness of others sharing my body. I met him after work.

About halfway through the session he had a knock at the door. I was surprised he answered the door and even more surprised by who was there. There was a female and male police officer that had come to help me over to the hospital. Dr. Wilets had felt that I was a definite threat to my well-being and knew I would put up a fight over his suggestion that I go into the hospital again. He couldn't have been any more right in his thoughts.

I attempted to argue with his decision and reluctantly followed the police officers down the elevator and walkway to the hospital. Along the walkway, the destructive alter tried to run but was retained by the officers. A struggle ensued and continued until they got me to the ward.

I was placed immediately in one of the isolation rooms for my own safety. Dr. Wilets reassured me that this was going to be a short stay if I agreed to cooperate. He had placed me on a 72-

hour mental health hold. At that time I was feeling very confused and hurt by his not trusting me. I didn't understand the degree of the threats that this alter had imposed upon him. He had no choice but to take this action.

He admitted me to St. Joseph Hospital psychiatric ward as a result of continued complaints of distortion in time and amnesiac events. The alter had also taken an x-acto knife and cut me several times on the foot.

Over the course of the hospitalization, there was evidence of multiplicity; however, Dr. Wilets was a little conservative in the diagnosis and listed it as atypical dissociative disorder. I had complained of being in different ego states with episodes of amnesia between them. Prior to this time I had also been diagnosed as having a complex seizure disposition and they were not clear as to whether this had any influence on these episodes.

He talked with a number of my ego states while in the hospital and had hoped to get a better understanding of how destructive this alter felt and what her true intentions were. It kind of backfired on him. She acted out a little but then got scared off because she was no longer in control of the situation. That's how she was; she had to have the upper hand on the situation or would disappear from the scene.

The hospitalization was brief as promised. Just a few days. Not a lot of ground got covered, but at least I regained some control over my feelings and was not in imminent danger any longer. At least for awhile.

This little surprise from Dr. Wilets scared some of the alters terribly. He had become somewhat of a threat to their control issues. Trying to explain the way things were was not easy, because of my lack of co-consciousness at times. Control is a big issue for many of the Group members. They pulled back and were very hesitant about making any appearances in the sessions that followed.

He saw what had happened and suggested that he try a new angle on my therapy to prod some of the alters into showing themselves. He suggested using hypnosis. I remembered one instance when I was in junior high when there was a magic show and hypnosis was used. I was one of the guinea pigs for the act but found myself having to fake the hypnotic trance because I didn't relax enough to be pulled under the trance. I told him that there may not be a level of cooperation that would be conducive to being drawn into a trance. Regardless, I wanted to cooperate and allowed the sessions to begin.

I did obtain a hypnotic trance. Initially they were strained at best, but as time progressed I found it easier to relax and succumb to the trance. Alters did come out and speak their mind. Reluctantly at first, but soon gained enough courage to be uninhibited.

I had a very slight co-consciousness to these sessions. The words seemed to flow from the alters. I had no viable control over what was being said. Dr. Wilets would discuss what had come from the session. I was somewhat surprised with some of their remarks.

Once the alters again felt safe with Dr. Wilets and understood that he really did care, hypnosis was not necessary, except with extreme memories or feelings of guilt. Soon they came forth whenever they had something to say. At first the alters had no names. They were types of people. Soon they wanted their own identities and no longer wanted to be recognized specifically for their talents, even though that's still how I tend to recognize them.

Keeping track of who is who has become harder of late because so many of them are crossing over to others' boundaries and job functions. At first I thought I had about 10-12 alters. This then grew to about twenty. Now I don't have a clue as to how many alters or fragments of alters I have. New ones keep popping up and claiming some territory. I welcome all my alters and treasure each and everyone of them, but life is real confusing. They aren't afraid to make their presence known anymore.

New talents evolve with every life situation I encounter. I feel I spend most of my time on auto-pilot and the one who knows what to do steps up to the plate and gains control of the situation as warranted. Their actions don't always come without flaws, though. Some step up without a clue as to how the situation should really be handled. They feel the bravest at the time and have the best level of confidence for the task at hand. Many days I draw a complete blank as to what went on because so many alters had a handle on helping me get through that day's events.

This is how things work now. It wasn't like that earlier in my therapy. There was no control. Everyone was vying for their fair share of time out to accomplish their own predetermined goals. Things got real messy at times and I found myself backed into corners from time to time with what seemed like an impossible way out. My life was a tangled up mess. Dr. Wilets thought the only solution was integration. MPD was not widely accepted when I received my diagnosis. Doctors were still learning about how to treat it. It wasn't until I wound up at the National Institute of Health in Bethesda, Maryland in 1986 that the renowned doctor in the treatment of MPD, Dr. Frank Putman, had suggested that there was another option available to me. That option involved a level of cooperation and communication amongst the entire Group.

I have grown up a lot in the past few years as my manic-depression has been brought under control by the right medication. Thank God for the progress medicine has made in the treatment of this illness. Dr. Wilets and I have concluded that my alters have greater difficulties with control and cooperation when I am depressed or manic. When I have been in my mood swings is when I have ended up out of control, confused and a threat to my own well-being.

Before I go any further describing how my therapy progressed from the point of diagnosis, I feel you need to understand how my life evolved into such a state of torment and confusion and then how I climbed out of my deep hole of despair to lead what I hope is a newly rejuvenated and focused life.

MY EARLIEST MEMORIES

It is so hard to speak of your birth if you don't remember it. How many individuals do remember that glorious event anyway? There's a lot I don't remember about my childhood, but I'm sure there's much that normal human beings don't remember. Then, again, there are certain memories which are as vivid as if they had happened to me just yesterday. I may jump around a bit in telling my story, but that's the way my memories come. One memory often leads to others and sometimes I get sidetracked.

As I'm told, it was a mild December afternoon when my mother's water broke and she went into labor. Labor was long and hard for her. When it was evident that I wasn't going to make a speedy entry and come that evening, the doctor gave my mom some morphine to kill the pain and give her some rest. Actually, it did just the opposite. It made her very ill. She vomited all through the night and became very dehydrated. With all the upheaval that was going on, I turned a few times. When my mom was finally taken to the delivery room, she was taken with an IV in her arm. They were afraid I may come breach. The spinal they attempted to give her didn't take, either. Well, at the last minute I turned again and came out the right way. I was born on Wednesday, December 15, 1954 at 2 p.m.

I was born the second of three children. I had an older brother, Roger, who was almost two years older than me. I was the first girl. In fact, at the time, I was the first granddaughter born to my dad's parents. Despite all the problems during labor and delivery, I was a healthy and normal baby as far as everyone could tell.

I was born in the small western community of Sheridan, Wyoming to Eric and Harriet Newman. I was normal, yet again, I wasn't. I was a very quiet baby. So quiet, in fact, that I rarely cried out. Not even when I was hungry or my diaper soiled. My mom was always checking on me and waking me to see if I was okay. I slept a lot as a baby. Even though I was quiet, I observed a lot of what was going on around me when I was awake.

My mom said I was an exceptional baby. Other than this great disposition, I guess I had the same wants and needs of any baby. I was very precocious at an early age. I was walking and feeding myself by the time I was one. I was forming sentences and in daytime training pants.

I almost had to be this advanced, because I sensed something different about my mom. She was getting big, and rightly so, because eleven months after I was born, I had a new bouncy, crying baby sister.

Suddenly, I felt deprived of my mother's attention. I was no longer the central point of her attention; it all seemed to be going to my sister, Karla. I was on my own and had to learn to fend for myself. It was expected even more of me since I was so independent and as advanced as I was. I seemed to have sensed the birth coming and knew I would be left a lot by myself. Something kept drumming into my head that I was going to have to go it alone. Besides, it's not an easy chore to keep track of one baby, let alone two. This was my first experience in survival.

I didn't allow myself to go totally unnoticed. I made my presence known by wanting to help with my sister and occasionally demanding that her bottle was "my bobble."

My parents had two houses when I was born. We lived in the smaller one and rented out the larger one to two different families until Karla was born. When she was born, we moved back into the big house and took over the whole house. My parents then rented out the smaller house in the back.

My parents were both self-employed with a gas station and rent-a-car franchise. They soon provided limousine service from the tiny 2-flights a day airport and were on call at all hours; especially in the winter when weather caused flight delays and layovers. Needless to say, I grew up with babysitters.

I continued to remain quiet while around other people and pretty much to myself. I seemed sad most of the time but was not alone because I had some real and imaginary friends to talk to or just have around when I did need some company.

As I search back into my childhood, I remember my first friend coming to me when I was about 2-1/2. We lived in a town where we had an annual All-American Indian Days celebration every August. I was intrigued by all the pageantry and mystery of the Indians.

I had the voice of a wise old Indian man come to me. I don't think I was intelligent enough to understand what he said, but I just remember a warm and loving presence about me that comforted me and made me feel cared about. It was as I grew up and became a little older that he came back and explained how and why he chose to appear to me.

He introduced himself as Whispering Owl. He was an old Medicine Man of the Cherokee Nation. He said he saw me in a vision and found me to be a very sad and lonely child that needed some wisdom in how to cope with my surroundings and family situation. From that point on no matter how lonely I may have felt, I was no longer alone. I had someone I could talk to and share my feelings. Someone who somehow understood and had great patience with me.

He was like a grandfather to me. He was one of my best friends when he was around, but would go away for long periods of time. He would tell me stories about how the Indians and settlers used to live. He almost made me wish I was one of them. I often liked to pretend I was an Indian or cowgirl.

As I grew up, I never had the proper influence to develop strong people skills. I was so used to being by myself that I didn't know how to respond to others. There was always an ever present sense of discomfort around people and other kids.

Don't get me wrong. I did have friends as I grew up, but would never consider any of them close. They were more like comrades that helped me get into trouble or do things that were not proper. Because the trauma of being around others was so uncomfortable for me, I developed additional alters that would allow me to cope with being around people.

One of these alters was Mike, the tomboy of the Group. One of my few male alters. He fit in with all the guys in the neighborhood.

A boy my age, Rusty, lived a couple blocks away and was my best real friend. We played often when I was big enough and able to leave the yard. His folks had an old storage shed that we'd climb up on and just sit and talk or jump off of. We would sing "Take Me Out To The Ball Game" and jump off the roof. We would do it with our eyes shut, hand in hand and backwards. Fortunately, there never was a sprained ankle or any broken bones.

We spent a lot of time over at the school yard playing on the fire escape, collecting pigeon feathers, or climbing on the old boiler building. We did this when I was big enough to climb the one story building. I would get a verbal scolding for doing this. It was hard keeping it a secret from my parents, because the building had a red roof which would rub off on us and our clothes.

Johnny and Rusty were Mike's best friends until one day when I became more than one of the guys. The boys knew I was a girl. One day, they invited me over to Johnny's house to play cops and robbers in the basement. I was the one who got caught. During the interrogation, they made me strip down to my underpants and then tied me to a chair. I fought them for the longest time, but they convinced me it was okay and they wouldn't tell anyone if I promised not to. I was seven about this time. It was the breeding ground for a new alter, Sally. It is unclear if anything else transpired beyond that point. I'm sure Sally or Monique know and they are keeping it a deep dark secret for now.

Our friendship changed from that point on and I distanced myself from them. It was something that was bad enough to cause a friendship to diminish. Somehow, I could never face them again.

It wasn't long after this event that I discovered my sexuality. I spent many of my summer evenings alone on the old swing set in the back yard. We called them the "monkey bars" because they had a double bar across the top which you could climb around on. Most of the time I'd just climb on top and lay across the two bars and watch the sun set. In the fall I'd watch the geese fly south for the winter. One day, as I was playing around on them, I discovered a very wonderful thing. If I would hang from the bars and pretend I was climbing a rope, a very special sensation and tingling would go through my body. This became a regular ritual when I was by myself and no one was around to see what I was doing. I did this often because it made me feel real good. It wasn't until I was older that I learned what was happening to me was that I was having a woman's orgasm.

Mike resorted to playing with my brother when he needed manly companionship. He climbed trees by himself, and jumped at every opportunity to go to the mountains with my father to go fishing.

My protectors The Big Guy and Chrissy also appeared before I was in grade school. Our parents got called away to the airport one stormy night and didn't have time to find a baby-sitter. The lady next door wasn't home so us three kids had to stay alone.

I always had a fascination with thunderstorms. They scared me, but intrigued me at the same time. I would always count to see how far away the storm was. That night we had a horrible thunderstorm. We were fine until the lights went out. We finally found a flashlight, but were afraid and went out to the front of the house on the step and huddled together until mom and dad came home. For a three or four year old, this was a terrifying experience to face alone.

When TV's came out in the 50's, my dad bought the first one in the neighborhood. It was something new to do, but I didn't spend a whole lot of time watching it. I would watch it more in the evening when it was dark and there was little playing to do. When I did watch it, I got very involved and intrigued with what was going on during the program. I got more into TV as time went on and took everything very seriously. On nights when my parents weren't home, my brother and sister would talk the baby-sitter into letting us watch a late, scary movie. I was usually afraid to watch them since I believed a lot of what I saw to be real. I never had nightmares that I can remember, but it did make me a little frightened of the dark. However, as I got older, I understood what was real and what wasn't, and even enjoyed watching the scary movies. In fact, I usually preferred to watch the movies or longer lasting programs. Shows that you could really get into. They became fantasies of mine. They still do. I rarely cared for watching cartoons. I would watch them only when it was Roger or Karla's turn to watch what they wanted. Often, I'd go off at these times and play by myself.

I had other memories in that big Victorian home. Some were good and some were not so good. Each time I found myself alone or feeling like an outcast, I called on my newfound friends. My Sorority of Survival. It had a lot of places to play and go to be alone. It made things easier when I wanted to play with my friends. My mom wasn't around to ask me who I was talking to. I shared a room with my sister. We had a deep, claw-foot tub that was almost big enough for me to swim in. We also had two porches. The front one had a little room off it where we stored a lot of our toys. The basement had one big room that the furnace was in and three small rooms, of which included a canning room. We used it just to store canned goods. I overcame the fear of the darkness and cold of the basement in exchange to be alone.

I was not a healthy child when we lived on Fifth Street. I did not like food. I was always protesting having to eat. I guess I had an iron deficiency or something. I had to go to the doctor regularly for shots. I despised them. I would always run and hide when I caught wind of what was about to happen. One time I was so adamant about not going that I was going to hide so no one would find me and I would miss my appointment. Before, I had hidden in various places in the basement. In the dark where I was terrified. But nothing was as terrifying as those big needles. Always I was found out. This time I tried a different tactic. I searched high and low for a new place to hide. This time I hid in the china closet at the foot of the stairs. It was a good place, my mom looked for the longest time to find me. I did miss my appointment, but I paid for it. My perfect hiding place was found out and I got a spanking that was almost as bad as the shot. I did end up getting the shot anyway.

I rarely got into trouble when I was a little girl. I was generally patient and obedient because I knew I'd get a spanking if I wasn't. I was more helpful than destructive at the 18 month to three year old age. The one thing I would get punished regularly for though was not eating. My parents would not let me get down from the table until I ate what they told me to eat. There were many times that I bribed my sister to eat my food when my parents left the table. I promised her that I would do her chores if she would eat my food so I could leave the table. When Karla, my sister, was not around and I was in kindergarten, I could not go to school until I ate my sandwich or soup. I was tardy numerous times. My dad would usually drive me the three blocks to school in tears.

Because of my deficiency, I had a tendency to get real sick when I caught a cold. When I got the measles and chicken pox, I was real sick. I scratched myself until I bled. These sores then turned into big scabs. I was often sick at Christmas time. Karla and Roger were jealous because I got 7-Up when I was sick and they didn't. This did not help with their acceptance of me.

We did some things that kids were not suppose to do or that our parents did not approve of. We were scolded, but I'm sure not any differently than other kids in those days. I was terrified of my parents so I went out of my way to please them. My father took his belt to me just twice. That was all it took for me to learn who was the boss. My mom did most of the punishing. Her favorite punishment was to smack you hard with a wooden spoon or a yardstick. She broke many a yardstick on us kids. My brother got the worst of it. Just seeing the welts on his leg or arm was enough to run terror through my bones. They controlled me through intimidation.

Other than being forced to stay at the table, I rarely got scolded as a small child. As a rule, my parents didn't really like punishing me because I was so good. I'd generally do as I was told then go off and play with my siblings, friends or self and be content. One of my belt lashings came when my mother found that I had cut all the beads off an old Indian papoose carrier she had received from an Indian couple.

The other time my dad took his belt to me was when I was in the second grade. Some of the neighborhood kids had discovered some metal caps that fell from a train. My parents threatened me with severe punishment if they ever caught me over by the train tracks. This was one time when I was invited to participate with the other kids. I went knowing fully well that I would be punished if my parents ever found out. I got so wrapped up in the activity that I was late coming home for dinner. My parents were extremely worried about me. In addition to getting the belt, this was the first and only time my parents ever grounded me.

I did get into some minor trouble one time by going through a neighbor's trash cans with Rusty and Johnny before breaking apart. I would also get scolded for crossing the big street in front of our house because it was a main street and had a lot of traffic. I would also venture a block away to the river that ran through town. It had a steep embankment and my parents were worried that I would slip and fall in. The scoldings were not usually more than a way to get some attention, so I did this often. It was the only way I could get my parents to show me they loved and cared about me.

I did do some things my parents never found out about. When I was five or six, my parents let me go to the grocery store three blocks away. I would buy one or two things for my mom when she asked me to go. What she didn't know, was that on about a half dozen different occasions I would steal some candy or gum. I don't know why I did it but just did. I wanted the candy or gum and could have bought it with the spare change my mom had coming, but didn't do it that way. I still don't understand why I was compelled to steal it.

My parents had several businesses going. They owned a gas station, Avis Rent-A-Car franchise, and on occasion, the city taxi and limousine service. They were always meeting people and gone a lot. They had to be on-call at all times to meet the airplane which was often off schedule in the winter because of weather. In the summer, they would drive people out to local dude ranches and up into the mountains. They would also have to go after their cars when they were dropped off in other towns. My parents even rented a car once to Prince Phillip of the English Crown.

As young kids and because our parents had a lot of responsibility with their business, we were assigned chores at an early age. I remember doing dishes while standing on a stool. I wasn't even big enough to reach over the sink, and I was tall for my age. We were given adult responsibilities that should have come much later. My childhood was lost early on. We also had to keep our room clean and work out in the yard and garden. We had lots of trees in our yard so when fall came, there were plenty of leaves to rake. This was one chore I looked forward to, because it afforded me an opportunity to play while I worked.

When I grew out of my friendship with Rusty and Johnny, I turned to adults in the neighborhood. I was mature enough at an early age that I associated well with the older people. I really liked helping some of them in their yards or just listening to their stories. A couple who lived across the alley from us had a big yard and lots of bushes and flowers in the back. They even had a fish pond where they kept giant goldfish and had some frogs that would sit on the lily pads. I would help them in the garden or even help feed the fish or clean the pond. Sometimes we would just sit around the fish pond for hours and talk or watch the fish and frogs. I was even there in the fall when they got their winter shipment of coal for their furnace. I would help shovel it into the basement.

There was also an old gentleman who lived across the street who had a peg leg. I would visit him for hours and he would fascinate me with stories of the old days in Sheridan and the west. He'd talk about the mountains and real cowboys and Indians. One day he had what I was told was a heart attack in his car in front of his house. This was my first experience with a human death. I was sad, because I had lost a real good friend.

An old widow lived next door. She was like another grandmother to me, my brother and sister. Sometimes she would get to baby-sit us. She was neat. She would bake us cookies to have with our milk. She also let me help her with her garden in the back yard. She even let me help paint part of her house once. This would have been work to most kids, but I got a lot of joy out of it. She lived in that house for a long time. She was nearly 100 years old when she died just a few years ago.

Another prominent adult in my early childhood was the lady who would come in and help my mom keep the house clean and laundry caught up. She would baby-sit us on numerous occasions. She did most of the baby-sitting until I was eight years old. She was nice and kind to us. She would play with us or let us go off and play by ourselves. Whatever kept us content.

In addition to being sickly, I was quite clumsy as a little girl. I was always tripping over things or falling down. I always had cuts and bruises on me somewhere. I was running down a small hill one time and tripped and fell at the bottom and got a big bruise on my hip. The bruise seemed to last forever. My mom was so concerned that she took me to the doctor. He said I may have bruised the bone or chipped it. To this day, if I run into something with that hip, I have an excruciating jab of great pain.

The worst tumble that I took happened one day when I was playing jump rope in the driveway in our back yard. We were playing chase. I was going so fast that I caught the tip of my toe on the rope and ran straight into the door post on the garage. I had glasses and was in the second grade at the time. I bent and put a big dent into my new glasses. I had a headache that would not end and was dizzy for quite some time afterward. I had a small cut over my eye. My mom called the doctor. He said I probably just got a mild concussion and should lay down with a cold compress over my forehead.

Mike was quite a tree climber, but he was also quite a daredevil up in the tree. He would try to go to great heights and sometimes would slip on the slick branches and get scratched up from time to time. On another occasion I stepped on a rake that was laying with tines up and got a small puncture wound on my foot and got hit in the face.

One Christmas, we nearly lost our Christmas tree. I was standing on a table helping hang some tinsel when, suddenly, I lost my balance and fell into the tree. The whole thing fell with me on top of it. Fortunately, only a few balls were broken and none of the lights. I was more embarrassed and frightened than hurt.

My mom seemed to be sympathetic and comforting in these moments. It isn't clear to me, but I may have been more careless than usual at these times knowing that I was going to get some attention. At no time do I think any of this was premeditated, but I won't go so far as to deny that an alter may not have been deliberate with accidents from time to time.

I was jealous of my brother at Christmas. He seemed to get all the really neat toys. He got a train set with a tunnel, town scenery and crossing lights. He even got a race car set one Christmas. To say the least, Mike spent a lot of time in his room playing with his toys. He didn't mind it, either. In fact, I think he liked having someone to play with who really appreciated his toys.

I remember going to visit my dad's parents a lot when I was young. They lived at least a mile away from our house. When I was in school, my parents would let me and my sister walk down to their house alone. We would talk a lot, but usually I would spend more time with my grandfather in his garden, or in the garage just watching him. He would let me pick strawberries and carrots from the garden in the summer when they were ready. We would sit on the back porch eating them. My grandpa was the first one to introduce me to smoking. We were sitting on the back steps one night and I asked him why he smoked. Both my parents smoked and I was curious about this activity. He said that I could try it for myself and see what I thought of it. Well, I didn't like it very much because I got tobacco in my mouth. This was before filtered cigarettes were around. It was hard for me to understand why people did smoke when I found it to be so awful.

My mom's parents moved into the house out back when I was just starting school or in the first grade. They moved from Billings, Montana. It was fun to have them. My grandmother was a great cook and I would often go over to their house for cookies and milk after school. My grandmother had an old piano that she would let me play sometimes. My grandfather had a way with animals. We had a lot of squirrels in the neighborhood. He had a real attraction to them. He had tamed a number of them to the point that they would crawl up his leg and take nuts right out of his hand. I really liked to watch him with the squirrels and would sit real still out on the sandbox with him.

We had a blonde cocker spaniel when I was born. Her name was Sandy. I didn't get too attached to her, but did find her to be company at various times when alone. My first experience of loss was one cold, fall evening. She had been let outside. My dad was going to have to go to the airport and had the car warming in the street. There were leaves under the car and the heat from the engine warmed the leaves. Sandy crawled under the car. Sandy was still outside when my dad went to leave. It didn't occur to him to look for her. As he started to take off she tried to crawl out from under the car and he ran over her. I was real sad, but don't remember really crying a lot. I guess that was because I hadn't learned how to become really attached to anything yet.

Not too long afterward, we got another cocker spaniel. This one was black and his name was BoBo. My grandfather did not like this dog because he liked to chase the squirrels. My grandfather was always chasing him off or spraying him with something. I did not like my grandfather for doing this at all. I thought he was very cruel and thinking only of himself. Needless to say BoBo ran away one day and we never saw him again.

We also had a beautiful white cat at one time. I really liked that cat. She got down in the basement and became lost. I thought I heard her in the back storage room behind our furnace. We never found her. She may have died wedged in the duct work of the house. The meowing stopped after a couple days. Despite my fear of going in that back room I would go there from time to time in hopes of finding her.

I really liked animals. They were great silent companions. They would not hurt me or scold me or tell me bad things about me. They didn't expect me to do things for them other than to love them. They gave me love back in return.

Most of my play time was by myself. I don't remember where my sister was. I do remember a few occasions playing with her, but for the most part I have very few memories that include her. I think I had a great resentment toward her coming along and taking my mother's attention away from me.

I rarely played with dolls. Sometimes I played with stuffed animals. I would play house with them. A lot of time was spent in the basement playing with Legos, tinker toys, and log cabin blocks. The basement was dark and a place I would hide from others. I also spent a lot of time in the sandbox. Mike loved constructing things. There may have been another alter at that time that helped him. Maybe it was Bonnie. Mike made another alter friend about this time. Her name is Peggy. She looked up to Mike and attached herself to him like Velcro. She idolized him.

Bonnie and Bobbie spent a lot of time drawing and painting. They are twins. These two were my early artistic alters. They were very creative. These two came across a beaded papoose carrier that an Indian family had given my parents when they bought a car from us. I was so young at the time that I had no concept of its potential value. All I saw was the beautiful beads. I wanted to make an Indian headband and necklace and found this to be a great source of beads for them. I proceeded to cut the beads from the leather for my projects. When my mom discovered what I had done, I was punished severely. My dad belted me and I was sent to my room without dinner. This was a hard lesson that taught me to hold the highest level of respect for other's property.

My parents went to a lot of meetings and conventions because of their rental agency. Following one trip to New York, they returned with a gift for my sister and me. The "in" thing in New York and latest craze was Barbie and Ken. To keep us from fighting, they bought one of each. Since Mike was dominant at that time with all my tomboyish activities, I, of course, got the Ken doll. I was very jealous of my sister's Barbie because she had beautiful hair and lots of beautiful clothes. My Ken doll was just a boy doll with plain clothes. He had fuzz for hair that eventually wore off. His arm also kept popping out. I don't remember whether I was too rough with him or he was just poorly made. I wanted to play with the Barbie doll, but from the earlier bead incident, learned to respect my sister's property and never tried to take it from her. I would occasionally play with my sister to have some sort of exposure to this beautiful doll.

Our family would go on outings to the mountains numerous times during the summer. My dad liked to go fishing, and so did Mike. My dad, brother and I had our own fishing poles and would go off fishing while my mom and sister would stay near the car and fix a picnic lunch for us. We used to take an old Volkswagen beetle to the mountains. It got good traction going up the treacherous mountain road. It was a scary road because it got real narrow on one corner near an old spring. It was barely wide enough for one car to get through. The cliffs along the road were real steep and didn't always have trees there to protect you. Anyway, back to the car. My sister and I would usually fight over who got to sit in the storage compartment behind the back seat. Usually we both would get back there for awhile. One time when we were on a fishing trip, my dad decided to go cross country in the little bug. Well, he came to a little gulley and tried to cross it. We got both bumpers high-ended and were stuck for some time. That was a scary trip because we thought we'd never get out of our predicament. Somehow, late in the afternoon, my dad got things figured out and we were on our way. My parents argued about it the whole way back. My dad seemed real calm and matter-of-fact about the whole incident.

I was a good student in school. All my teachers liked me. I guess that comes from being so mature and able to get along with adults. I seemed to get along better with older people than those of my own age. My kindergarten teacher gave me the highest marks for everything. This included areas of language, social, expression, health, work and mental. I got high marks for even playing with the boys, because I was at least socializing. My teacher wrote on my report card, "Michele is doing very well. She has many interests – she plans well and is able to finish what she has planned." Going to school was fun because I could express myself in ways there that I couldn't at home. I was introverted but my teachers usually overlooked this because I was so outgoing in other aspects; mainly my talents.

In first grade I got good marks for everything but reading. Even then, I was always improving steadily. I got my first A's in first grade, too. That was in art. Her comment was, "I have surely enjoyed having Michele in my room this year. She is a fine youngster."

Second grade was a bit more challenging for me. I initially had difficulties with reading, language and arithmetic. By the end of the year, though, I was doing very well with everything but knowing my number facts in arithmetic. Comments from this, one of my favorite teachers, was "Michele is a very good student and splendid citizen." Also, she wrote, "Michele is working with the upper third of her class in all subjects except Science and Social Studies. She is doing average work in these areas." and, "Michele has exceptional work habits, so she is an excellent student. I have enjoyed having her in my Second Grade."

In first and second grade Mike would again play with the boys during recess and tried to out-perform the other kids in gym class.

I obtained great respect and admiration from the teachers and school staff but not from my peers. In a school full of laughing, playing kids, I was alone. No one to really call a friend. My only friends were the adults around me that I came in contact with.

I got to join Brownie Girl Scouts when I was in the second grade. This was a real help to get me away from my wanting to be alone and away from people. I made a lot of new friends my own age. The girls and leaders respected me for who I was and my talents. This was the beginning of a very strong devotion I would have towards something that helped me become a well-rounded and independent person. I took the Promise and Laws literally.

THE BIG MOVE

One day shortly after school started of my third grade year, my dad came home and gave us the news that we were going to move. He felt we needed a higher social stature than we had.

We were going to move up on "the hill" where most of the prominent people in town lived. My dad had gone out and found and made a contract without any consultation with the family. A big fight ensued that evening. It was the second worst fight I remembered to that point. So, we moved away from the big, neat house.

The first fight that I remembered took place in the kitchen. My mom to this day denies what I remember as the way it happened. I don't think I would remember it so vividly if it hadn't really happened. My mom and dad got into a shouting and shoving match. What about I don't remember. My dad shoved my mom against the refrigerator and cupboards. She tells me she had broken her finger before that fight and it hadn't healed. I don't remember that. All I remember was that during that fight, she cried out in excruciating pain and her little finger was bloody and the bone was showing through the skin.

The fight over the move was just a shouting match to the best of my recollection. My mom didn't put up too big a fight. She just kept arguing where we were going to get the money and how could we afford to live up there. She was really glad to be moving up in the world even if it meant having to work much harder at the business.

My mom belonged to a local temple of the Daughters of the Nile and was going to be queen in 1965. It would be embarrassing to her to still be living in our old house. She wanted a nice place to entertain the women and people she would get to know from this. She knew it would be tight and lots of work, but realized it was something she would enjoy.

The house we bought belonged to one of the owners of one of the two big furniture stores in town. My dad bought the house with all the furniture, so our move was not that big a deal. We just packed up all our personal belongings and moved. I don't remember the actual move. I just remember being in one house then all of a sudden in the new house. The house was modern and the furniture was luxurious. We had a piano and a xylophone and two fireplaces. There was a shuffle board in the den. The living room had tables with marble tops.

My mother moved the home office into the bedroom in the basement. Karla and I shared a double bed in a pink bedroom upstairs. Roger was in the bedroom next to ours, and our parents were at the end of the hall off the bathroom.

I thought this move would be a great opportunity to make some new friends starting in a new school and all. The excitement of the possibility of friends didn't change my social skills. I was still mainly a loner, shy and intimidated by the other kids. I wasn't outgoing enough to initiate conversations or to give myself permission to join in games with the other kids.

I took up orchestra and violin lessons in hopes of fitting in with some of the other kids. My dad used to play a pretty mean fiddle. At the same time, my mom had enrolled me in piano lessons with a teacher that lived about 4-5 blocks from us. I don't know what made them think I was musically inclined. I just remember banging on the new piano. They took this for a desire to want to learn. This brought out a new alter, Susan. She managed to fake her way through these lessons and gain some recognition. It also brought tears. She didn't know music and notes. She learned to play mostly by ear and just faking it. I got into trouble on numerous occasions by continuing to play the piece and not turning the page to where the notes were. I wasn't much for practice, either and this got me into trouble.

Susan became frustrated with the piano lessons and violin after a couple years. By the time I got into the sixth grade, she decided she wanted to try to get recognition another way and took up the trumpet. This time she made a better attempt at practicing and learning her music. The big push for taking up the trumpet was to be able to play for the flag raising before the school day started. All the trumpet players in the band at school took their turn playing revelry. My first attempt was not so successful, because the air was cold and my mouthpiece was not warmed up. It was an embarrassing first showing. I was given the tip of keeping the mouthpiece in my pocket as I went to school so it would be nice and warm and easy to play. This worked. I continued to play for about three weeks. By that time the six month trial rental was up on the trumpet. I had to decide whether my parents were going to have to buy the trumpet or whether I would quit. It was decided that I would give up the trumpet if they would buy me a guitar. Susan would teach herself to play.

Once again at this new school I received high grades and the respect and admiration of the teachers. I got along great with them and they favored me in the classroom. The other kids did not like this. At least that's how it seemed. They were always teasing me.

Until I got in the third grade I weighed less than my younger sister, Karla. Because of the constant nagging and intimidation from my mother about not eating, I started to eat what I was told to avoid any punishment. I began gaining weight. So much so that the kids teased me because of it. My eyesight was also bad and I had thick glasses. The boys called me names like German Tank and Cyclops. They were cruel and it caused me to draw within myself more.

One boy decided to really lay into me and tease me to the max. I wasn't going to sit back and take it any longer. I chased him all over the playground and around the building a couple times until I chased him into the boys bathroom. I got into trouble for defending my ego. Chasing him was inappropriate behavior.

Despite my increased weight, I continued to maintain a high level of agility and physical fitness. I did not earn the Presidential recognition for physical fitness but did receive the standard physical fitness award. I played dodge ball with the big kids. Often I was able to end up as one of the last ones in the pen. I walked to school every day except when the weather was real bad or cold. It was about 15 blocks to school, plus I had a big hill to go down. There were about 120 steps from the bottom of the hill to the top.

The hill was great in the winter for sledding. I learned to slide down the hill on my two feet without a sled like the big kids. I was proud, but still unable to win friendships by all my abilities.

As an attempt to obtain new friends at the new school, I joined that school's Girl Scout troop. Once again my perfectionistic overachiever made a strong showing. I think this alter's name is Shelley, but I'm not so sure she was the only one with this kind of behavior. I don't think she is totally responsible for all the achievements I've made through the course of my life. It became a game to see how many badges and accomplishments I could attain.

I did make some friends of other overachievers, but they never really became close friends. In fact, instead one girl, Wendy, that I wanted to recognize as my friend, really became a childhood opponent. We were friends to a degree, but were actually always competing against one another to see who could do more or win more. This lasted through the years that I was in Sheridan.

One day after school, while in the sixth grade, she and some of the guys were teasing me. There was snow on the ground. They threw rocks at me as I was climbing the steps up the hill. I got hit and it hurt. It made me very mad. I took off after them and chased them up the rest of the stairs and around the back yard of my old kindergarten teacher's house. I finally caught up with Wendy, grabbed her and flung her down in the snow and mud and proceeded to beat up on her. We still remained friends but at quite a distance. We were in so many activities together that it was not going to be easy ignoring her without dropping out of sight altogether. Her camaraderie was too important so I let bygones be bygones.

Our family life changed with the move. We upgraded ourselves into a new status level and found ourselves trying to keep up with the Jones'. My parents tried to give us whatever we asked for as a way to replace any love. They were with the business at all times of the day and night. They built an addition onto the back of the gas station for the office and rent-a-car headquarters. My mom was no longer at home when we got home from school. We became latchkey kids without the key. You see in those days we didn't have the crime you now find in neighborhoods. The back door was always unlocked.

I felt a new level of tension evolve in our home. I didn't understand it. Everyone was changing into strangers. I even took on new identities. My brother was starting to go through puberty or something his first year in junior high. My parents were around less and less and thought we were old enough to take care of ourselves. Little did they know what was going on behind their back.

My brother had started to take his sexual experimentation beyond himself. It started out slowly with a little prodding. It would happen on nights when my parents would go out for dinner or have a late plane to meet. By this time he had moved into the bedroom in the basement and I into his old bedroom. He would sneak up in the dark and crawl alongside my bed. He would reach under the sheets and begin stroking my body. It started out slowly with just fondling at first. Before long, he was crawling inside my bed with me, rubbing his body against mine. Before I knew what was happening or could say anything, he had me engaging in intercourse.

I was terrified at first, but began sensing this as one way to receive love and attention from a family member. My brother was accepting of me for what I could give him. Little did I think he was using me. My feelings were too clouded to see what was really going on. New alters evolved to cope with this new experience. I was terrified of what was happening, but starved for the attention. I needed to be held and loved no matter how it came. Soon these visits became a game to me. The actual sexual act was not the turn-on. In fact it was a turn-off whenever I thought about it. I knew it must have been wrong because of what little I knew about sex and stuff. It was the secrecy and anticipation of him sneaking into my room that turned me on.

These visits occurred fairly regularly when my parents were not at home at night from the time I was going into the fifth grade until I started my periods in the sixth grade. I quickly put a stop to these visits when I learned that I could get pregnant.

Those alters that had established themselves from these games were sensing additional needs for attention and arousal. I took my new sexual experiences and tried them out on my sister. Sally would tell how she could make Karla feel good and discussed how we could explore each other's bodies. This would go on during the days when our parents were at the station and my brother was still at school. We would strip and explore each other's private parts and practice kissing and caressing one another. This maybe lasted for six or nine months.

When this ended, those new alters were lost and turned inward for their arousal and exploitation. When they decided to show themselves, I was out of control. I found their acts revolting, grotesque and sadistic. They were so starved for outside attention that they drag our poodle in on their fun and games. Monique is the sadistic one. She would put the dog on the bed and force her to lick our genitals. The dog resisted at first but soon became addicted to this act as much as she was. The dog would lick intensely and at times attempt to bite. This threw her into ecstasy.

When that bored her she had to find new and creative ways to excite and try to bring her to orgasm. She began putting any and everything she could find or think up my vagina. This included Ping-Pong balls, candles and bristly hair curlers. She would even try to put two or three tampons inside my vagina at one time.

Then, to top all acts, Monique coerced Mike to come out and pretend he was raping her. This is a feat that is hard to perceive unless you were caught up defenseless in the middle of it. Two alters in a host body working up a sweat. I would just disappear and hide in some dark corner of my mind till they were finished.

This goes on today. I still view sex as very repulsive and can't see how people can partake in something as lewd as this for such little pleasure. I will never understand and don't care to. I accept that all humans have certain natural needs and desires that must be met, I'm just glad there is someone else inside me that gains such pleasure from these acts. All the power to them, but I will continue to run and hide whenever these burning desires surface.

This incestuous behavior was not the only changes that occurred when we moved. Other tensions developed between my parents. I didn't understand then, but now feel it was because they were living beyond their means. My parents would socialize and party with other visible people in the community. My mother and father began to argue.

The arguments became regular around the house. I also learned that my father was becoming an alcoholic. We kept our booze in the cupboard by the telephone in the living room. I regularly heard my dad come home during the day and get into the cabinet for a quick shot. It wasn't long before he was even attacking the cupboard early in the morning. I smelt alcohol on his breath at all times.

The fights became more physical; people were being pushed around. Us kids were stuck in the middle. My mom would antagonize my dad and egg him on into an argument. My dad was a big man, but I really looked at him as a big teddy bear; harmless. My mom had a way with pushing people to their limits. In addition to pushing each other around, my dad would blow up at the dinner table and throw food at my mom. Of course, my sister and I got to clean up the mess. My dad really tried to restrain himself against hurting anyone. In his fits of rage, he would resort to shoving the furniture around. Lamps were knocked off tables. One night my dad gave the long coffee table with a marble top a swift kick. He knocked it over and broke the marble.

When the arguing got to be too much for me to take, I would run screaming and crying to my bedroom and slam the door as hard as I could. I did this in hopes of getting their attention and to hopefully distract them. It never seemed to work until it had gotten to the point that I had done it so many times and with such force, that the door jam ripped from the wall. It distracted them all right, but also got me into trouble.

I loved my dad very much because I felt he understood me. I identified with him and the frustration he must have felt in the constant nagging of my mother. She was extremely domineering.

I didn't approve of everything my dad did. In fact he embarrassed me much of the time. He walked around the house in just his T-shirt and without any underwear. I walked in on him countless times when he was in the bathroom because the door was not shut. He would sit in the dark smoking his cigarettes. He grabbed at my mom's breasts in front of us kids and in public. He would grab at waitress' butts in restaurants. He would swear and use vulgar language in the house and in public.

I was scared for my dad. During the summer when he would have too much to drink, he would sometimes decide to go to the mountains to go fishing to get away from my mom. I was terrified that he might have an accident. Mike and Peggy would drum up enough courage and offer, no insist, they go with him. Remember now, Sheridan is a small cowboy community of only around 10,000 people at this time. Streets in the town were not all paved. Roads in the mountains were all dirt. The road up Red Grade was single lane in some places with sheer drop-offs from the edge of the road. It was real treacherous if two cars should meet in these places, even when the driver is sober. We always made it up and back in one piece. This is more than any kid should be expected to endure.

When the fights would get bad at night, my dad would have a habit of taking off for the gas station to sleep it off and get away from my mom. Once again, Mike and Peggy stepped in and insisted he let them go with him. We would let him go back into his office. I would dust or clean the office while he slept. He would always usually fall asleep with a cigarette in his mouth. This is what scared me. I knew how easy it would be for the place to catch on fire. Being a gas station, should it ever catch fire, the outcome could be fatal for not only my dad but devastating to the neighborhood and community.

Mike and Peggy were not the only ones who loved my father. Bobbie and Bonnie had a deep fondness for him. So did Susan. You see, my dad was the one who argued with my mom and allowed Susan to buy the guitar. Bobbie had taken the Famous Artist Institute's test when I was in junior high. A representative of the Institute came to the house one day to sell us a Famous Artist's study course. Bobbie begged and pleaded with him to buy it for her. He obliged. Dad would let Mike and Peggy wash cars at the station and paint the fence around the property. This may have been work to most kids, but was a joy to them, because it was something to repay him for his kindness. My parents rented parking spaces behind the station in a vacant lot. They had paved the lot and put up parking blocks. Dad let Bonnie paint the customer's names on these blocks.

As I got older and my parents spent more time away from the house, my responsibilities grew. By the time I was in junior high, my sister and I were sharing in the housework and cooking. We alternated weeks dusting and vacuuming and doing dishes. We each helped with cooking breakfast and starting dinner. In the winter we shoveled the sidewalks and in the summer we mowed the lawn. I was also on garden patrol cause I liked to see things grow and had a small vegetable garden. My sister and I kept up the house because my brother spent all his free time down at the gas station learning how to become a mechanic. He started pumping gas and working on the cars when he was in junior high.

I still spent much of my time alone; however, I did make some friends in the neighborhood. Of course they were not the popular kids in the neighborhood. There was a girl younger than my sister and me, Jan, who lived next door. Her parents owned a construction business and were gone a lot, too. I did some baby-sitting when I got into junior high. It wasn't so much a job because we had fun playing together. Most of the time was spent at her house. I didn't have her coming over to my house very often because I never knew what the situation would be.

Debbie was another friend. I did some off-the-wall stuff with her and her older brother. This is where I learned any bad habits I may have picked up. I did some experimentation with adult activities. We would steal cigarettes from our parents and practice smoking in their basement. We had a makeshift clubhouse in the basement. We also played with fire and lighters. I also swiped candles from the cupboard. We would test our tolerance to pain by dripping hot candle wax on our skin. We started by dripping it on our hands then progressively onto more sensitive areas like our arms and legs. We would see who could stand it the longest.

Debbie's older brother, Greg, would occasionally join us. One day he came in when we were smoking. He told us that we were doing it all wrong. He showed us how to inhale and swallow the smoke into our lungs. When I tried it, I nearly turned green. That was the last time I smoked when he was around. Debbie was my sister's age. When I went to junior high, I tried to find another group of friends.

The friends I made were also kids that tended to be smarter than the average kids. They were certainly less than popular. Despite that, I never really got close to anyone. In fact, I didn't go out of my way to find them or be around them. They kind of migrated towards me and claimed *me* as *their* friend. I learned to tolerate them just to get positive marks for my social skills. I rarely played with them after school.

Other than my school activities and escapes to the basement with my poodle, Sheri, when at home, I involved myself completely in my Girl Scouting. In seventh grade, my Cadette troop saved enough money and planned a camping trip to Canada. We were to be gone for two weeks the summer before my eighth grade year. My sister was in the troop but didn't go. She didn't like camping and the outdoors like I did. I was having a great time until I got an excruciating toothache. We had already made it to Canada when it hit. I didn't know if I would get home. I didn't have any money to pay for a dentist on the trip and it wasn't in our plans. I didn't want to disrupt the troop's plans, so I didn't let the leaders know just how much pain I was really in. Fortunately for me, one of the leaders had a medical emergency at home so we had to cut the trip short. Boy, was I relieved.

The first thing I did when I got home was have my mom make an appointment with the dentist. I despised going to the dentist, but that was the only way I was going to find relief. I found out that my tooth had abscessed. I needed to have a root canal and large filling in my tooth. The pain at the dentist was nothing like the pain I had on the trip.

I excelled in junior high. Every spring there was an awards ceremony. I received numerous awards for my academics, music and art. Bobbie and Bonnie were prize art students. Art was my favorite subject. I also did well in Home Economic. Susan sang in a music ensemble with 10 other girls. We performed a lot at Christmas and sang at other schools and meetings.

Bobbie and Bonnie worked together on a number of art projects. They entered some poster contests and won them. One was a safety poster and I won some money for it. Other pieces of art won awards at the annual junior college art fair.

My art teacher signed me up for a special art seminar at the junior college with a famous artist. Bobbie learned how to finger paint with oils. The painting she did was framed and hung in the school office. A representative of Encyclopedia Britannica was so impressed with the painting that she wanted to buy it. She paid me $25 for it.

Another alter appeared in junior high. Her name is Katherine. She is the author in the Group. In fact it is with her skill and cooperation that this story is being written. She became editor of the school newspaper. It received a national runner-up prize for a series of articles done about lung cancer, smoking and drugs. I got my picture in the local town paper for receiving the award.

I was in an accelerated math class. This class also managed to get some of the popular kids in it. They were always pulling pranks on the teacher. She was unable to control their behavior. One day in the spring they brought in matches, were striking them and throwing them through the air in class. This was unacceptable behavior to me and I was extremely embarrassed by the whole ordeal.

The following week things got even more out of control. One of the kids found an old package of hot dogs. We had a test on that day. The teacher left the class during the test. This kid pulled out the hot dogs and started throwing them around the room. I wanted to get up and leave. I didn't want to be recognized as a part of this class. The teacher came back in the room after hearing all the ruckus. She scolded everyone and went down to talk to the principal. She came back and said that everyone was going to have to come in after school. I decided I would not come in because I played no part in their practical jokes. Besides, that night after school was when the newspaper was coming to take my picture.

I felt guilty because as it turned out, I should have gone since the principal came afterward for the award presentation. I was embarrassed and just hoped that she didn't know that I was a part of that class.

I couldn't get away from the teasing in junior high. Actually, it wasn't so much teasing but a crush that one of my classmates had on me. The Beatles song, Michelle, came out that year. This guy followed me around the school singing the song. He also had a habit of punching me in the arm. I told him to leave me alone and threatened him. When this did not work, I would chase him and punch him in the arm and shove him against the lockers. This was not the proper behavior for a young lady. I got in trouble when caught; he didn't.

All during my childhood, I was taught that it was not appropriate to show or express my anger even though my parents regularly engaged in such practice. I had a lot of stored up anger and frustrations between what was going on at home and at school. Finally, one day in the eighth grade, I could not take it any longer. I had to blow off steam somehow. This is when Kim evolved. (Kim represented herself early on as Chrissy. Everyone thought Chrissy was the one with self-destructive behavior.) One day shortly after this incident in math class, I was sitting in my science class. I was severely distracted and not paying attention to what was going on. The next thing I knew, I was scraping the back of my hand with my comb. Before all was said and done, there was an "N" carved in the back of my hand. This wasn't good enough for Kim. A few days later, she took the comb to my other hand. This time she carved an "M."

I was able to deal with what had happened until my mom noticed the cuts on my hands. Boy did I ever have trouble trying to explain what happened. When I finally managed an explanation, she didn't know what to say. Her immediate instinct was to punish me and make me feel completely guilty and embarrassed by what I had done. She sent me to my room without dinner to make me think about what I had done.

Once again I withdrew and isolated myself from others. I hid my hands from everyone until the scratches had healed. I wanted to talk to someone about how I was feeling and to try to find out appropriate ways to express my frustrations and bottled up emotions. We had a counselor assigned to the school. I had a girlish crush on him, but was too embarrassed to approach him to ask for help. I didn't want this man that I had a crush on know the real misery I was in. I just kept to myself.

Toward the end of my eighth grade year a new guy came to the school. I developed a real infatuation for him. I thought about him all the time. I followed him around school and learned of his schedule. I watched him from a distance whenever I could. I even went to a dance in hopes of drumming up enough nerve to ask him to dance. Instead, I just melted into the wall. That summer before high school, I woke up to a news report on the radio about a boy being shot the night before. It turned out that Kelly had gone joy riding in his mom's car. He hit another car at the drive-in and left the scene. Someone had gotten the license plates and reported it. He was so scared that he came home, got his dad's gun, went to the basement and blew his brains out. I was in shock for days.

That wasn't my first exposure to loss, though. That April, after an extensive illness and severe bout of rheumatoid arthritis, my grandmother passed away. I was not very close to her, but cried quite a bit. I did spend a lot of time at their house when we lived on Fifth Street. My sister and I would often walk down to their house after school when my parents had plans in the evening. They baby-sat us when my parents would go on trips before my mom's parents moved in behind us. I couldn't stand to see her in so much pain when she became crippled and bed-ridden. We still did go to visit on a regular basis. I would always go outside to get away from her moaning and complaining.

That same summer the doctors had confronted my father about the severity of his alcoholism. They gave him an ultimatum. If he didn't do something about his illness, it would consume him and ultimately do him in. His liver was severely damaged. My parents were mortgaged to the hilt. There was no way he could come up with the money for a rehab center. Besides, he was still in denial about his alcoholism. Finally, my brother came forward and said he would give him $800 of his own money to go to a center in Minnesota.

With strong objections, my dad did agree to give it a try. He was there for a week. He was so addicted to the booze, that he couldn't stand it any longer. The center was way out in the country and cabs would not come out when a patient called. My dad packed his suitcase and walked away from the center. It was a five mile walk to town. He was that adamant about getting away from that place and back home.

During the short time he was there and before he left, the doctor gave us what information he had about the illness. My mom was given an option of divorcing him if he didn't change his ways. She would not leave him no matter how bad things got. She was going to stick by his side.

Reading this material opened my eyes to what was really going on with him. I really started to feel sorry for him. I came to realize how my mom's nagging and prodding just drove him to drink more. I soon began to side with him during the arguments. I also learned that a lot of alcoholics have a depressive nature which compounded problems. For the first time I came to the conclusion through my identity with him that part of my problem could possibly be depression. I didn't know at the time that it was hereditary, but often felt that I could feel the pain that my dad was feeling. It wasn't until later in understanding my own manic-depressive illness that this identity would become even closer. I can now see that he was also manic-depressive and obsessive-compulsive.

As and eighth grader, other national and international Girls Scout opportunities opened up to me. I applied for a number of camping activities. I was selected to attend a Wyoming Conservation Camp and was alternate for a Covered Wagon Trek. This made for a busy summer for me and my alters. At least I got away from the home situation which was becoming quite unbearable.

I made a lot of friends at Conservation Camp. The other girls seemed to be quite accepting of me. I jumped in with all the activities and participated to the fullest. No wallflower here. Susan took her guitar and had a good time singing at the campfires. Mike got to help build a dam and be around wildlife. We went on an excursion that took us on an air boat ride across swamp lands in a goose banding project. We also got to go to a wildlife preserve.

One afternoon in July, I got a call from the Girl Scout Council. One of the girls and the first alternate were not able to attend the Covered Wagon Trek and they wanted to know if I would be able to get packed and be in Tensleep the next day. I said I would have to check with my parents and get back with them. My parents said I could go but they would not be able to take me up the mountains to the base camp. I called my troop leader and she and her husband agreed to take me.

By the time I got up to the base camp, everyone was there. In fact the actual check-in day was the day before, so everyone had had a chance to get to know one another. I kind of felt like an outsider trying to play catch-up with what had gone on so far. Girls at this camp came from all over the U.S. I think there were twenty counting the two leaders. We also had a father and son team who were the wranglers and wagon drivers.

The next morning we loaded all our gear into the back of the covered wagon and left on our trek. This camp was to last about two weeks. Each day, we would travel from 10 to 12 miles. The wagon was drawn by two big team horses and had the framework of an actual old covered wagon. The only modification that had been made was that the wooden wagon wheels had been replaced by rubber tires.

Each morning of the trek, we would get up at dawn, prepare breakfast, break camp and load our gear in the wagon. We were on the trail by 8 or 8:30 a.m. We trekked through the Wyoming Rocky Mountains like the pioneers once did. We had tents, but most of the time we slept out under the open stars unless there was a threat of bad weather. We would stop along the day's travel about noon or one o'clock for lunch and reach our campsite by 4 or five in the afternoon.

One day I was busy with a number of chores. Before I knew it, camp was down, including the latrines being filled in. The next thing I knew, the wagon was loaded and we were on our way. All of a sudden, I felt a strong urge to go to the bathroom. I had no time to find a place in the trees to take a leak. I was afraid if I did, they would be out of sight by the time I was ready to join the group. I had no choice but to hold my water.

The day involved a fairly strenuous trek. It was rugged, but we were moving quickly through the mountains. All I could think of was how bad I had to go. The steep climbs seemed of little concern or labor. No matter how bad I had to go, something told me I would fall too far behind the group and be lost in the wilderness. It wasn't even a consideration to ask the group to slow up so I could relieve myself. I didn't want to appear weak. I had to keep going. I kept telling myself that I could hold it till we stopped for lunch. As luck would have it, we had an extra distance to go before we would break.

Finally about 1:30 we came upon a meadow. This is where we were stopping for lunch. Great! I didn't think I could go one step further. As I looked around for a place to relieve myself, I noticed there was no cover or trees in the area. There was a stream with a slight embankment. I was still very modest and had to find the right place where no one could see me. I was in absolute agony. Finally I said, hell, and just dropped my pants. It seemed like I went on forever. I must have peed a gallon of fluid. From that point on, I made a vow that I would never again make myself go beyond a strong urge to relieve myself.

Except for one other accident, this was a very enjoyable experience. We were going to go on a field trip to an old mining camp and would make the trek a short day hike. We were informed that the campsite we were at the day before the side trip would be a two-day campsite. We got back from the mine early the next day. The wrangler told some of us that we could ride the horses if we wanted to since they weren't tired out from a long day's journey. We jumped at the opportunity.

These horses were team horses mind you. Much bigger than any old quarter horse, and bigger than any horse I had ever ridden. To top it off, there were no saddles. I had to ride bareback. No problem, I had ridden Mr. Hobby's pony bareback when I was much younger. I could handle it.

When it was finally my turn to ride, I had to have a boost up on the horse. I rode alongside the other girl who got her turn. The girth of the horse was so big that even with my long legs, I couldn't wrap them around him. No problem as long as I kept the horse at a walking gait. It was a very enjoyable ride until I made the turn to head back for the camp. The horses were hungry and ready to get back. All of a sudden, they took off in a dash for the camp. I did my best to hang on, but it finally got to be too rough. The horse stumbled and off I flew. I came down with a hard thud. I swear I must have shook the ground. My pants filled with sand and I was quite dazed. I don't know whether I hit my head or not, but it took me awhile to figure out where I was and what had happened.

When the leaders saw the horse come back without a rider, they came down the road to find out what had happened. They found me staggering along and came to help. I landed real hard on my tail bone and was limping a bit. I must have had a concussion because I felt quite numb and disoriented. I got sick after dinner and went to bed early.

I was stiff and sore the next morning. The leader asked if I wanted to ride in the wagon. I wasn't going to let them know how bad I felt and told them that I would walk behind the wagon with the rest. To be honest, I was embarrassed by my inability to hold on to the damn horse. I was still trying to gain everyone's acceptance and didn't want to come across as a weakling. Many of the girls on the trip were juniors and seniors in high school, and I felt like I just never really fit in. They all seemed so much more experienced than me.

It was the summer of 1969 and was a history making time for mankind and the United States. You see, while I was on this trek, the American astronauts and Apollo 11 mission were landing on the moon.

The moon landing was scheduled for our next to last day on the trail. We were to be picked up outside Tensleep on the Girl Scout's National Center West plateau. We were coming out of the mountains onto hot, dry plains with cliffs.

The day before the landing as I was walking along the trail, Peggy saw a snake run across the road. She got Mike to pick it up. Not long after he picked up the garter snake, the wrangler's truck came up the road with a leader and a couple of the girls in it. I stood in the middle of the road waving the snake in the air. The girls were terrified. They rolled up the windows and sped past me. Not long afterward, Mike decided to put the snake down because it was getting slimy and started to smell. I continued on to meet up with the others at that night's campsite. When the girls saw me coming, they got back into the truck and rolled up the windows. I could not convince them that I no longer had the snake. All of a sudden I heard a loud rattle. I must have jumped three feet into the air and landed in the back of the truck screaming. They knew for sure then that I must have had the snake. I was hysterically trying to tell them that I didn't have my snake but that there was this big old diamondback rattlesnake in front of the truck. We all started screaming at that point.

I caught a glimpse of that sucker as he slithered off. He must have been at least four or five feet long. We warned off the other girls as they came down the road to be careful that there might be rattlesnakes in the area. When the wranglers got to the site with the wagon, they got out their shotguns and checked out the site. They didn't find any snakes, but did find a mouse nest that looked like it had been intruded upon by a snake. There were baby mice scattered all over the ground. Needless to say, that night we pulled out the tents and everyone slept inside and didn't venture very far from the campfire.

My parents didn't come up to get me to bring me home. One of the other girls on the trip was from Sheridan. My mom had called her parents and asked if I could get a ride back to town with them. I was a little disappointed that my parents were too busy to spend some time with me. At least when I got home, my dog was glad to see me.

Junior high was just a two year school. For the ninth grade, I went to the high school. For the second time, I was in the same school as my brother. By the time I was in high school I was quite large. I was overweight and had large breasts for my age. My brother was popular and a star athlete at the school. He didn't want anyone to know I was his sister. He ignored me whenever we passed in the halls.

I was embarrassed by my size in gym class. I avoided the showers like the plague. I was very modest about my body and didn't want anyone to see me because I was so much different than the other girls in my class. I would leave my bra on when I went into the shower with my towel wrapped around me. I would go in and get my arms and feet wet so that I could get credit for my shower. If I didn't get my shower credits, I could fail gym.

I was very athletic, despite my size. I was also very competitive. I would usually be pitted against Wendy for intramural finals. She usually won, but from time to time she slipped up and had a bad day. Fortunately we were on the same intramural basketball team. We won most of our games.

One winter day during my sophomore year, when we had a semi-final game slated, I had an unfortunate mishap. It was a cold and snowy day. My brother had given my sister and me a ride to school. I was in the front seat. My sister was in the back. We both shut our car doors at the same time. I didn't realize what had happened until I tried to turn and walk toward the school. I was stuck. My thumb was caught in the back door. I panicked and didn't know what to do. Finally I was able to get across to my brother that I was stuck and needed to have him come unlock the door to release my thumb. I felt nothing. After my thumb was freed, the blood rushed to the tip and began throbbing to an unbearable level.

I was in shock and didn't know what to do. I finally decided to go to the office to ask them what I should do. They called my mom and said that she should come get me and take me to the doctor. I had to endure the pain for a couple hours until I could get in to see the doctor. The doctor shaved the nail to allow the blood to spill out to relieve the pressure. I was fine until I saw all that blood. I turned as white as a sheet and got very light-headed. Needless to say, I had a splint put on my thumb. I was bound and determined to play in that basketball game. A sore thumb was not going to stop me. As it turned out, I made more points in that game than any other game I played in all season.

I got interested in other things my freshman year. New alters also evolved at this time. First there was Karen. She came to be when I decided to try out for the speech team. Because of scouting I had developed leadership skills and had developed some confidence in speaking in front of other kids. But, this activity was more than just leading a discussion in front of friends. It meant performing in front of strangers and adults. This caused me to shutter. What if I messed up? What would people think? God, I knew I would screw up. Not Karen. She was strong and bound and determined not to give up. Yes, my hands shook and my voice quivered, but she never gave in. I specialized in oral interpretation, specifically dramatic interp. I did try humor and poetry, but it just wasn't for me. I went to what seemed like all the meets.

I traveled a lot on weekends during the season. The closest school in our class was Gillette which was 86 miles away. We made several trips to Casper, Cheyenne and Billings, Montana. I got to know the roads well. It was an escape from the fighting and strong emotions at home. I gained some acceptance and new friends from my teammates. I really liked my speech coach. I never placed at any of the meets I attended in four years of speech competition, but kept coming back for more because I was challenged by it. I did make it to some final round competition, though.

Karen had a tendency to choose selections that expressed pain and suffering. I think it was her way of letting out a little cry and found it a way to express the pain and suffering we were all feeling. Her first selection was focused around Melanie in childbirth in *Gone With the Wind*. The primary selection of choice in successive years was variations of the prose about the trials surrounding Auschwitz and the concentration camps during World War II. She really got into the horror and suffering of the Jews.

I experienced some excitement during one return trip from Billings. It was dark and we were driving through the Blackfoot Indian Reservation, when out of nowhere a car crossed in front of the bus. We hit it, but not hard enough to render the car unable to drive. The Indians in the car tore off across the fields to a farmhouse. Because it was a school bus and the accident occurred on government land and the highway, we had to wait for the authorities to come and investigate.

I was setting on the back of the bus facing the farmhouse. I got into an investigative mood and watched the farmhouse with due diligence. I acquired a keen sense of vision in the moonlight. I saw movement around the farmhouse and reported it to the speech coach and authorities. They sent a reservation patrol car over to the farmhouse and apprehended the suspects.

During the wait for the events to unfold, I also watched the skies. I saw a meteor and found my personal constellation. This night I dubbed the Seven Sisters as my own constellation. Wherever I go and when I am out at night, I always look to the skies for these stars.

One other extracurricular activity I partook in to gain some acceptance by the other kids, was Pep Club. This was the only way I could "rub elbows" with the popular kids. I was able to get some recognition and acceptance when the members found out that my brother was one of the star players. They must have thought that by being friends with his sister, would get them closer to the star himself. Little did they know just how distant we were to one another. At least I started to feel like a part of something. Francie was the alter that evolved from this interaction. I so wanted to be accepted by the other girls, but didn't know how to act or react around them. Francie came along with her happy and carefree personality. She could laugh, joke and carry on with the others like she hadn't a care in the world. I like to refer to her as footloose and fancy free. She knew how to be an active participant, and sometimes came across as the life of the party.

Again, Girl Scouts played an active part of my freshman year. I was an older scout eligible for new adventures. During the summer I was an assistant leader at troop camp for some Juniors and also an aide at Day Camp for Brownies. At day camp and troop camp new alters were born because it wasn't a situation where I was just an older scout having fun with the younger girls. I was a leader, and the girls looked up to me for showing them what to do and make decisions for them. They looked for guidance as well as a friend.

My teacher alter evolved out of this. Her name is Carol. She has one thing that I have very little of — patience. She never raises a voice and accepts everyone for who they are and doesn't think less of them for any shortcomings.

My mother alter also evolved at this time. She is Alice. Alice has a firm, authoritative personality, but is also very loving and caring. She can be stern like my own mother, but is warm and also accepting of others.

Things had not changed that summer. The fighting and arguing continued. Summers, I was home or at the station during the day and spent more time around my parents. I was right in the middle of their daily rituals. I still had a tendency to side with my father. I even drummed up enough courage from time to time to be vocal at blaming my mom for driving my dad to drink. She would just yell at me.

That fall of my sophomore year, my whole life changed. One October day, I came home from school and found both my mom and dad at home. This was highly unusual. My dad looked different. He didn't look well at all. My mom informed us that she was taking my dad to the hospital. He had developed an acute case of jaundice. He was all yellow. I was concerned but figured he'd probably come through this. My dad was a strong man. I never remembered him ever being home sick in bed.

The next day his condition had deteriorated severely. He had lapsed into a semi-coma. My mom said we could go to the hospital to visit him that night after dinner. When we went she told us not to expect too much. When we saw him, he was just lying in bed staring at the ceiling. I don't think he knew us. I spoke to him but got no response. I still had it set in my mind that he would come through this. My mom never really informed me just how serious it was.

I went to school the next day as usual. About 10:30 a.m. as I was sitting in study hall, I saw my aunt's Bronco come down the street and turn into the school parking lot. I knew something must have been wrong and asked to be dismissed to the office. When she came in she was very solemn. I asked how my dad was doing. Had he gotten worse? She just looked at me and said that he was not suffering any longer. I kept asking her how he was. Finally, she informed me that my father passed away the morning of October 26, 1970. I choked. "No!" I screamed. It can't be. My dad is strong, he isn't dead. He can't be dead. He is going to get better. I just went numb. I withdrew totally inside myself.

My aunt took all us kids home that day. She stayed with us while my mom was making arrangements with the funeral home. Mike and Peggy were devastated. When I got home, I went into my room, shut the door and just started balling my eyes out. I cried for what seemed hours and then days. I couldn't believe that my dad gave up; that he was not going to be with us any more. I didn't come out of my room except to go to the bathroom. I wouldn't even come out to eat. My mom came in and tried to talk to me and explain that we all need each other right now and asked if I wouldn't come out to be with the family. Friends and neighbors came by for the next few days before the funeral. I wouldn't come out to visit or share my sorrow with them.

My dad was raised Catholic but hadn't been a practicing Catholic since he and my mom got married, but the priests knew our family. My mom was able to convince the church to bury him. The priest tried to talk to me and said he could see how badly I must have been hurting and my loneliness. He tried to cheer me up by asking me to find some scripture that I felt would be appropriate for the service. I spent the rest of the day with my Bible.

We buried him on October 30. I stayed out of school all week. I didn't want to go back to school. I was confused, sad, and thought my red, puffy eyes from crying would never clear up. The fighting was over, but I was alone. More alone than I had ever felt before. I felt different from the other kids and like I was even less a part of the community than felt previously. I didn't know what to do with myself. I tried to keep up with my activities, but my heart wasn't really into things.

Later that fall or early the next spring, Johnny's mom passed away. I had nothing to do with him for years since that incident when I was young. Now, we had something in common. I had some company with my feelings and emotions. I never talked to him about how I was feeling, but just to know that I wasn't alone in my feelings of loss were reassuring. I kind of picked myself up after that and regained some courage to go on with my life.

Things were tough. My mom was trying to run the business by herself and was depressed over the mess my dad had made of everything. She tried to get everything in legal order, because she had decided to try to sell the business. It was too much for her to handle without even the little support and partnership she had had with my dad.

STARTING OVER

My mom had a sister living in Billings, Montana with some kids our age. She and her husband convinced my mom that she should sell the business and house in Sheridan and move herself, me and my sister to Billings to be closer to them. Grace was an older sister, but closer in age to my mom than the sister in Sheridan.

I wasn't too sure about this but very open to the idea of getting a fresh start with things. I was going to hate starting in another school, but didn't have too many friends that I would be sad about leaving.

By July, my mom had a buyer for the business and within a few weeks someone interested in buying the house lock, stock and barrel. Even our dog. My mom said there was no way we were going to be able to take Sheri with us to Billings. I cried a lot over this, because Sheri was my dog. She saw me through good times and bad. She waited for me while I was away during the summers.

I was also very angry with my mom, because I knew she really didn't care for pets, but rather just allowed them for the rest of the family's enjoyment. She must have thought that her life was now empty, so ours was going to have to be the same. She had no one else to fight and argue with. That must have been a real blow to her ego.

Well, early August, my mom, sister and I packed our belongings. The house would not close until mid August so we just took some clothes and essentials and headed for Billings. My brother was going to start college that fall and decided to stay in Sheridan and attend the junior college there. He had gotten a basketball scholarship and felt that was what he wanted to do for the time being. My mom was not happy about the idea, but soon became accepting.

We spent not quite a month living at my aunt's house. Just before school started, we found a 2 bedroom duplex about a mile from the new high school. It was the school my cousins attended so I would at least know someone there. My mom had made enough money on the house and business to buy new furniture and put her back to school in a business course and to support us for a year.

For this new start, I had gone on a diet and lost some weight in hopes of having a more acceptable appearance and giving me a better chance to make some new friends. I wasn't where I wanted to be but was pleased with the results.

I tried to get active right away and joined the speech team and Pep Club. I also got active in art classes. These art classes got the creative juices in Bobbie and Bonnie flowing again.

Bobbie had a painting class where she did some acrylics and oils that really expressed my true feelings and sorrow. One painting was a portrait of my father using greens and blacks and placing him in a big teardrop. Another was not to make sense until I was diagnosed as having MPD. It was a woman's head nailed to the barren desert floor with muscular humanoids hammering away at the skull and breaking off pieces. It was around that time that I remember losing control over my mind. I felt bits and pieces of my mind were being robbed by other beings or voices. Sometimes I felt I was out of control with my thoughts.

I found it difficult to get into the Pep Club routine. My cousins played sports, but cheering them on was not the same as my brother. I didn't know these kids at all. In Sheridan, I had grown up with everyone and knew most of the kids on the various teams. I tried to be enthusiastic, but I guess more than anything else, it was a way to feel like I belonged and was a part of something.

I went to speech meets and Karen did her thing. I don't remember this one year as well as the two previous. I know she used a lot of the same interp cuttings I had in Sheridan because they were new to this region. I got a mixture of ratings on the Auschwitz trial.

My heart, though, did draw to my art. Bonnie did a wire sculpture of an old sailing ship. She cut and twisted several hundred pieces to form the hull and sails. She must have had over a hundred hours tied into that piece. It was my pride and joy of the year's accomplishments.

All was going well until around Thanksgiving time. My grandfather Wilder had suffered a stroke. He was not recovering from it. By Christmas he had given up. On December 26, he passed away. I remember being sad, but never really cried over his death. I guess I had cried my tear ducts dry with my father's death. I don't even remember the funeral.

My grandfather was prominent in bringing ranching to Montana and was well known in the ranching community. I didn't particularly favor him, but I was very proud of having him for my grandfather. He was a very stern and rugged man and I could see where my mom got her hard edges.

Early that next spring, a stranger came into our lives. He was not a stranger to my mom because he had done business with her in Sheridan. He had rented cars from us on numerous occasions. His name was Roy Scafe and he was from Denver, Colorado. He had heard about my father's death and learned that my mom had sold the business. He got her new address from the people who had bought the business from my mom. He had business in Billings and came to pay his respects.

Roy and my mom went out to dinner that evening. I don't know what they talked about, but soon afterwards, my mom started getting long distance phone calls from him on a regular basis. At first I didn't understand what was going on. Actually, I guess I didn't want to acknowledge what was going on. My mom was falling for this guy.

By April, she announced she and Roy were getting married. In February, my brother announced he was getting married in June to the girl he went to his Senior Prom with. Wow, what a blow. Two very prominent parts of my life were going to bring strangers into the family. This news did not set well with me. My mom had talked to my brother and decided she would get married right after my brother and Linda returned from their honeymoon.

I couldn't understand my mom. I knew almost nothing about this man. It had been only a year and a half since my father's death. How could she fall in love with someone so quickly unless she was never really in love with my dad? All sorts of thoughts began racing through my head. I really began to hear voices then. I was confused and hurt. I sought help from the school counselor.

I tried to devise a plan where I could stay in Billings my senior year on my own and not move to Denver. I worked out budgets, how I would get a job; everything. The counselor was of little help. He tried to explain that I would become accepting of Roy and that it was not practical for me to follow through with my plan. He thought Roy sounded like a real stable guy who cared for my mom.

I couldn't deal with it any more. My mom and I got in a big fight one night over this. I locked myself in the bathroom. The next thing I remember, I found myself in the medicine cabinet reaching for a razor blade. I don't remember feeling suicidal, just deeply hurt and abandoned. Before I could stop myself, I was making slashes along my wrist. They weren't deep, but they did draw blood. Actually, they looked more like scratches. I couldn't believe what I had just done. I was disappointed in myself but somehow felt relieved of some pressure and anger.

I wore a band aid on my wrist for the next week. If kids asked what had happened, I just told them a cat scratched me. I didn't even tell the counselor what I had done.

Finally I came to terms with this marriage. The new start in Billings was not all that great. In fact, it was a little disappointing. By accepting this marriage, I would gain an older sister. Maybe someone I could talk to. Maybe my third start might be a little better than the last. As they say, "third time's a charm."

THIRD TIME'S A CHARM

Shortly after school was out my junior year, we packed up our belongings once again. After the movers came, we drove to Sheridan for my brother's wedding. We stayed at my aunt's apartment. My brother was married June 17. My mother and Roy were married June 22, after Roger and Linda returned from their honeymoon. My sister, Karla, and I drove back to Denver after the wedding with our new stepsister, Sue, while our parents went on a brief honeymoon.

The summer was an interesting one. There were long periods of getting to know Sue and becoming familiar with new surroundings. Sue was a sophomore in college and was just home for the summer. We became friends, but never close enough to really share all my secrets.

With this marriage, I had also gained a step-brother, but at the time of the wedding, he was sitting in jail. I knew his name and that he existed, but never really heard them talk about him. Since their marriage, I have seen him only twice between prison sentences. He is now serving life in a federal penitentiary.

I also got to know my new father a little better. I learned he was a Materials Manager in the Denver office for Shell Oil. He did a lot of traveling to oil well and field sites. His hobby was rebuilding old antique Fords. He had completed two when he and my mom got married.

That summer I was filled with mixed emotions. I was excited for another new start, yet still very apprehensive to this whole ordeal. I did lose some more weight over the summer and get to a point where I felt halfway good about myself.

Early in July, I got a call from the Girl Scout leader I had worked with in past summers at troop camp. She wanted to know if I would like to come up to Sheridan and help out again that summer. It took some real convincing, but I talked my parents into letting me go. They said they would buy me a bus ticket to get up there. Mike, Peggy and Susan were very happy with this. They loved camping, scouting and campfires. Susan took her guitar and prided herself in playing the campfire songs.

August was very uneventful. I rode my bike to the park, watched cars on the highway that was half a block away, and laid out in the sun.

Before long, it was time for school to start. There were some problems with transferring some of my class requirements. The schools in Denver had different educational priorities. All told, though, I was fairly happy with the classes I ended up with. I had a photography class, art class, speech class and was able to get on the school yearbook. I had a Social Problems class in which I got very close to the teacher. She became sort of a confidant of mine. She knew my step-sister quite well. I also had a biology and English lit class that I wasn't too terribly crazy about. Reading was not a favorite pastime of mine.

I had always liked taking pictures, but my photography class brought out a new alter. Her name is Elizabeth. She has a way of seeing inner beauty in everything she photographs. She was out a good deal of the time on our trip to the Pacific Northwest. I think over the course of eleven days, she must have shot at least 25 rolls of film. I pulled off the road in the most obscure places and took side trips that could very well have gotten me lost. Needless to say, I think she is good. She also has a great eye for composition. Because of this, I was soon promoted to Photo Coordinator for the school yearbook.

My Biology class was quite interesting, literally. Much better than chemistry or regular science classes. My class project was even interesting. It involved testing the intelligence of rats versus mice. I built an elaborate maze and documented time it took for the rats and mice to go through it, if they did that. The rats were very inquisitive and were bound and determined to find a shortcut to the food. My female rat had one litter of babies, but they never survived because she ate them.

The mice couldn't get over the wall, so they were stuck finding their way through the maze. They didn't do that well. The only thing they did well was have babies. The son got the mom pregnant and I ended up with a litter of baby mice, too. Only this time, the female did not eat the babies. When the project was over, I donated all the mice and rats back to the science department.

I do have an analytical side to my Group, but no one stands out as being overly scientific. Most of our experimentation and mathematics seem to be worked through by trial and error. The alter that best seems to fit this bill is Shelley.

Bobbie loved my art class. It gave her a chance to be creative but had some structure to it which Bonnie helped her with. This class was a lead for my first paying job.

That spring of my senior year, my art teacher had gotten a request from a local production studio for help in blocking in color on an animated television commercial. Bobbie jumped at the opportunity to get paid for her artistic talents. I started the job in early March. It was a commercial with a Princess and the Pea storyline for toilet paper.

The job went well and Bobbie did good work. About midway through the project the company moved its headquarters, and not long afterward the head artist on the project quit. The first commercial was too jumpy and needed smoothing out which would require almost three times the number of picture cells. One other high school girl was working on the project with me. It soon was dumped in our lap to do these new drawings and paint the cells, too. It required a lot of overtime, but she and Bobbie got the job done. Bobbie even added her own personal touch to the little angel. She put a nose on him. They were still using that little angel on the packaging for the toilet paper after I got out of college.

This job ended up on a sour note, though. The company was in financial trouble and I never got the last three hundred and some dollars that were due me. It was a great experience, regardless.

The other big project involved creating an Honor Banner for outstanding students at Denver South. The school colors were purple and white. Bobbie and Bonnie created a huge purple banner with fringe and hand cut out each of the recipient's names in white felt and glued them to the banner. This was a major undertaking because it easily had over 100 names on it by the end of the school year.

I also competed on the school speech team. Again, nothing spectacular, but Karen did compete in a local public speaking oratorical contest and get second place. Enough points from speech meets were earned to obtain a Degree of Excellence in the National Forensics League. Karen was pleased by that.

That fall, Karen also had her debut on stage. She had a walk-on part in the school theater production of Camelot. She was in one of the magic acts.

All in all, it was a fairly good year for everyone. I also got recognition from students and teachers alike. The popular kids would talk to me and invite me to participate in some of their activities. The teachers and some students honored me by selecting me as an outstanding Rebel Rouser. This was a distinct honor and privilege and usually went to students who had attended the school all three years of high school. It rarely went to someone who had been there only one year.

Despite the year being good, it wasn't without problems. I found myself emotionally unstable and experiencing a considerable amount of depression or the "blues." In the spring, my Social Problems teacher coordinated a program with Bethesda Community Mental Health Center on psychodrama. It was the newest rage in therapy. She asked if I would create a poster for the school advertising the program. Bobbie put a very nice poster together.

I decided that maybe I could learn something from this program and attended. I saw how psychodrama could loosen up all the bottled up rage that was inside of me. I talked to the presenters after the meeting and they suggested that I come over to the center to discuss it further. I did start going over to Bethesda, but don't remember really getting involved in any psychodrama therapy. I guess I was too embarrassed by how angry I was, and too ashamed by how hurt I was over what had happened in my life so far. I did participate in group therapy.

My mom was very reluctant about me going there and let me know it. She did drive me there for my appointments, but I could just sense her discomfort in the thought of me talking about my feelings. She knew I was having difficulties in adjusting and thought maybe things could get straightened out with me. I believe she thought I still had problems adjusting to her and Roy. Little did she know that was only a small part of it.

There was no question as to where or whether or not I was going to college. That decision was made my junior year setting in the counselor's office. I had decided that one way or another I was going to Arizona State University in Tempe. Spring of my senior year I had filled out the applications and taken my SAT test for acceptance. Before spring break, I got my acceptance letter and that I would be allowed to enter with honors.

The big trick was to find out where I would get the money to attend school. Roy and Mom would help me but I had to contribute to the expense. I got the idea of joining Air Force ROTC and thought that maybe I could get a scholarship. I wanted to be sure of my choice and begged my parents to let me go down to the school on my spring break. They agreed. I had an aunt and uncle living in the Phoenix area and I could stay a couple days with them.

I left snow in Denver and got to Phoenix which was experiencing some major flooding. That didn't stop the thrill and excitement of the trip. I fell in love with the campus at first sight. I got a big knot in my gut that said "no matter what it takes, you are coming here to school." Actually, it was all my alters who were telling, no, shouting that this is where they wanted to be.

I spent time at the financial aids office, housing office and ROTC headquarters. It didn't look too promising for an ROTC scholarship, but with Mike's persuasive prodding, decided I would still go into the program. After all, I did like flying and planes. With class catalog and financial aid forms in hand, I came back to Denver.

Once the paperwork was completed and sent in, it was just a matter of time. Just before school got out, I got word that I was being awarded a school loan to attend. I was elated and filled with excitement. I now had to get down to business and find another summer job to earn money for expenses. It was not going to be cheap, because I had declared myself as a commercial art major, and art supplies were expensive.

That summer before college, I got a job at the Denver Dry Goods Company. It was a department store in the Denver area. I split my time in two positions there. During the week, I packaged up merchandise in the shipping department for mailing or delivery to customers. On the weekends, I was a sales clerk in the domestics department. The pay was not great but did give me something to start the year off at school. It also gave me exposure to working and dealing with other people.

FUN IN THE SUN

I couldn't wait for August to come that summer. It was hard to believe that I would be going off to college and have an opportunity to live my own life. Mom and Roy drove me down for the start of school. Because of campus policy, all female freshman students under 20 years of age were required to live on campus. I didn't mind it. I was assigned to Manzanita Hall. It was a new high-rise dorm. My room was at the end of the hall on the seventh floor.

I got there about the time that many of my floor mates did. I met my suite mates. They were from back east. My roommate, Terry, didn't check in until the day before school started. She was a junior. Her parents lived in the Phoenix metro area but she wanted to be on her own, so she elected to live on campus.

Terry was rarely around. She was taking a heavy load of classes and worked nights at a bank. She was in bed when I left for class and came in after I went to bed. She also had a boyfriend that she spent a lot of time with. We did some sharing the few times we were actually in the room and awake together, but pretty much had our own lives. She did have the nasty habit of smoking, but was courteous enough to smell up the room with pipe smoke rather than cigarette smoke. At least it was a sweet-smelling tobacco. She even gave me permission to smoke her pipe if I got the urge. Mike took her up on it from time to time when I was down and bored.

My freshman year, I was enrolled for 17 hours. Throughout college, except for summer school I usually carried 15-17 hours. My grades suffered a bit from all these hours. At least from what I was accustomed to getting. I got my first C's in college. In fact, my sophomore year, I ended up with a D in a Trigonometry class.

My freshman year, I took a lot of art, AFROTC and general studies classes. First semester was tough, because I was having to adjust to a whole new way of life.

Bonnie and Bobbie enjoyed my studio art classes, but found the grading criteria a bit difficult to understand. They had dreaded sketch book assignments that had to be completed for a grade. All the assignments faired quite well except for those. They were intrigued with the knowledge gained from the art history classes, but found that the tests were extreme and very difficult to study for. Slides of art pieces were shown on the screen and I was suppose to write an essay about that particular piece. Hundreds of slides were shown between tests and it was difficult to learn enough about every single piece.

Mike was thrilled to death with Aerospace Studies. He learned about the history of the Air Force, planes and major battles that involved the Air Force. Again wanting to gain acceptance and a sense of belonging to something, Mike decided to join an AFROTC organization. The organization was called Silver Wing and was an elite group of cadets that were hard core in their goals.

I attended the organizational meeting for the fall pledge class. There were about fifteen of us at that first meeting. The Silver Wing members spelled out what was involved in the pledge program and what was expected of the pledges. This was going to be a very rigorous and disciplined program if I decided to accept the challenge.

Mike and Shelley couldn't get enough. They were eager to jump in with both feet. I was surprised with Shelley's enthusiasm and that she wanted any part of it. She is quite the disciplinarian and I guess she thought she would stand by Mike and give him that extra push to go through with it.

The AFROTC cadre thought highly of the Silver Wingers and they seemed to shine through as the leaders of the underclassmen. I definitely wanted to be a part of this and have the opportunity for that kind of recognition.

Women were more readily accepted into the ROTC program by then, and there were two other women who decided to give the pledge program a try also. The pledge class met once a week formally, but the pledges had to go through a twice weekly check-in to be tested on the material and discipline of the program. We were also encouraged to meet as a class informally to help one another with the material and drill procedures we were expected to know.

Most other freshman women were pledging sororities by this time. Not me. I wanted to be one of the guys and was pledging a fraternity-like program. I guess I always did seem to go out for something a little out of the ordinary.

The pledge program was very difficult and rigorous. I sure was glad that I had lost all that weight and was in good physical shape. We drilled for hours, ran and had to stand on the wall at attention for long periods of time. This program was very much like what the cadets at the Air Force Academy went through their first year. There was a lot of hazing and intimidation that went on. The actives did everything they could think of to break you down and ridicule you for your weaknesses.

Mike faired very well in the program by memorizing the material we were given and keeping up with the rest of the guys. He was not going to let anyone break him.

That year, the annual ASU vs. UA game was going to be held at ASU. When the University of Arizona came up for the game, they would always pull some prank and color or vandalize the big "A" that was on the butte behind the stadium. On those years, Silver Wing took it on to guard the butte before the big game. This was the first big test for the pledge class, because it was really the class that was suppose to guard the butte.

The pledge class prepared for this and climbed the butte at dusk the night before the big game. We were going to stand watch the entire night. Little did we know that not only were we protecting the butte from U of A students, but we were playing King of the Mountain with the actives that night. In addition to our primary responsibility, we were, under no circumstance, to allow the actives to take possession of the butte. The game was on.

Each pledge took their position at key posts around the "A" and toward the top of the butte. We stood guard and confronted anything that moved. Mike posted himself toward the top and back side of the butte. Many an active tried to impede on his territory, but he was very alert and able to capture all that would attempt to cross his path. Unfortunately, by about 4 a.m. one of the actives did get past one of my pledge brothers and capture the butte. Even with that done, we were still to stay on top till daybreak.

Adjusting to being away from home for the first time and a number of other issues presented themselves to me that fall. The pressures of the pledge program and the classes I was taking compounded all my other emotions. It was also close to the time of my father's death. I found myself wandering campus alone late at night, walking for hours in search of something. Voices of my Group kept telling me what to do and think. On weekends, I would climb the butte to do my studying in silence.

About mid-semester I was getting very depressed and lost. I went to see one of the school psychologists. He worked with me the best he could but found his hands tied when my depression got deeper and I was really feeling hopeless. He suggested I go to the Medical Center and see the school psychiatrist. She might be able to put me on some antidepressants.

I went to see Dr. Bohn and see if I couldn't get some better help to get me out of the hole I was in. She prescribed some Elavil. It helped to soften the edges a little but I was still hopeless and confused. I couldn't concentrate on my studies and was becoming concerned about my grades.

One night, I was hearing all kinds of voices and could not get any peace. I walked the campus for a couple hours. I then came back and turned my radio on real loud to try to drum out the internal noise. I was in a bottomless pit with nowhere to go. The next thing I knew, I was taking a handful of the Elavil that the doctor had given me. I was desperate, but not suicidal. I just wanted to get rid of the voices and get some sleep. I don't remember how many I took. I did get to sleep, though.

I woke up with one heck of a hangover. I had the shakes real bad, too. In fact, I was scared by how I was feeling. I went to my first class but couldn't stay awake. I went over to the health center after class to see if I could see Dr. Bohn. I had a little wait but did get in to see her. She was very concerned about my overdose gesture. She suggested that I come into the infirmary for a couple days to recover. I complied. I was embarrassed, but felt safe. I got a lot of TLC when I was there. Something I really needed at that point. My pledge brothers found out where I was and that I wasn't feeling well. They all came to visit me. Some of the actives even came to visit me. I was embarrassed and didn't tell them why I was really there. I just told them that I had been studying too hard and my system got run down. One of the actives brought me a little white stuffed dog to keep me company. For the first time in my life, I felt cared about and that I really had some friends. It was a wonderful feeling, and did wonders for my recovery.

I continued to take the antidepressant and see Dr. Bohn for a couple months after I got out of the infirmary. She felt I had some deep seeded problems and was not happy when I told her I thought I was okay and would not be seeing her any more. She thought I had serious problems dealing with my anger, separation issues and hadn't quite resolved my father's death. I also quit taking the Elavil, because I felt my depression had gone south and it wasn't needed any more.

For the first time in a long time, I felt rejuvenated and had purpose in my life again. I had one more real test in the Silver Wing pledge program that November. The pledge class was to go on a desert survival training weekend. We had been learning how to navigate with maps and compasses and were going to be put to the test.

We got out to the campsite by nightfall. We had some drilling to do once camp was set up. The actives also gave us a tune for which we had to come up with a pledge song. They also tested us on our unity that evening.

The next morning we got up early. We had to assemble a solar still before the day's activities. Once that was completed, the pledge class was broken up into three platoons of three people. By this time, there were nine of us left in the program. Each group was given a set of coordinates that would lead us to the next set of coordinates and only one quart of water to last for the whole day. We had to carry our backpacks with us on the hike. We were suppose to meet up at a point with the whole pledge class by nightfall. An active went with each group just in case they could not find the next set of coordinates.

Everyone did meet up about 5:30 that evening, just before dusk. We were given one last set of coordinates. The actives had taken our pledge symbol, which was an empty bombshell, the night before during the drills. We were told we would not be allowed back at camp until we had regained our pledge symbol. The new set of coordinates led up the side of a small mountain. We all climbed the mountain and proceeded to look for the pledge symbol. It was dark by the time we got up the mountain and found it difficult to locate the pledge symbol. When we did find it, we found that the actives had defaced it and filled it with sand. We were given explicit instructions not to empty out the sand.

Actives were waiting for us near where the pledge symbol was. We were informed that the final test this weekend was a little exercise in escape and evasion. We had to find our way back to the campsite and not get caught. If we were caught by an active, we would be interrogated and placed in a concentration camp of sorts as POW's. We were given a window to enter the camp freely five minutes before and after the hours of 11 p.m., midnight and 1 a.m.

The pledge class started out together, but as we got within a couple miles of the campsite, broke up. It's amazing how well you can see at night with just moonlight. We could not use flashlights for fear of being caught. It was a real challenge to miss all the cactus that was in the desert.

I got to within sight of the camp a little after midnight. I knew some of my pledge brothers had been captured from the sounds I heard in the area. Mike laid low in a dry wash to survey the situation. As it got closer to 1 a.m. he slithered to the camp on his belly. It looked as though only a couple actives were in the actual campsite. Mike waited till five minutes before one and when the actives' backs were turned, dashed into the camp to the campfire. They argued, saying that he didn't get in before they saw him. How could anyone walk right up to a campfire with people standing around it and not be seen? The object was to get into the campsite five minutes before or after the hour, and Mike had done just that.

By that time, only one other pledge brother had not been found or made it in. He had ten minutes. All the other pledges were being held in an old dry reservoir basin in the POW camp. The actives took me over there to show me what could have happened to me. The guys were shoeless and stripped down to their underwear. They had not gotten any food or water since their capture and were being interrogated to test the unity of the group. Some extreme hazing was going on.

I was accused of not being a unit member by not allowing myself to be captured, too; however, I sensed they were a little glad that I was not captured, because their plans didn't really involve a woman. My only pledge sister still in the class, Alice, had been caught but only about a half hour before I came in and they hadn't quite decided what to do with her.

My one pledge brother still out, made it in safely at 1:10. By 1:30, the E&E exercise was over and everyone was allowed to come back to the campsite. We were offered water. The actives had confiscated all our food, but offered us cold beans or grapefruit. Grapefruit was just the right thing for a dry, parched mouth. Not! I had some anyway because I hadn't had anything to eat all day and very little to drink.

Not long after the desert training, I met Carol, an Angel Flight member who was dating one of the Silver Wing actives. She felt sorry for the way we were being treated and came to our aid. She helped my pledge class pull off some unified pranks against the actives. Carol also became a very good friend. In fact she became what I could call my first real friend. I could confide in her things that I couldn't tell anyone else. She lived in the dorm on another floor so we spent a lot of time together.

Final Boards for Silver Wing were held the first Friday in December. I thought that night would never come. It was an all night hell night of sorts. We were really put to the test for what we had learned that semester and then some. We had wall sessions where we were drilled thoroughly. If we didn't answer properly, we were to do push ups or assume the position holding our ankles that would allow the actives to take a pong paddle to our butts.

We had all our dress uniforms for the final board in front of the officers and cadre the next morning in one of the classrooms. As we were off on a scavenger hunt on campus, the actives were busy in the room making a mess of things. They stacked the desks, threw our clothes all over and in every corner, sprayed shaving cream in our shoes. Boy was it ever a mess. They gave us two hours to clean up the room and be dressed and ready to meet the Board. We were not allowed to leave the detachment to get a clean uniform. They did have an iron there for us to use. It didn't help the guys who had shaving cream on their uniform. I was lucky and only my shoes got the brunt of the shenanigans.

My eight other pledge brothers, sister and I made it through our Boards and were all made actives of Silver Wing. This must have been the hardest pledge program on campus that fall. I couldn't have been any prouder of Mike and my Group for getting me through it. There were any number of times when I really thought about quitting.

In addition to the pledge program, the AFROTC detachment had an excursion to Las Vegas to the home of the Thunderbirds. We flew there on an Air National Guard refueling tanker with passenger seats. We got to observe a mid-air jet refueling on the way over. Only the top students in the detachment were allowed to go. I was one of them. We got there on a Friday afternoon. We had that night and Saturday night to see the sights of Las Vegas. This was my first ever trip to Las Vegas. We stayed in a little offbeat motel on the strip. We did go back to the base Saturday morning to tour the headquarters and see a small performance before the Thunderbirds were off for a show. We got to meet and talk to the pilots.

I did a little gambling but mainly took in some of the shows that only had a set number of drinks for the cover charge. I was playing a couple slots in the lounge at one casino, waiting for the show to start when Mark Lindsey, one of the performers from Paul Revere and the Raiders, brushed by me just before the show. My first close contact with a performer. I was on cloud nine all night.

The trip back was a bit exciting. I sat by the window over one of the wings. I didn't have anything better to do but watch out the window. Not long after we took off, I noticed some oil dripping along the wing. I watched it for some time and noticed that it was more than just a little bit leaking out. I mentioned it to one of my cadre. He told the pilot. They began to watch their gauges. Before long, they were informing us that they were going to have to shut down one of the engines. Luckily this plane had four engines. We flew the rest of the way back to Phoenix on three engines. To top it off there was a lot of turbulence. I felt I was going to be sick. When we got back to Phoenix, we had to circle around a couple times. I didn't know if I could hold it. Boy, was I ever glad to get on the ground.

Spring semester went much better. I had a lot of good new friends and a true sense of belonging to something for the first time in my life. My grades were back up to where I was accustomed to them being. I got all A's with the exception of one B in Art History.

My art classes allowed Bobbie to be a lot more creative. My English class was a composition class. Katherine really loved it. She had some set assignments, but also had opportunities to do some creative writing. She did one piece of prose from atop the butte that really got in touch with what she saw and felt. I really liked it and wish I had it for my collection; however, the only copy I had of it was in a journal that was loaned to a therapist. He ended up losing the journal; so he says.

That spring I also started dating a guy for the first time. He was one of the Silver Wing actives. He said he really wanted to date me in the fall but it was not proper for an active and pledge to be dating. His name was Bryan. He was a very funny fellow and great cartoonist. He had his work floating all over the detachment. He was on a scholarship and going to be a pilot.

Bryan's folks lived in Scottsdale and his dad had a small two-seater Cessna. Bryan had his pilot's license already and took me up flying on numerous occasions. I really liked Bryan and we got along well. I really respected him.

We dated for a semester before we got sexually intimate. Before that, there was a lot of heavy petting and fondling. I was really scared after our first time, because we used no protection and I wasn't on the Pill. Sally and Bryan were drinking quite a bit and things just got out of hand. I was really concerned about getting pregnant the first time I ever did it with someone since my brother. Carol, my friend, told me about a pill that would kill the sperm before they had a chance to fertilize an egg. I went to Planned Parenthood and got a prescription for the Morning After Pill. Soon afterwards I made an appointment at a doctor for a physical and to get a prescription for birth control pills. What happened that night was not planned, but I knew that once the ice had been broken, this activity would become part of our relationship. Sally was hungry and I didn't think I could hold her back any longer.

By the time I was a freshman in college, my weight had dropped from the 185 I was at right after my dad's death down to 145. I was looking real good, because I was quite tall. The Silver

Wing actives selected me to be their queen candidate for that year's Military Ball. Each group and class had a candidate so I had six other candidates to contend with. The queen is usually a junior or senior so I knew I didn't have a strong chance, but I was selected as second runner-up.

I was Bryan's date and he was one of the more popular guys in the corps. I looked great and felt great. This was a feeling I never wanted to lose. For the first time I was accepted and admired by others for who I was. There were no put-downs or bullies to deal with here.

The summer after my freshman year I went back to Denver. I got a job in a restaurant called the Yum Yum Tree. It housed nine small restaurants under one roof. I worked in the German restaurant preparing salads and serving food and ringing up customer orders. It was a long summer, mainly because I allowed myself to be scheduled to work split shifts. I would work the lunch bunch, then go home for a couple hours and come back to work the dinner crowd. Oh, well, it was a job and I didn't have to look very long before getting it.

That summer Roy bought an old Volkswagen Beetle for me to drive to and from work. He decided that he would allow me to take it back to school that fall. He wouldn't permit me to drive it back by myself because he didn't think it would make the long road trip. Instead, we towed it down to Arizona. It was nice to finally get some wheels and not have to rely on everyone else to help me get around.

My sophomore year, Carol and I moved into a room over at the College Inn. At that time it was owned by an off-campus company and was located across the street from the campus. We had our own private outside entrance to our room so it was easier to have boys in our room. It was a coed housing facility. We worked out a code in the window to let each other know when we had our boyfriend over and didn't want to be disturbed.

Living off campus, having a car and a boyfriend, and being active in extracurricular activities had a distinct influence on my grades. Shelley was not getting enough time to do the studying. I had also changed majors for the second time.

During spring of my freshman year, Bobbie got fed up with the arbitrary system of grading in the Art Department. She worked hard on the projects but sometimes could just not satisfy the teacher. If she did, she wasn't satisfied with the results. I looked into changing majors. I decided to get into something a little more disciplined with some precision to the work. It wouldn't be all creative and open to personal taste. I decided to get into the Engineering Department and major in Industrial Art. Bonnie loved this. It was her turn to have fun. This major lasted through the summer when I did some more research on the classes I would have to take. I was going to have to take Calculus and Engineering. These were definitely not strong areas for me.

When I got back from the summer, I talked to Ken, Carol's boyfriend. I told him I wanted to stay with something that had a creative angle to it but was structured. He told me about his major. He was majoring in Physical Geography. He explained about the mapping discipline known as cartography. I became intrigued and thought I would give it a try.

I kept most of the classes I was pre-enrolled in but added one Geography class required for the major. That fall I was taking Photography, Geography, Algebra, Arithmetic Theory and Industrial Wood Processes. A little something for everyone. The photography was for Elizabeth, the geography for Bonnie and Diane (the new alter who really got deep into the geography thing), math for Shelley and the shop class for Mike. This semester our grades did a flip flop from the last. I got all B's except for one A, and that was in Mike's shop class.

During the fall in my Aerospace Studies class, I was selected as Cadet of the Month and given a jet ride at one of the training bases in the area. I went out to the base, was dressed in a flight suit and given a parachute. I was wearing glasses at the time and couldn't wear them and the flight helmet at the same time, so I couldn't see where or what we were doing in the air. When I went up, the pilot had me pull some G-forces and did some barrel roles and loops. It was great but I was getting a bit queasy. The pilot put me on 100% oxygen and that helped. He gave me the stick to do some flying. I had to put my nose right into the control panel to keep it straight and level since

I couldn't see. I did get to do a couple turns. Mike was ecstatic over this and in seventh heaven. This was a thrill to match all thrills. In fact everyone in my Group was excited about the ride. I'll never forget it.

After that ride and the experience of not being able to visually experience it, I decided I would check into getting contact lens to replace my glasses. I did get them. I started out with soft, but within a few months had to change to hard. My eyes generated a lot of protein build-up on the soft lens that made my vision blurry. I couldn't keep the lens clean enough. They didn't have enzyme treatments that were over the counter then. I had to take my lens into the doctor's office to have them treated. The hard lenses took longer to adjust to, but I managed.

At the fall Silver Wing Dining-In, I was elected to be Silver Wing Commander the next semester. This was a real honor. Not only did my fellow actives recognize me for my leadership skills, but the cadre held a lot of respect for the leader of this group. Not only was it unusual for someone who was not going to be a pilot or navigator to hold this position, but I was the first woman in the history of the organization.

Second semester Carol and I moved further off campus to an apartment. We took in one of her friends as a third roommate to help with expenses. This was a real test for being on my own, because now I would have to cook for myself if I was going to eat. I never really got very close with Carol's friend, Sandy. She had a bedroom to herself while Carol and I shared one. We also had a kitten that we found towards the end of the first semester. That was one reason for moving. Also, to have a bedroom with a door that shut and could give us privacy. That way, when our boyfriends came over, we wouldn't be embarrassed or have to feel obligated to get lost.

That spring, I had a physical out at Williams AFB for qualifying for the AFROTC officer training. My eyes were so bad that they would not allow me into the program as an officer candidate. I could enlist after college, though and possibly work my way up the ranks. I was not going to go through college to become only an airman. No thanks.

By the summer, my GPA had dropped to 3.06. The only A I got was in Aerospace Studies. I got a C of all things, in Equitation (horseback riding), and this was something I loved to do. This class was more than just horseback riding. I had trouble identifying the lead my horse was on. Peggy really loved this class despite the low grade I got. I got my very first D in Trigonometry. It was too much for Shelley. It was a math that had precision, but was not accomplished through trial and error like she was accustomed to. She loves working with figures but trig was a whole new animal that she could not relate to. I should have dropped the class, but was willing to sacrifice my GPA for not having to take another math class.

Just before school was out for the summer, I answered an ad for summer help in sales. I figured I was good at selling Girls Scout cookies when younger, and wouldn't have any problem with this job. Besides, it promised you could make some real good money. I went to see what it was all about and came away signed up. It was for doing door-to-door book sales in communities east of the Mississippi. The company hired mainly college students for the summer. Those from the western U.S. were sent to the east and the eastern students to the west.

By taking this job I would miss Carol and Ken's wedding. They were getting married shortly after school got out. I was suppose to be a bridesmaid. Carol was extremely disappointed over this. She didn't hate me for it, but did bring a distance to our relationship. A new alter stepped in and pulled me in another direction. Carol was the best friend I ever had, and I should never have done this to her.

This job required me to leave for training in Nashville three days before the wedding. Whichever alter appeared to get me to take this job bailed out early that summer when things didn't go as planned. The job must have turned out to be more than she had bargained for.

A lot of things that I was doing was seeming quite random at this time. I would jump from thing to thing and not seem real organized at doing anything well. I was losing a lot of time. That's because I was not real co-conscious to my alters at that time and really didn't realize how much control they had. In fact, I really didn't know it was anyone other than myself that was doing all the things I was doing. Everything seemed like a blur and just happening. It is only now, in my therapy and understanding of them, that I can put alters with certain acts and accomplishments and troubles.

When I got to Nashville, I would soon learn that hard-core sales was not something that you learn selling Girl Scout cookies. A lot of play acting was involved and you had to be firm on your grounding. This was not me. I made it through the week of training, barely. I got my assignment. I was going to Lexington, Kentucky. The heart of the Bible belt to sell Bibles and sex education books. What a combo!

I met up at a minister's house with the girls who were going to be my three roommates. The minister had a friend that had some apartments in town that they rented out. We went to take a look the next day. We ended up with a cheap basement apartment near the university in Lexington. It was a two bedroom and furnished quite poorly. The furniture in the living room was quite run down and very lumpy. The beds were propped up on bricks and the closets were steel lockers. It had a gas stove and refrigerator and one bathroom. Regardless, we made do and called it home for awhile.

The first thing we did was split up the town as to what we were going to cover. Not being familiar with Lexington, we didn't know where the best neighborhoods were. The minister did give us some general information that helped us to disregard the real poor neighborhoods. In training, they recommended that we try to buy a cheap bike if we didn't have a car. I didn't take my bug. I left it back in Phoenix with Bryan's folks so was on foot. I didn't locate a bike to buy until the second week.

I was not real good with my sales pitch. Like I said, the alter that got me into this left me high and dry by the time I got to Lexington. It was difficult to back out at this point. I did the best I could. I took a lot of rejection that summer. Fortunately, I had a lot of experience with that. I met a lot of neat people, though. I spent more time talking and getting to know the people rather than selling books. If I happened to sell some books it was by sheer luck and not my selling skills. A month through the summer I was asked to spend a couple days with my team leader because the company felt I needed to see how a real pro handled the customers. My sales were pretty pitiful. It looked easy by the way he did it, but he was all bullshit. I wasn't like that. I could not lie or lead people on like he did. It just wasn't in my nature.

When I got back to my territory, I tried a few of his tactics with little success. Like I said, it wasn't me. I did find myself getting angry and telling off a few rude customers. Not long after I got back, two of my roommates became quite ill. They had come down with mononucleosis. We were not eating and sleeping properly and it caught up with them. They decided to go home to recover. Because of my sales being so poor, I couldn't afford to pay a share of their rent to stay in the apartment. We were only paying $160 a month, but $40 and my groceries were barely all I could handle. I decided to bail out. I called my parents and they said they would buy me a plane ticket back to Denver for the rest of the summer. They would not allow me to go back to Phoenix until school started. I took them up on their offer.

If ever given this kind of opportunity again, I'm sure I would pass it up. I'm just not into hard core sales. I like a personable approach. In looking back on this experience, I'm not totally dissatisfied for having it. Despite the rejection, it forced me to get out around total strangers and to make the first connection with them. I got a hell of a lot of doors slammed in my face, but I met a lot of interesting people along the way. I would never do this again, but feel I am a better person from having had the experience. One thing, though, I have become a real hard ass when it comes to door-to-door salesmen or sales people trying to sell me over the phone. I know their routine and I'm not as gullible as I once was.

The summer was half over when I got back to Denver. There was no way I would be able to find a job for six weeks. My mom informed me that her church was looking for an assistant cook to help up at church summer camp. It was a two week camp up in the mountains near Bailey. Mike and Peggy jumped at the opportunity. Elizabeth was excited to. My mom said how pretty it was up there. Elizabeth was able to take a number of pictures of the scenery and people up there. Susan was even excited, because they had evening singing sessions. Carol and Bobbie liked it too, because they got to help some of the kids with craft projects. It didn't bring in a lot of money, but I got a very warming experience and feeling from it. It even kind of brought me back to God. When I got back to school, I found a church that I felt comfortable in attending on a fairly regular basis.

That fall I had to find a new place to live, because my best friend and roommate had a new roommate, her husband. I checked out some new apartments that were going up about a mile from campus that spring. They were finished in time before school started. With more rent to pay, I was also going to have to get a part time job during school. I checked out the new apartments and decided to rent a furnished studio there.

With my summer experience, I was not hesitant at all to mention that I was looking for a job. A couple who had three kids were the managers. They happened to be looking for an office secretary. I asked if they would consider me for the job. I got it and started the day after I moved in. My job was to show apartments, type up rental agreements and take rent payments.

The complex allowed small pets because the managers had a dog. We got rid of the cat that we had when Carol and I were roommates. I went to the dumb friends pound and fell in love with a little white puppy. She was a poodle mix. I had to bring her home. I named her Toshi. This was a new experience for me. I had had pets (dogs) before, but never had they really been all mine. I also had no experience at house breaking a dog, but I managed. I got her so well trained on newspapers, that I had to be careful reading the Sunday paper on the floor. We became the best of friends.

That fall I was enrolled in sixteen hours of classes and was working twenty hours at the complex. This was on top of my active participation at the AFROTC detachment. I was no longer in the program, but I did join the women's auxiliary, Angel Flight. You did not have to be a cadet to belong. Many of the guy's girlfriends were in the flight. The initiation was nothing compared to Silver Wing.

I had returned to school also to have my first romantic jolt. Bryan was leaving me for another girl in the program. She was a freshman. To top it off, she was also joining Angel Flight. My heart was saddened by this because I really liked Bryan a lot. Having experienced love since then, I must say that I didn't really love him. We had a lot in common and had fun together. It just so happened that we were also lovers. I got over the loss within a couple months. I still kept current on his goings on, but looked to bigger fish in the ocean.

Diane really got deep into my major that fall. I was taking Geology, Landforms and Map Reading classes. I also took a class on Courtship and Marriage. I did not fair too well in this class. I got a C. Now that is embarrassing. No wonder I am still single and have never been married. I couldn't even get an A, let alone a B in a class such as courtship and marriage.

Geology really intrigued Diane. Learning about the development of the earth and mountains was a whole new world. I almost thought I was going to change my majors again, but figured being my junior year, it was a little late. Besides, I would have had to take chemistry and kinda figured not.

There were problems at the complex and the managers skipped town the end of the year. The owners brought in new management. I was out of a job. They also would not allow any new pets in the complex. I was able to keep Toshi because of a grandfather clause.

Right after Christmas break I went out to Williams AFB with some of the other Angel Flight members. We went to the Officer's Club. Some of the gals knew guys out there. I felt kind of funny because I knew no one and wasn't much into picking up strangers. That night, though, I did meet someone. His name was Ken. God, was he handsome. He was a pilot in the training program. He came over and sat down beside me and started talking. Before I knew it, we were dancing the night away.

Ken was a real gentleman. He didn't try to swoop me off my feet then run me off somewhere to get me into bed with him. He did ask for my phone number and if he could call sometime. I thought, yeah, I'm sure you'll call. I gave it to him anyway.

The following week, he called and asked me out. I was elated. Never in a million years did I think a good looking guy with manners would have anything to do with me. I was always brought up feeling inadequate or unimportant enough for anyone, let alone someone as good as he seemed. We went out to dinner and a movie and had a very enjoyable time. This time he asked for nothing more than a kiss. I obliged. All along I was feeling this drive inside. I bet Sally must have been fit to be tied when she still didn't end up in bed with him. It didn't bother me one bit, though.

Our dates were distanced. We saw each other every week or two. He was really dedicated to his pilot training and didn't want anything to get in his way. Sally, in the meantime, would go out to the Club to pick up guys on a regular basis. She didn't really pick anyone up as much as she got to know some of the guys real well. They invited her to some of their parties. That's when she would pick up guys.

Sally had a keen way of flirting with the guys and luring one into a bedroom. She would get him all hot and bothered and play games with him. Then when he couldn't stand it any longer and was ready to tear both our clothes off, she would calmly say, that she usually doesn't do this with guys. That she has had sex with only a few special men and that he should feel privileged that she is giving in to him.

I believe my masochistic alter, Monique, came out at some of these parties, because she had a way of being very overpowering of the men during sex. She loved to have total control of the situation and loved to tease the guys till they were ready to explode and/or try to rape her. This excited both of them; the so-called struggle that ensued was the real turn-on. Sally just liked good, clean sex. Monique loved to go down on the guys and do oral sex.

Ken and I finally ended up in bed by about our fifth date. Some of my alters thought it would never happen. He was great in bed. Myself, I just faded into the woodwork. Sally was in seventh heaven with him. He was creative, yet gentle; very civilized.

Ken finished up his pilot training that spring and was transferred to Oklahoma. We kept in touch. We would see each other when he came back to Phoenix with flight missions. His parents lived in Scottsdale, so he had another excuse for coming back. Again, I really liked Ken very much but never felt that gut wrenching tug that I got when I was in love. I guess I always thought he was too good for me and a dream. I did feel more romantically toward him than Brian.

That spring semester all my classes pertained to my major. I had a class on Arizona Geology. That class took a weekend trip to the Grand Canyon. We stopped at many of the road cuts and looked off over the plateaus at the coal deposits. We discussed the evolution of Arizona. It took all day to get to the canyon.

The class met the next morning at the rim. The trip down into the canyon was awesome. Diane found numerous outcrops of rocks with fossils on them. It was a long, hard trek and many of the students got heat exhaustion. I managed okay, though. That night class members walked to the rim and viewed a phenomenal sunset. Elizabeth was there with her camera. We even saw a Doberman give birth to a litter of puppies. Made me think of Toshi. She was back at the apartment. One of the guys from the detachment was taking care of her. I wasn't going to let her have pups, though. I had her spade when she was old enough.

About March I found an ad in the paper for another job. It was at Globe Discount in Mesa. It was a large discount department store. It was about five miles from campus. I applied and got the job. I started out learning the registers and worked as a cashier.

Shortly after I got the job at Globe I was going out to an air show at Luke AFB. It was fairly early in the morning. I noticed crop dusters spraying the fields. I also noticed a truck with a trailer of cotton and another car pulled off the side of the road in front of me. As I was getting closer, I noticed the car pull onto the road and drive off. I also noticed the truck start to pull back onto the road. I figured since the car had gone on down the road, so was the truck. So, as I got closer, I pulled into the oncoming lane to pass him since he was not going very fast.

Boy, was that a mistake. You see, the truck was not going on down the road, but rather pulling into the driveway on the other side of the road. By the time I noticed what was really happening, I had two choices. I could hit the truck at the trailer hitch or try to speed up and go around him before he got across the road. He didn't even see me coming. Just before I got to a point to go around him, I saw a big drainage ditch on both sides of the driveway. I now tried to make it into the drive before him. It didn't work. He hit me on the passenger side nearly tearing my wheel completely off. I had slowed down when I knew I wasn't going to get around him. At that point everything seemed to be going in slow motion and there was no way I could stop the accident from happening.

I came to a thump of a stop. I was hung up and going nowhere. I didn't get whiplash or anything but a big bump on my leg. I was really shook up. I got out and staggered around. All of a sudden, I didn't know where I was. Everything was a big, bright blur. I was still in shock by the time the sheriff's department arrived. I couldn't talk. It all seemed like a dream. I couldn't defend myself with my story. I just stood there and let the woman who was driving the truck give her spleel.

Here I was stranded on the other side of nowhere out in the country. I was about 20 miles from my apartment and about 4 miles from Luke. The deputy offered to take me to the base if I was sure I could get a ride home from some friends that were there. I knew a lot of Angel Flight and Arnold Air guys were going to be there and that one of them would surely take me home. We were working a hamburger stand at the air show that day. Somehow I just couldn't get into the scene and just wandered around until someone was ready to leave.

Needless to say, I was without a car for about a month. Major damage was done to the front end and suspension system. For the next month, I rode my bike the five miles to and from work.

I decided to stay in Arizona that summer and continue to work at Globe. By late summer, I had been moved over to the layaway department. I had proven my skills on the register and demonstrated my responsibility as a hard worker. I would be in charge of watching the fitting rooms, doing all the paper work on layaways, put the merchandise away and take payments. I was also eventually trained on how to do the reports for the department.

I also decided to attend summer school. One of the courses was a six hour class on field methods that was required for graduation. First summer term I took a class on Money and Banking and got a C in it. No wonder I had financial problems later in life and ten years later ended up taking out bankruptcy. The other class I got a B in. It was a Religious sociology class.

I had to take a week off from work that summer because my field methods class had an assignment that took the class to California. We went to the Oceanside and San Diego area. We mapped the avocado groves and San Diego's lower downtown pleasure shops. It was very interesting. I enjoyed my instructors and classmates. They were a lot of fun.

One night after a long, hard day in the field, some of us loaded up into the school car and drove to Oceanside to a bar that some of the guys knew about. It was a topless bar. Mike went with the guys so was not embarrassed at all. He was just one of the guys, after all. Sally went, too. She hid behind Mike for awhile until she started to get turned on. She loved to dance, and seductively at that. She pulled a couple of the guys into the corner of the bar and started dancing with them. The manager didn't care for this distraction and said that if I wanted to dance, I was welcome on the stage. The guys got a big kick out of this so she said he was on. Only Sally was not going to remove any of her clothes. She had a tank top and shorts on and took her shoes off. The music was great and Sally danced for two songs. The guys were stunned yet excited. All eyes were on me for a change.

I had a good long talk with my professor on the way back and asked for his advice on where I could use my education and training. I also asked if there were any other classes I should take that would help me with a cartographic career. He suggested I take some graphic art classes that taught me about printing and the production of the maps I would make. I thought, "What a great idea. More art classes." He also suggested that I might take some computer classes.

When I got home, I went over to Ken and Carol's to pick up Toshi. They had been taking care of her while I was in California. I was stunned when I got her into my sights. She had a leg-long cast on her front leg and a plastic collar around her neck. Ken asked that I not get too excited, and that she was okay. He explained what had happened. She had made a mess in their apartment and he went to scold her. Toshi jumped up and backwards into a doorway and broke her leg. She had a collar around her head because she had chewed through one cast already. I was embarrassed that my dog was not the perfect angel, but also angry for what happened.

She looked so pitiful, but was a terror on three legs with that cast. She got along just fine. In fact, when I took her out for walks, she would tear off into the field way ahead of me to chase the birds. When she got mad at me, she would come up and give me a whack with her cast. She was cute, but this little cuteness set me back about $500.

I signed up for a printing class that fall and intro to computer science. The computer class ended up being more than I could comprehend at that time and withdrew. I had a Cartographic Design class that I had to do some work with computers. The final project in the class was to build a map using the computer. I was going to create a map of Colorado showing all the major ski resorts with a skier on the map where they were located. This was back in the days of keypunch. I had over 175 cards in my stack. The only thing, is it wouldn't print. I got a border around the map and a title, but no map or skiers. I went in to see my professor and student aide on several occasions and they couldn't tell me where my problem was. Because I couldn't get my final project to print, I got a C in the class. Diane was bummed out by that.

I really liked my printing class and thought I would do a quick minor in graphic design. I ended up taking an incomplete in the class because I didn't have my final portfolio with project summaries done by the end of the semester. I also had a special project I was working on.

One of the geography professors who was writing a book found out that Bonnie was taking a printing class and said he would pay her to draft a map and print it up for him. She agreed. The map took a little longer to do than expected. That's why she didn't get it done before the end of the semester. Because of the incomplete and the two C's and A that I got, my GPA dropped down to 2.98. A real blow to my self esteem and ego as a good student.

To be honest, I don't know how my grades were even that good. It seemed like I hardly studied. I would study for tests for what seemed like hours and take good notes, but feel like I hadn't absorbed a single thing. I went into many tests with the idea that if I didn't absorb it the first time I read it or heard it in class, I was never going to learn it.

I don't know whether it was from school, activities and working 25 hours a week, but I had a real problem my senior year. Actually it started the last part of my junior year. I had the hardest time staying alert in class. My mind and ears were tuned into what was going on, but my eyes would roll back in my head as if I was falling asleep. To try to adjust to this, in certain classes I would try to contribute to the discussion. Before I knew it, words were rolling out of my mouth and I didn't seem to be making any sense at all. I felt I was in the heart of the discussion, but was actually making a fool of myself because it seemed like I had absolutely no control over what I was saying. If this wasn't the weirdest thing. This was one point when I was beginning to think I was going crazy. I don't know whether it was alters trying to adjust to this phenomenon or what. All I know, is it was not a very comfortable feeling at all.

Around Thanksgiving, I got a call from Ken. He had been transferred to a base in California and moved to Riverside. He wanted to know if I could come out and visit over Christmas. I told him I had plans to go home for Christmas but would make up some excuse to come back to school early and then drive out to see him. I told my parents that I had to be back at the store and that I could only get a week off. Besides, they were letting me off at the busiest time of the year, Christmas.

When I got back to Tempe, I had a surprise waiting for me. Someone had broken into my car and stolen the engine. What a shock. How could something like this happen when you have a policeman living in an apartment that faced the parking lot?

I called my parents and they in turn contacted the insurance company. I had a police report made. It delayed my trip by a day. I was not going to give up my trip to see Ken over a little incident like this. After all the formalities were taken care of, I went out and rented a car to drive to California.

I left for California the next morning about 5:30. The trip went well. I did get tired. This was the first long trip I had taken by myself at the wheel. I got into Riverside late in the afternoon.

It was good to see Ken again. He took me to the base and showed me the big jet that he was assigned to flying all over the world. He also took me flying over the San Bernardino Valley. We went to a discotheque one night. Sally had a sexual marathon with him. We must not have come out of the bedroom for a whole day. It was a visit that ended almost as quickly as it appeared.

The trip home did not come off without incident. I had rented a little Chevette. It really moved down the highway. I had been playing leap frog with another driver for several miles before coming upon Palm Springs. All of a sudden I looked in my rear view mirror and saw flashing lights. I slowed down and pulled over, but the patrolman passed me. I felt a quick burst of relief because I knew I had been speeding. When I got further down the road, I saw the patrolman had pulled the guy I was gaming with over. I thought I had really lucked out by not getting caught. Not! As I pulled up to where the patrolman was, he saw me and motioned me to pull over. He had tagged me, too. I was sure I had been going over 75, but he gave me a ticket for going 68, because that was what he clocked me at. Fortunately, I didn't have to go back to California to appear in court. The ticket ended up costing me $25.

My bug was out of commission for about a month. The auto shop had trouble finding a good rebuilt engine for the car. The only one they could locate was a Baja Bug engine. I was not too keen on having a souped up vehicle but needed to have my wheels back. I let them do what they had to do to get it back to me. It never seemed to be the same after that. My car felt like a stranger and little things kept going wrong with it.

I went to White Mountain for a wedding over Spring Break. I got a vapor lock about 20 miles outside of town and had to flag down some help. On the way back over the mountain, I lost the greatest portion of my brakes. Needless to say, I didn't take long trips after that.

My final semester in school had me taking some interesting classes. I was so into flying and planes, that I thought it would be neat to take an Air Traffic Control class. It was a little more technical than I could understand. I got a C. I had three classes in the Graphic Arts department and got A's in all of them.

My final geography class was in Remote Sensing. Like my Cartographic Design class the previous semester, it was a graduate level course. I faired better in this class and got a B. I did an interesting study on the fauna of the desert. I had Cary, one of my pilot friends from the detachment, fly me out over the desert. Elizabeth did some infrared photography of the vegetation and water sources.

The spring was fairly uneventful. Sally was up to her sleeping around. I don't have a clue as to how much she did do, because of my memory lapses during these episodes. To be truthful, I hope I never figure it out. I am too embarrassed by her conduct and don't like to admit that any of my alters are promiscuous.

I did my best that spring to locate a career-based job in the Phoenix area. I promised my parents that if I did not have a job by graduation, I would return to Denver with them. I had to abide by their wishes, because I came up empty.

I was excited about graduation until my mom hit me with a blow that would shatter my excitement. She informed me that I would not be allowed to bring Toshi back to Denver with me. I argued and threatened to not go back to Denver, but her level of intimidation had not dissipated while I was away at school. She had a remarkable way of making me feel guilty if I did not abide by her wishes. She said I was obligated to abide by their wishes since they had spent all that money on my education.

I cried hard–very hard–for a day. I took long walks with Toshi, wishing that I had the guts to just run away. I finally got up enough nerve to call Cary and cry on his shoulder. His father was a veterinarian and might know someone who could give Toshi a good home. He made me a promise that he would personally find a new home for her, and would not let her wind up in the pound.

I was also informed by Roy and my brother, who had come down for graduation, that I would not be allowed to drive the bug back to Denver. It was literally a wreck and unsafe on the streets, let alone the highway. We packed it up and towed it behind my parent's car.

Graduation was on Friday, the 13th of May, 1977. Fortunately, I was not a superstitious person, or I would have thought my future doomed from the start. On the contrary, I was eager to get out in the world and find a new life as a young professional.

BRAVE NEW WORLD

I took a couple days off upon my return to Denver before starting to look for a job. I had no transportation when I started my search so had to have my mom drive me around. I agreed to live with my parents and rely on them for transportation until I could get settled in a new job and start bringing in some money.

A couple days into my search, I found an ad in the paper for a map drafter for an oil company. I talked to Roy about it and asked how much work he thought was in it. I couldn't figure out why an oil company needed a map drafter. He said that oil companies rely quite extensively on maps and suggested that I check into it. It might be a very good job.

I called that day and had an interview set up for the next morning. It was with a company that was in the top ten of the Fortune 500's.

I went in for the interview. I was first asked to take a small drafting test. I don't think I did as well as I could have because I had never really been tested on my artistic talents before. Nonetheless, I went into it head first and completed it satisfactorily. Jim was the supervisor for the department. He was a personable guy and made me feel real comfortable. As I was going over my qualifications, he noticed from my resumé that I had been honored in *Who's Who in American Colleges and Universities*. This made for a direct hit and feather in my cap, because his daughter had also been selected for this when in college. He knew right away that I must have strong work habits and dedicated to the job at hand. I left the interview on a very positive note.

Jim called back that afternoon asking if I would like the job, and when I could start. I said right away and he asked if I could come in the next afternoon to fill out my new hire paperwork. He said the job paid $900 a month but was also based on hourly wages, so it could be more when overtime was needed. This was about $100 more than I had expected. Later, I would learn that oil companies took good care of their employees and paid them well.

I actually started on the following Monday. Jim wasted no time in giving me work to do. I was a bit slow at first trying to get into the flow of things and putting my talents to daily use for eight hours. I was just accustomed to working 2 to 3 hours a day on art and cartography projects. I had a tremendous amount to learn about this job, but went into it with a positive and open mind. I picked things up and adapted quickly to what was required of me. I was eager to learn as much about the industry as I could. I found it quite fascinating and exciting.

It didn't take long for me to prove myself to Jim and the company. Bonnie and Diane were ecstatic and had found a place to call home. Not more than a month after my hiring, Jim started giving me more than one assignment at a time. I was fairly quick at getting the work out and was always going to him asking for something else to do. As work came in that he thought I could handle, he immediately gave it to me. It wasn't unusual to have three or four projects at one time on my table. I had a natural tendency to know how and when to work on something and juggle things around so all my deadlines were met.

Living at home and having my mom drive me to and from work every day was getting to be a real drag and embarrassing. I was used to coming and going on my own schedule and not accustomed to having to rely on someone. By September, I had enough money for a down payment on a new car and was eligible to join the company credit union. I began shopping for a new car. I spent about a week in this process and became quite confused by all the choices. Finally, one night I went to a dealership and picked out my new car in the dark. It sort of reached out and grabbed me and said, "Take me." I got the loan approved and a week later was once again independent.

There was added expense and costs involved in owning a car of my own that I hadn't experienced before. I now had to pay for parking downtown, gas, taxes, license and insurance. When I was at school, all I paid for was gas. These added expenses were worth it, though, to have the freedom it provided.

When at college, I was a Girl Scout leader with Carol. We had a troop of Cadettes. That summer, I got in touch with the local Girl Scout Council and offered to be leader for a troop of Cadettes. There was a group of girls in my parent's neighborhood in need of a leader. I took on the troop. I had about seven girls who came to the first troop meeting that fall.

By late fall, I was ready to make my next move. I began looking for a place of my own to live. At first I thought about getting an apartment with my sister because she was living at home, too. She was working in a nearby Penney's store. We spent some time looking, but she found out that she might be transferred to Boulder and thought she would hold off. I couldn't wait any longer, so decided to look on my own for a one bedroom. I found a place a couple miles from my parent's. I made a deposit and signed a lease. I moved the first of November.

Cary, the guy who took Toshi and found her a home, was coming through Denver before he started pilot training. I told him that I didn't have a bed yet but he was welcome to sleep on the floor. We had a good, strong platonic relationship. I did get my waterbed the day he arrived. He helped me set it up. Cary stayed for a couple days. It was nice to visit with a school buddy. He encouraged me to get out and involved to meet new people.

I was still in touch with Ken after moving back to Denver. He was glad to hear that I had gotten a place of my own. He said he had some vacation time coming up in February and wanted to know if he could come visit. I said I'd love to see him again.

Ken also encouraged me to get out and make some new friends. He suggested that I try skiing because he would like to go skiing when he came up. I told him there was a ski club in my part of town and promised that I would go on some trips and learn to ski. Little did he know that this suggestion would soon mark the end of our relationship.

As promised, I went on a ski trip in January. I was bound and determined to take up skiing so bought skis and equipment right after Christmas before I went on my first trip. The day of the trip I got on a bus not knowing a sole. I was sitting beside a window by myself when and guy asked to sit next to me. I told him he was welcome to. His name was Gene.

We ended up talking to one another the whole way up to the ski resort. As it turned out, he also worked for a major oil company as an engineer. We found out that we had a lot in common professionally and personally. He offered to teach me how to ski that day.

Gene was quite patient with me. I had a rather negative skiing experience before college and was a bit paranoid to get on skis again. He stuck with me as I fell off the lift and slid down the mountain. I told him that if he wanted to go off and do his thing after lunch he could. He said that he thought I would improve after getting some rest at lunch and some food in my stomach. He was right. I wasn't quite as pitiful after lunch. He stuck with me the whole day through.

Upon the return to Denver, some of the people on the trip decided they would go to a local bar for some dinner and drinks. Gene asked if I wanted to go. I said, "sure, why not?" As we got ready to leave. Gene said he had a good time with me that day and wanted to know if he could call me later in the week. I thought that would be great and gave him my phone number.

He called about three days later and we talked for almost an hour. He asked if I would like to go out with him on Friday. I accepted. After dinner and a movie, he brought me back to my place. We sat on the couch and started talking. He soon started kissing me and fondling me. I was not going to let Sally come out on our first real date and come across as an easy pick-up. I held her back. I told him I was not ready to get involved just yet and needed more time to get to know him.

He came back with "patience is a virtue," and said he would respect my wishes. I appreciated that and it made me respect him.

It wasn't long and we started dating regularly. After about four weeks, I gave Sally permission to do her thing. I felt this guy was worth keeping and I didn't want to lose him just because I didn't care for sex. He had needs and Sally had needs.

A couple weeks before Ken was planning on coming out, I had to make one of the most difficult calls to a guy. Always, it had been guys who would break off with me. It was now my time to break off with a guy I liked very much and had good memories with. I had to be realistic, though. Ken was in California and I would be lucky to see him a couple times a year. Gene was here and now and able to directly satisfy needs and desires.

We went on several ski trips that spring with the ski club. We usually did something Friday night after work and then I'd spend most of the weekend with him. He had a small townhouse in Aurora, not too terribly far from my apartment. I met a lot of new people who were his friends and he got me active with other people. Kind of pulled me out of my reclusive shell.

By April, I was doing something every night. I also joined a softball league with Gene. If I wasn't with my scouts, or bowling or playing softball, I was with Gene.

I was still feeling good about the way I looked and felt. I was having the time of my life and had some of the best self-esteem I could ever remember. I felt so confident about who I was that I tried out for the Pony Express in May. They were to be the cheerleaders for the Denver Bronco professional football team. I loved to dance but didn't take the choreography directions very well. I was dropped from the group on the second cut.

Sally and Francie were having the time of their lives with all this attention and time out that these activities and my relationship provided. Bonnie and Diane did their thing at work during the week. Gene loved photography, so Elizabeth took to him right off. They would go on camping trips or drives to the mountains to take photographs.

Monique even got into this relationship with her domineering and controlling sex. Gene would go absolutely crazy when she would go down on him and give him a blow job. She even enjoyed swallowing the semen when he came. Yuck! How appalling. No complaints from Gene, though.

Gene and I took some vacation time over the 4th of July. We flew to San Francisco to see the sites and tour the wineries in the Napa Valley. This was my first trip ever to the San Francisco area and wowed by all the things to see and do. We drove to the Napa Valley. Along the way, Monique would turn Gene on as he drove. She even went down on him a couple times. Later, I would hear about a woman who had done this and caused an accident. The couple were killed. When the paramedics arrived, she was still down on the guy.

That same month, Gene and I flew off to Los Angeles for a weekend. I stayed at his mom's house. We attended an art festival and went to Disneyland.

Gene sold his townhouse the end of September 1978 and bought an old Victorian home in the City Park neighborhood. It was a predominantly black neighborhood. My rent was going up so I found an apartment in Central Denver that was closer to his new home.

By fall I still had my scout troop. Instead of bowling, I took a stained glass class and belly dancing. I also worked the national Girl Scout Convention.

In October, Gene and I flew with a tour to Seattle to see a Bronco game. We saw a Washington University vs. ASU game the day before. We stayed a little longer than the tour and saw the King Tut exhibit and took the ferry over to Vancouver Island. We toured the Butchart Gardens and took a gondola up to the top of Vancouver's Grouse Mountain.

That Christmas I decided to play the 12 Days of Christmas. On each of the twelve days before Christmas, I gave him a gift with a number of items he needed corresponding to that day. This is how the Twelve Days of Christmas went: 1 tie rack; 2 down booties; 3 torso warmers; 4 lbs. of slide storage; 5 tubes of toothpaste; 6 boxer shorts; 7 bars of soap; 9 odds 'n ends; 10 buttonholes; 11 pair of socks and 12 cans of beer.

In January I had more to think about than just Gene and me. Toward the end of the month, Roy suffered a severe heart attack. He survived but was in the hospital for three weeks. I was really scared about losing him. I had grown to love Roy and consider him my father.

Gene gave me someone to talk to who would listen and not condemn me like my mother. Things were not going well at work and I was doing a lot of complaining, but he would listen patiently and give me the kind of caring feedback I was in need of.

Morale was real low and there had been numerous shake-ups. In the spring of 1979, I got so fed up after an incident that I quit and went to work for another oil company for three months. One of the guys told me to "fuck off" in front of the whole department and a couple geologists. Things were out of hand and I didn't think that kind of treatment was justified. Some of the guys were back-stabbing Jim and I was standing up for him. They didn't like this.

One of the exploration groups were moving to another building and they wanted a drafter to go with them. Jim valued me too much in his department and was going to send a less-qualified drafter over there. This was too much for me to take after all the hard work I had done. I needed some recognition. That's why I quit for only $50 a month more.

It wasn't long before I was just as unhappy at the new job. The supervisor's personality just didn't fit with my standards for a superior. I kept in touch with some of the people back at the first company. Things quickly fell apart after I left. The guy they sent to the new building had bombed badly. Jim wanted me back and was willing to let me work at the other building. I was not surprised when he called to offer me more money to come back to work for him. The drafter I had been talking to suggested I not come back for pennies and that they were willing to make it worth my while. I named a price that was $300 a month more than I was making at my new job. Jim called the next day and asked how soon I could be back to work, that they were willing to meet my request.

I really enjoyed the people I worked for in the new building, but had my work cut out for me. I had to redo a lot of the mistakes the other guy had made along with preparing all the exhibits for that department's annual budget meeting. I worked some long hours. At least I got paid overtime for it and was worth it.

We were in the peak of the oil boom days and the company was experiencing growing pains. We got word that fall that we would be moving into a new building the next spring. All the departments would be back together again. A new company would even be formed. We would have both divisions housed in the same building.

Gene and I joined a bowling league downtown that fall. I also enrolled in two classes at the University of Colorado at Denver. I took a Real Estate and a Business Law class. I also took the exam for admission to graduate school. I was thinking about getting an MBA to help advance myself with my job.

I hid in a closet in my mind throughout this wonderful relationship the others in my Group were having. They would go overboard and spend all kinds of money on Gene and to do things with him. For Gene's birthday that year, the Group took him to dinner at his favorite restaurant...in San Francisco! I flew the two of us out there for the weekend. On top of it, I bought him a new 19" color TV.

Yes, I even allowed myself to break all my moral standards and moved in with him that November. He said he wanted at least six months living with a woman before he would decide to marry her. I was so terribly and madly in love with this guy, that I was willing to do anything to keep this relationship going. I truly felt I was ready to make a real lifetime commitment and fantasized about it constantly.

For my birthday in 1979, Gene had rented a condo up at Copper Mountain. We were going up for a weekend of skiing and romantic encounters. The trip was cut short. That morning as we got up to the top of the mountain, there was an emergency message for Gene back at the base of the mountain. I told him to go ahead and ski down as fast as he could and that I would be down as soon as I could. He was still a much better skier than me.

When I caught up with him at the base of the mountain, I found him solemn and in tears. He had just gotten word that his mom was killed the night before in a car accident. She was in Phoenix. We immediately packed up and came back to town. He was really shook. He was an only child and he had lost his father a few years back.

Alice, my mother alter, came to the rescue to try to comfort him and pull things together. She made some calls to his family to find out the plans. She then made plane reservations for the two of us to go to Phoenix to help with arrangements and for the funeral.

His mother was on the way home with her fiancé. They had just announced to the family down there that they were planning to be married. Out of nowhere came a couple kids in a truck. They had been drinking and ran a stop sign. His mother was killed instantly, but her fiancé died on the way to the hospital.

Gene was never the same after that. The boy that was driving was under age and would not be prosecuted as an adult. This made Gene very angry. He had a lot of rage built up inside him but would not talk to me. We grew more distant.

After six months had passed since I moved in with him, I asked him where our relationship was. He couldn't give me an answer. He was still lost. I needed to know what to plan for my future. I didn't know whether I should hang around with him or try to develop and pursue my career further. I couldn't continue to hang in limbo. I gave Gene an ultimatum. I told him he was going to have to make a decision about us or I was moving out. He did not meet my deadline so I moved back home with my parents shortly after Easter.

Gene did not like the arrangement of me being with my parents. We couldn't do anything at their house and it was difficult for me to spend the night at his place. My parents knew we were sexually involved but let me know they would not approve of any hanky-panky while living under their roof. Sally and Monique were having to get creative with their time.

By summer, Gene was coming around a little. He thought that maybe I should look for someplace else to live. He offered to help me buy into a condo or townhouse. The search was on. After spending about three weeks looking on my days off, I found a place that suited my needs. Gene agreed to give me the money for the down payment. He had already gotten some money from his mom's estate and thought it would be a good move to bring us back together. I closed that August on my two bedroom condo at Oak Park. Gene and I gave it a royal christening that night after I closed. It seemed that things were going to be back to normal.

I did some decorating in the condo before moving in. Once I got moved, Gene and I seemed to be back on better terms. He did seem a bit distant, though, and we didn't spend quite as much time together. He was looking at selling his Victorian and buying a Denver Square on the other side of City Park.

During the fall of 1979, I joined my company's local Civic Action Program. I had also joined the American Institute for Design and Drafting. In addition to my other activities, I had meetings and luncheons with these organizations to fit into my busy schedule. Even though Gene and I were once again seeing each other regularly, we had really toned down the time we were spending with one another.

In May, I was invited to attend an all-expense paid trip to Washington, D.C. with the CAP group. This was my first trip to the capital city. I rubbed elbows with politicians and was wined and dined.

Karla was getting married in June. I was jealous. She met Larry about the same time I had Gene, and here my baby sister was getting married before me. She certainly was not superstitious, because she got married on Friday the 13th. The day following her wedding, Gene and I left for Oklahoma to attend his family reunion.

Work had become real stressful. Morale was at an all-time low. A lot of shake-ups were happening throughout the company. Jim had been replaced. He was still there, but in a less obvious supervisory position. I had applied for his job, but a guy, Nenad, from California was selected for the job. I had been promoted to Lead Geologic Drafter after the move. I was having problems getting the people under me to listen to me, because after I would instruct them to do something, Nenad came around after me and told them to do just the opposite. They would talk nice to my face like everything was okay, then go into Nenad's office and stab me in the back.

In addition to my responsibilities as Lead, I had taken on the task of indexing and filing over 3500 maps that were setting in wardrobe boxes after the move. I was Lead and Drafter by day, and Librarian at night. The overtime money was great, but played hell on my relationship with Gene. We barely got to see each other on weekends. I was in a manic swing at this time and driving myself into exhaustion. By late September of 1980, I was worn to a frazzle. I was ready to snap.

Fragile, Handle With Care

Mid-September my mania started to take a dive. I was falling into a depressive episode. Things were becoming hopeless. I lost my energy to continue at the pace I was going. My mind was becoming distracted and unable to focus on the tasks at hand. I felt I was just going through the motions of life. I was losing a purpose to live. I was extremely frustrated by my job, and relationship with Gene and my mom.

I had gone to the human resources department to discuss the issues in the drafting department. I tried to explain how I was getting mixed messages from Nenad and had difficulty performing my job with the way he was handling the department. He would be nice to me on the floor, then call me into his office. He would then begin to shout and argue and put me down. I would get angry and shout back at him. One day, it sounded almost like two cats in a brawl. We were nearly at each other's throat. When it was all over, he reached across his desk, grabbed my hand and kissed it, as if to say he was sorry. After it was over, some of the people who heard what was going on remarked that they were afraid they might have to call an ambulance before it was all over.

I think Nenad respected me for my knowledge and abilities, but at the same time felt threatened by me. He knew I had applied for the position and that I may have resented him. He was bound and determined to prove to me he was in control, when on the contrary, he was very much out of control.

Employee Relations referred me to a company psychologist, who in turn, referred me to a local practitioner. The company psychologist was hired mainly to counsel employees on drug and alcohol abuse problems and not so much on other social problems.

I had been keeping a diary at this time, and after a few visits loaned it to him in hopes that he would get a better feel for what was going on with me. Little did I know at that time, I would never see it again. This was a journal that I had been keeping off and on since my freshman year in college. I treasured it. It had some of my poetry and prose in it, also.

The entry on September 21 mentions my seeing the therapist and giving my journal to him. It also mentions that I had been out of town that weekend to attend my cousin's wedding in Billings. I was on a fasting cycle at the time and really conscious of how much I was weighing and eating. Eating was making me nauseous.

I went to Billings with my mom. We drove up on Saturday and I flew back on Sunday after the wedding. My mom tormented me the entire time we were together. She saw that I was not eating and began to torment me over that. She has a way to make me do things when I don't want to. I guess I was still fearing the thought of being punished if I didn't do what she said. She didn't like what I had done with my hair and argued about what I was going to wear at the wedding. I was really glad to get on the plane and get away from her.

Gene picked me up from the airport that night. He was sad and wanted some sympathy because he learned that day that his grandmother had passed away and his family did not call right away. I was really feeling at that point that my purpose was to comfort and do what everyone else wanted. There was no "me" anymore. No one seemed to care if I was feeling bad or hurt.

I had injured or sprained my thumbs playing volleyball during the fall and had received some Tylenol 3 to take when the pain got a bit more than I could tolerate. Sunday, I was really not caring about anything or anyone. I was feeling real turmoil on my split mentality. Part of me was being driven to get on with things while another part was ready to pack it all in. I got the first thoughts of overdosing on 15 Tylenol 3 pills this night. Things were starting to become bizarre. I was deeply confused and my life felt just like a movie.

On Monday, I was really feeling out of control. I was light-headed most of the day and experienced void feelings and thoughts. I was just numb. I didn't think I had control over who I was or what I would do. I was living a bad dream.

Tuesday, September 23, things got to be too much. I lost total control. Kim slipped in and took the Tylenol. The entry in my journal was made right after taking the pills. I mention that I was not really feeling suicidal, just desperate. I was feeling nothing and just going through motions. I didn't feel like I had any purpose any longer and that my motivational drive was gone. It didn't occur to me that I had alter personalities. I wasn't really aware of this illness at the time. I just felt everything stemmed from fluctuating moods. I just mentioned that I felt I was constantly battling with conscious and subconscious parts of me, with the subconscious usually winning out.

In my journal, I wrote, "I think that's why I do things that I really don't understand. Logically, they're illogical, but I do it anyway — like take those tablets. I was feeling better than yesterday, and kept telling myself 'no' to such thoughts, but something else takes control and says, it's OK, nothing's going to happen."

Not long after that entry, the drugs began to kick in. I was feeling very lethargic and losing perspective on what was going on around me. My hearing was going numb. In fact my whole body was going numb. I was not feeling any pain any longer. I was moving into a state of euphoria. I was getting scared that there was more to these drugs than anticipated. I left work and immediately took a bus to the doctor's office.

I got to the office and he was not there. I went into the bathroom and threw up. I mustered up enough courage to tell his receptionist and assistant what I had done. They called the poison control center and then insisted they take me over to Presbyterian Denver Hospital. I was scared, numb and did what they said.

While in the emergency room, the doctors had me take some ipecac to try to get me to throw up some more. They decided to have me stay over night for observation. I was having trouble urinating so they catheterized me. The doctor's report on admission stated that I had borderline personality with some depressive features but was not suicidal. I expressed feelings of hopelessness and trouble with work, my boyfriend and relationship with my mother. Fortunately, the Tylenol had not reached a toxic level. It was just a bit over the cap on the therapeutic range.

The next morning before I was dismissed, my doctor and a psychiatrist came in to talk to me. I guess I was more than what he wanted to handle. I explained how I felt I had no control over taking the pills. I was sorry for the trouble I had caused but found myself still very confused and lost. Dr. Nelson, the psychiatrist suggested that maybe I take some time off from work and check myself into a hospital for some professional supervision. They would make arrangements for me to check into Mt. Airy Psychiatric Hospital the next day for an evaluative stay.

My mom hadn't come back to Denver yet, so I called my sister. She was living in Broomfield with Larry, her husband. Gene went out of town the day I overdosed, so I couldn't call him. Karla came down and got me from the hospital. She took me home to get my car from the Park 'n Ride and to put some clothes together to go into the hospital. We went back up to her apartment where I spent the night.

The next day she brought me back down to Denver to the hospital. I had no clue as to what to expect. During the check-in, they went through all my things. They took everything in glass or with sharp edges away from me. I was placed in a locked ward. It was coed. The rooms were like dormitory rooms at school.

On admission, I was reported to be cooperative but anxious and having depressed thoughts that were preoccupied with a boyfriend problem and being unloved and rejected. My dress was neat, posture was tense, and facial expression changing. I had a cooperative attitude with an anxious, inappropriate and depressed mood. My speech was logical yet controlled and soft.

I thought my stay would be for a week, two at the most. Was I in for a surprise. I stayed at Mt. Airy for a month until my insurance ran out. They were not sure of my mood stability and had me transferred to a community mental health hospital. The final discharge statement from Mt. Airy read:

"Initially remained aloof and didn't become involved with staff; complained about mistreatment by other people — expressed anger and disappointment in other people. Showed little evidence of any ability to be psychological minded, to use confrontation, nor showed much evidence of observing ego functioning. When these tests were responded to appropriately, patient went into rapid and marked regression with multiple suicide threats and gestures. In and out of seclusion last two weeks. Behavior was angry, stubborn, rebellious and totally oppositional. Constantly accused others of being unfair to her and showed no willingness to look at her role in provoking behaviors to control self."

The following is my and the staff's account of what happened. The day of my admission, I had been battling a headache all day. My head would feel full of cotton and I would get a ringing, then muffled feeling in my ears. I was feeling very alone. Despite my problems with my mom and Gene, they were not there to help me through this.

SEPTEMBER 25, 1980
"Animated to response to interactions; conversation superficial while adjusting to unit; seclusive to room at intervals; working on needlework — good attention to detail and seeming proud of project sharing it with staff with enthusiasm; later in day room watching TV with gradual increase in interactions. Adjusting well to unit."

I did not meet my doctor the first day. I just knew his name. His name was Dr. Whittington and a staff psychiatrist assigned to my case. No one explained the routine to me. I was just thrown into a pen. I didn't know when or how often I would see my doctor. No one told me what the rules were or what my privileges were.

I was really feeling like I may not have made a wise choice to allow myself into this situation. I didn't want to think I might be crazy, but caught myself pondering the idea. The self-destructive tendencies I had engaged in was not normal. I knew that much.

My first night in the hospital was a very restless one. I probably didn't get more than a couple hours of sleep. I was having bad dreams of being in a black hole with people grabbing at me and telling me what to do. I got up and dressed the next morning at daylight.

SEPTEMBER 26, 1980
"Remained in day room most of shift; seems to remain on fringes with little interaction. Superficial with staff. Refused breakfast and lunch. Worked on puzzle and needlepoint. Took nap in p.m. - - Quiet and seclusive to self in day room. Latter part of shift talked about work. Seemed more animated and social late in shift. Still watching TV at change of shift. -- Remained up watching TV till 1 a.m."

Dr. Whittington came in to see me shortly after 7 a.m. The session lasted 30-40 minutes. What came out of it was that he thought I would need to stay in the hospital for 7-10 days. I told him that concerned me deeply. I didn't know what I was going to tell them at work.

Work was a major topic of discussion during that session, even though I found it very difficult to verbalize my feelings. All I knew was that I had many bad feelings about work and what wasn't getting done. I was frustrated and very angry. I had difficulty thinking about it rationally.

My thoughts had me feeling like life was a real struggle and I was merely existing from day to day. It was a hard fight and I was tired of being black and blue. I felt like I would never heal. I was finding it harder and harder to cope with reality.

Suddenly, I found myself with a lot of time on my hands. In fact, I was getting bored. I didn't know how not to work. I worked a bit on crewel work (staff permitted me to check out my needle) then spent some time on a puzzle. I finished it in one day and it was only half done when I started. I started a second puzzle and got much of it done.

My first full day in the hospital was not uneventful. One of the other patients got upset because she wanted to see her doctor and leave. She got hysterical and the staff had to all go down on her, fold her arms and legs and take her off to a more restrictive ward.

My appetite was still almost nonexistent. I helped prepare some food for dinner on the ward but didn't eat anything. My stomach just rumbled, ached and cramped when I would eat anything, so found it easier to just not eat.

My sleeping and dreams were fairly disturbing so I found it difficult to go to bed that second night. My dreams ended up being reenactments of what I have seen and heard with an awkward twist to them. That was why I had trouble distinguishing from what was real and what was a dream.

SEPTEMBER 27, 1980
"Related more warmly today and not inappropriate in affect. Describes some feelings of estrangement and visual distortion with and without derealization. At times she feels 'light-headed like my head is expanding and then in an empty space' plus on two occasions has fainted. Will get EEG."

Dr. Whittington came in on Saturday. He usually saw patients just Monday through Friday. I expressed my concern over all the weird sensations I was having with my body and questioned whether something physical may be contributing to my depression. He didn't balk at the thought, but rather suggested I be put through some tests starting on Monday.

I tried to open up a little more to the staff that day. I was getting the idea that that was how things worked in the hospital. I figured if I was going to get out in a short period of time I was going to need all the help I could get to work things out.

Gene came by the hospital that night. We had some courteous chit-chat then got into a very heavy discussion. I could tell by his eyes and avoidance of the subject that he might be seeing some other woman. Finally he came out and said he didn't think he would be ready to get married for another 3-4 years and didn't feel he should limit his female socializing to just me. What a blow. Somehow I was kind of expecting something like that sooner or later. I'm just glad it came while I was in the hospital so I could possibly work through it.

Karla also called and told me that she explained what had happened to Mom and Roy. She said they were understanding and took the matter fairly well. In fact they were proud that I was able to reach out for help on my own.

By Sunday, I had completed three puzzles in three days. And these were not real easy puzzles either. They all had 1000 pieces to them. I had never been that good at doing puzzles before. It seemed like I could almost put them together with my eyes closed. I had developed a sixth sense for them.

Gene called that afternoon saying some flowers had been delivered to the complex office for me. They were from Jim. He wanted to know if he could bring them to me. He came by with the flowers and informed me that he thought he might check into getting some help with his problems and anger. I thought, yeah, right, I'll believe it when I see it. He called again later that night. It was like he wanted to tell me something but couldn't quite get it out. This conduct was really beginning to confuse me. Was he trying to make up to me or was he trying to tell me he wanted to break things off completely?

SEPTEMBER 29, 1980

"EEG -- Abnormal. The circuit is considered eplileptiform, and is viewed as compatible with paroxysmal disorder of the nervous system. No focal abnormalities were seen." Sidney Duman, M.D.

My tests began early on Monday. They drew blood early in the morning for a full thyroid profile. After lunch, they took me upstairs for an EEG. I had mud-like putty all over my head and hair. The test took about an hour and a half. I did doze off during the test until the technician woke me and had me breath heavy as if to hyperventilate. It was a real treat when the test was over, because he washed and rinsed my hair for me.

That morning, I had the dreaded job of calling Linda in employee relations at work. I tried to explain that I might not be back to work for a couple more weeks. I asked if she would relay the information to Nenad. She refused and said it was my responsibility to deal directly with him. I asked my staff person at the hospital if they would call and explain what was happening. He refused also. Shit! I did call him and he dealt me a strong guilt trip. He said Bob was on vacation, Bill was out sick and he had a number of slide changes that needed to get done. Yes, I felt bad, but it was things like that that stressed me to the breaking point. Needless to say, I was upset over the ordeal and very angry for the lack of concern Nenad had.

SEPTEMBER 30, 1980

"Patient still preoccupied with being a 'good patient' feeling that she must behave or 'you don't get out of here.' Affect is somewhat muted and patient is cautious in interpersonal transactions and not very revealing. She is generally superficial and remote. -- Pt. did not eat dinner...pt. talked of hopeless feelings and not wanting to try to work out problems any more. Pt. seems very depressed. Pt. asked to be keyed off the floor to go to basement for pop at 9:45 p.m. Was to be back in 10 minutes, but not back in that time and when staff person went to find her she said she would be on the unit by 10 p.m. which is when all patients have to be on the unit. Pt. did not return until 10:15 p.m. When confronted on this pt. said her watch was wrong. Pt. very gamy around this. -- Preliminary review of psychological testing reveals no evidence of psychosis. However, there are still some issues that are suggestive: relationship problems, arbitrary and at times autistic thinking, disturbances in sleep & waking cycle, very strong and sustained dysphoric states and annihilistic thinking."

Tuesday, things went from okay to worse. I woke up with a terrible headache. My head felt as though a vise was closing tighter and tighter and trying to squeeze my brains out. The back of my head was numb, and neck was stiff and tense. The rest of me was real blah and limp; I guess normal for being depressed.

I had an appointment scheduled at Dr. Whittington's office for some psychological testing. It started out with a bunch of personal questions asked by the attending psychologist.

He then gave me an inkblot test which I had a great deal of trouble with. I drew an absolute blank on many of the cards. This was very unusual for me. When I was younger, I would draw dots on paper and play connect-the-dots. I almost always came up with an image that resembled something, usually an animal.

The next part of the testing involved memory recall. I could not focus on anything he was reading. I drew a complete blank on a paragraph that I was suppose to repeat what he had read. Next, I had a written test that had me picking correlative statements and definitions.

The Grand Finale was a 500 true-false personality questionnaire. I got another headache halfway through the test. It made it even more difficult for me to concentrate. Because of this testing and the EEG the day before, I didn't have a session with Dr. Whittington.

That afternoon after the test I began to get more and more depressed. I was frustrated and felt like beating my head against the wall. Nenad called late in the afternoon and tried to lead me to believe he was sympathetic. I got the feeling he was more curious about what had really happened. He tried to hide it by asking about what work could be given to the temporary they had hired while I was out. I gave him enough information to let him know that what was going on at work played an important roll in my hospitalization.

As evening wore on I was feeling more and more lost. I just needed to get off the unit to be by myself without anyone watching me. I asked to go to the basement to get a pop. I didn't come back by the time promised and the staff came looking for me. Voices were telling me to give up and drop my facade of a happy, carefree person. I fantasized about quitting my job and find a dude ranch somewhere to work at, or to just buy a horse and find a place way up in the mountains to live as a hermit. Trying to gain acceptance from other people was too hard and I was getting to the end of my rope.

I also thought about reincarnation. I thought that in an earlier life I may have been a western woman like Annie Oakley or an Indian. I loved the out-of-doors and had a tomboyish personality. It is only now with my understanding of my system and Group that these thoughts and feelings make absolute sense.

OCTOBER 1, 1980
"Expressed feelings of wanting to punch her fist through a wall or window...she just gets used. When it was reflected to her that she could change this, she rejected the idea. Many 'I can't' statements. She wrote down some thoughts that she is having around the violent feelings. Then she offered to let this writer read her diary. We will talk regarding this tomorrow. Much of what she wrote today has to do with frustrations with not knowing who she is. -- Pt. and staff also discussed when it would be appropriate for pt. to ask for some time in the quiet room if she feels that she is losing control. Pt. and staff structured that she can ask to use quiet room if she feels she needs it and also if pt. looks like she is losing control. Staff may initiate movement to quiet room."

I had a bad night. I only got about two and half hours of sleep. I woke up very depressed and could not snap out of it for the life of me. By keeping busy with occupational therapy projects and my needlework, some of the depression subsided, but moved more towards anger. I developed a vision of shoving my fist through something. I was scared by the way the thought came because it reminded me of the way I felt when I took the Tylenol 3 tablets. When a destructive thought went through my head it became almost an obsession and would not go away until I acted on it. When I am depressed or in a semi-autistic state, I have no control over my actions. Anything could happen.

In my diary I wrote that I was confused, anxious and angry with myself. I was unsure of who I really was and that I lacked an identity. I felt like I was a prisoner of my own mind and becoming very weak for trying to escape. I had a feeling that these destructive impulses were all a part of a bad dream. If I saw myself act them out, maybe I would wake up from the dream. Besides, if it were really a dream, I wouldn't get hurt.

OCTOBER 2, 1980
"Pt. was able to describe clearly the dissociative state she had yesterday which is comparable to when she took overdose. She feels depressed and angry, then suddenly intrusive, obsessive thought regarding self-esteem which leads into consciousness; anxiety mounts to panic and suddenly she becomes 'numb;' anxiety disappears and she enters a dream-like state where she feels actions are

inevitable and she has no fear of pain. -- About 10:30 p.m. pt. came to nursing station asking to go to the quiet room because she was afraid she might do something. Feeling feelings she did not want to have. Stayed in quiet room about an hour. Got something for anxiety and went to bed. She could not express any reasons for her feeling this way."

I began to write in my journal about the feelings I was experiencing as they happened. I spent a considerable amount of time talking to my staff person about the difficulty I had dealing with my mother and her controlling personality. I was grown up and more than ready to run my own life the way I wanted to.

I seemed to be getting a lot of headaches while in the hospital. They ran across from temple to temple and at the base of my skull from ear to ear. The pain in the front seemed to jump back and forth like a Ping-Pong ball. I would become overly sensitive to sounds and then get a muffled and pressured ringing in my ears. My thoughts would become garbled and confused. My neck and throat become very stiff and tense, making my headache stronger. It was also very difficult to talk at this time. Kind of like when you get choked up in an emotional movie. I then feel real feverish, almost like I was on fire. Afterwards I get very quiet and still and feel like I'm suspended in a cloud.

OCTOBER 3, 1980
"Spent time staring out the window and at approximately 2:15 p.m. came to the nursing station and asked for time in the quiet room. Had a bed pad wrapped around herself and reported feeling cold. Then admitted 'keeping herself together' with this. Able to sit but seemed agitated and giddy. States the voices are telling her to punch a window out. States it's like a fight going on in her head. — One voice telling her to hit the window and another saying not to do so...Reporting fear of the impulses...Was encouraged to rest in quiet room. Complained of recent nightmares and difficulty differentiating reality from dreams over the past few days."

OCTOBER 4, 1980
"After lunch pt. approached staff stating she was having more and more thoughts of violence (ramming fist through a wall) which she couldn't control. Asked to go into quiet room. Did this with door open. PRN Vistaril given. -- Pt. spent about 4 hours in quiet room from beginning of shift. Declined to eat dinner but slept and rested during this time. Affect was sad/depressed and she stood at the windows for long periods of time. She started repeatedly pounding her fists softly against the window. She was given the message that she needed to talk, go to the day room or quiet room. She was walked to the quiet room by one staff on each side of her. She made no re-sistance. She talked in a whining, immature voice, wanting to know why staff wasn't helping her to feel better."

The handwriting in my diary on this day was rough and not as legible as the days before or after. I don't know whether someone else was writing it. It talked of hopelessness and frustration from trying to keep the obsessive impulses away. I feared losing total control and of really be-coming a loonie tune.

I didn't have much luck with putting my fist through the window. The windows were made of tempered glass and were not going to break unless something more substantial than a fist were rammed through them. Once again I failed. I think that by at least going through the motions, though, did have some affect on the voice and vision of the act.

OCTOBER 5, 1980
"Stated she hears a voice which tells her to do self-destructive things. Feels that banging on win-dows or walls would rid her of this tension once and for all. Conversation in 1 to 1 was filled with

hopelessness. Talked about past self-destructive behavior. Said her recent overdose was an impulse, sighting any previous thought about it. Talked also about the desire to break the window yesterday. Said her thoughts were racing and then '...the idea just formed...' and she couldn't get rid of it. Said the only anger she's aware of is anger at self for having the thought to break the window."

I was so mixed up and confused during this hospitalization that I did not know whether I was coming or going. The voices were those that I heard when younger. It seemed my alters would tell me what to do and I would obey. At first it seemed that I was carrying out their requests but now, in retrospect, I see I was not in control. I would clearly see the act being performed, but I was not in control. Someone else's mind was controlling my actions and just my eyes were the witness.

My mood swings at this time were also out of control. I would be up, down and all around the chart throughout the day. As mentioned earlier, I find that I am in less control of my alters when swinging between mania and depression.

OCTOBER 6, 1980
"Appeared angry early part of shift. Initiated several Ping-Pong games and attended RT — volleyball — fairly aggressive on volleyball court."

Dr. Whittington told me today that my EEG did display some abnormal indications. He had a neurologist come in and see me. I seemed to pass the Mickey Mouse exam with little difficulty. I didn't see how they could tell with that kind of exam whether you have brain abnormalities. Maybe I was just trying real hard to do everything right and not be myself.

I got very manic after lunch. I also felt like I had some aggressions and anger to play out. That's why I exhausted myself with Ping-Pong and volleyball. I may have also been getting some "cabin fever" from being cooped up inside the hospital. It did help me to wind down some.

By this time I was having a different opinion of the hospital. The confinement was seeming to bring out parts of me that were unpredictable. I no longer had an agenda for being a good little girl and getting out. I was not in control of my daily routine because of the hospital nor in control of my actions because my alters were not in control of my routine.

OCTOBER 8, 1980
"Angry and negativistic today. Up early looking nervous and agitated. Pass to baby shower night before. New cuts on hand. Responded by 'I might have hit something.' Seems depressed. Confused about what direction to take with problems. Staff shouldn't worry — she's not worth it. Pt. would not contract not to hurt self and doesn't look in control. -- At end of hall facing window with sad, depressed, angry affect. Answered questions in caustic, sarcastic, hopeless manner. Observed with superficial abrasion on right knuckles. Refused to tell staff when, where, how. Talked in hopeless/helpless manner. Said 'I signed myself in and can sign out when I want to.' During 8 p.m. rounds, pt. not observed in any visible place in room. Prior, had been sitting in bathroom in dark. Was found in clothes closet on floor clutching a light bulb. Started to tap light bulb provocatively on closet and getting harder and harder. Refused to come out of closet or give up light bulb. Given three choices: 1) come out and hand over light bulb and contract and stay in room, 2) stay visible in day room or 3) voluntarily walk to quiet room by self. She refused any of these. Staff tried to talk to her for 30 minutes. Pt. was folded and carried to quiet room with much struggling. She was secluded and restrained at 8:45 p.m. in full restraints. Pt. remained agitated. Kept pulling and struggling against restraints for 1-1/2 hours. Tried to pull or dislocate shoulder and restraints readjusted. Refused prn of Vistaril until 10:30 p.m. and put in diagonals (left arm & right leg). Out of diagonals at 11:15 p.m. Fine body tremors with chills observed at this time.

R_x: *9 p.m. - Seclude and restrain now and continue as needed through night for control of agitation and self-destructive impulses. Progress out of restraints when pt. able to maintain control. Continue Vistaril as prn for anxiety.*

I don't know what it was, but the struggle from fighting while being carried to the quiet room created a release for all the anger, anxiety and aggressions that had built up inside of me regarding that day's incidents. I never really had a way before to release the tensions inside of me. I now found a way, no matter how inappropriate. This discovery for resolution to my feelings set me up for the rest of my hospital stay. I had a lot of built up anger inside that needed to be worked through. Until I either got it out of my mind or resolved, I was not getting out of the hospital.

OCTOBER 9, 1980
"Ate breakfast and lunch in quiet room. To room for hygiene at 2 p.m. Slept off and on all day. Said felt somewhat better. Didn't want to set in day room and returned to quiet room. Talked about feelings. Didn't know where or why she was angry. Pt. had phone call at 3 p.m. Was asleep and not wakened. Earlier complained of being very tired. Right hand appeared swollen; soaked with neosporin dressing. -- Resting quietly in quiet room with door open. Affect drowsy and blunted. Under active but appropriate. Speech minimal, pleasant and cooperative. Agreed she had needed to struggle and that physical activity helped reduce agitation. Offered no complaints about being restrained. Refused dinner but more realistic and took fluids. Noted to have generalized tremor-like activity of head, neck, arms and torso, but not involving legs. Uninterrupted over period of 1 hour. Was difficult to arouse during this time but no evidence of loss of consciousness. Speech slightly slurred; no obvious disorientation. Complained of 'feeling hot.' Afebrile. Tremor appeared to increase when pt. aware of staff presence but also occurred during sleep and not aware of staff presence. Tremoring was at times accompanied by hyperventilation. When coached to breath slowly and deeply noted that tremors decreased with inhalation but increased markedly with exhalation.
   R_x: *Continue to seclude. Restrain only in event pt. becomes self-destructive or assaultive.*

I don't know what caused me to tremor. At times I remember sensing I was in some kind of fearful state of mind. No clue as to what I was afraid of unless, it was the fear of what I would do next. At other times, I would be shaking as if cold, but have a flushed feeling. Then at other times, there was no obvious reason for it. My whole body seemed to be out of control. It may have been some mild seizure activity, or as later learned in my therapy, pseudo seizures caused from the stress I was under. No explanation for it while I was asleep, though. It seemed as though I had lost conscious control of my body.

OCTOBER 10, 1980
"Affect flat with slow speech. During brief 1 to 1 expressed anger around her job and concern of not being ready for discharge. -- With doctor at beginning of shift. Followed by barricading self in bathroom with body against door. Door opened via reverse lock to reveal pt. had rubber band wrapped tightly around upper left arm and small puncture wound which pt. inflicted with embroidery scissors. Embroidery materials secured at nurses station. 4:20 p.m. pt. expressed hostility to staff and refused to walk to quiet room. Folded and carried per protocol to quiet room with much resistance. Full restraints applied. Refused prn remaining agitated and pulling at restraints. Refused dinner or fluids. 7 p.m. down to diagonal restraints (right arm & left leg). Sees conflict at work; rejection at work; inability to obtain different job; inability to work independently to avoid conflict. Major conflict of 'I don't know who I am. I don't know what I want; not worth time and money to continue to fight and feel shitty.' Restraints removed at 7:45 p.m. Up to bathroom but unable to void. Avoiding eye contact. Continues to refuse food and fluids. Closed seclusion main-

tained for pt. safety. Awake at 1:15 a.m. stating she wanted to go home, that she 'hadn't done anything wrong.' Whiny voice — eyes closed with no eye contact."

R_x*: Restrict to unit -- Level II (own clothes & unrestricted on unit). Moderate suicide precautions. Restrain and seclude prn. — Continue seclude/restrain prn for pt. safety; control of agitation and self-destructive and/or escape impulses. Cleanse arm wound as needed; no tetanus. Valium - 5mg. as emergency measure to decrease agitation. If agitation and self-destructive behavior and talk of leaving continue, doctor will initiate 72-hour hold.*

OCTOBER 11, 1980
"Pt. continues to be very regressed and suicidal. Will initiate 72-hour hold since pt. is quite suicidal. -- Remained in locked seclusion. Refused breakfast and lunch. Told about doctor placing 72-hour hold; was very hostile attempting to place blame for desire to suicide on staff. During talk, appeared to be agitated and become more vocal about her anger as to how others were responsible for her wanting to kill self. Didn't feel comfortable opening seclusion door. During one check found her lying on stomach, hanging her head off the edge of the bed, She said 'my world's upside down and so I am too.' -- Refused dinner. Pt. wanted to come out of closed seclusion for a half hour to walk around and said 'she would do whatever she had to do to be able to come out,' but this was said in an angry tone. Pt. continued talking in self-destructive manner and at one point saying that 'some people were into things. Hers was pain and that she wanted to put her fist through something.' Staff told her she didn't feel comfortable with her being out of closed seclusion. Pt. got angry and demanding and accusing toward staff. Pt. began banging and pounding head softly on wall. At 9 p.m. tore bandages off. As time wore on began banging head harder. Refused prn. Diagonals put on at 10:30 p.m.

By this time I was totally out of control of my behavior and actions. I really didn't know who I was or what was going to happen next. Kim was freewheeling it and becoming very gamy with the staff. She was sabotaging any hope for recovery.

I'm not sure, but I see this as her way of trying to get attention. Something I had been deprived of largely throughout my life. Acting out in her way was certainly getting a lot of attention from staff. She was just like a kid causing trouble just to get a rise out of the authoritative figures in her life; however, the games and trouble she was making were very serious and threatening in nature.

OCTOBER 12, 1980
"Pt. affect remained constricted, bland. Comment 'No future — wanted to die.' Voice was very loud and apparently angry but no change in affect. Made contract to be out of quiet room from 10 a.m. to 12:45 p.m. -- Continues to make contracts every 30 minutes but still saying she just wants to die and staff should let her. Pt. still doesn't seem to want to work at all on finding out what her behavior patterns are to enable her to control her depression and suicidal thoughts. Slept in open seclusion on 15 minute checks.

OCTOBER 13, 1980
"Whining, grabbing at sheets with eyes closed at 5:15 a.m. Would not acknowledge staff. Began rapid breathing. At 5:20 said to staff that she was awake and doesn't belong here. -- Affect initially sarcastic, hostile, flippant, though progressively more direct and appropriate. One hour out of seclusion and 1/2 hour open seclusion. Increased animation, organized. 'I've got to get as much in 1 hour as I can.' Increased mobilization and appropriate use of time with enthusiasm! Tested limits mildly. Returned to quiet room at 7:15 p.m. on own complaining of 'feeling ill' with fever. Slept in open seclusion.

This whining voice and comments of not belonging in the hospital must have been coming from Peggy. Peggy does not like hospitals. She thinks they are a place where people go to die. That's where my father died. In fact, she is scared of hospitals and doctors.

OCTOBER 14, 1980

"Pt. still gamy and bargaining, autistic and oppositional. Unable to make a commitment to remain in voluntary treatment so will initiate 90-day hold order. Because of poor progress in treatment so far, will request psychiatric consultation. -- Dr. W. -- When pt. told of hold seemed relieved and was very cheerful and cooperative throughout shift. Contracted and said not feeling like she wants to harm self, though says that somewhere in the back of her mind there might be thoughts of hurting self. -- Described self as being 'in a really good mood; keyed up.'

It seemed as though the confinement and control issues had caused my affect to deteriorate over the previous few days. My group and I have a real problem when I don't have some sense of control over my life. Everyone seems to have their own control issues and that is why I get real confused, because they all vary.

The court order was the first real evidence that they indicated I was a troubled individual in need of serious help. I knew I was troubled, but previously, the staff acted too matter-of-factly. I was just another pea in the pod. I wanted someone to listen and to take me seriously and help me understand.

I liked to have control, but was glad the staff and Dr. Whittington took it upon themselves to initiate some kind of plan. I was still concerned about whether or not I would have a job when I got out, but that seemed secondary to the issues. I needed to get my life back in order and find out just who and what I was and why I was plagued by the feelings and actions that had occurred.

OCTOBER 15, 1980

"Dressed in own clothes and contracted with staff. Affect pleasant, cooperative and engaging at times. -- Affect stable, calm and animated, pleasant. Behavior self directed, organized, interactional. Very receptive regarding staff contact and initiating contracts appropriately. Expressed sarcastic anger briefly regarding doctor not visiting today; noncommittal. Talked about previous self inflicted wounds on arm. 'I got angry at myself.'

OCTOBER 16, 1980

"Pt. angry and negotiating and doesn't really communicate. Says her mind is closed and resists therapy. Not clearly expressing suicidal intent but doesn't like new tranquilizer — drowsy, nauseous, feel 'feverish,' will DC. Again has insomnia, will increase tryptophan. -- Described feeling 'crowded' and 'overwhelmed' by all the people and noise in the day room and preferring quiet of her room. Spoke at length about progressively being sad, angry, withdrawn. Initially focusing on internal conflict of 'the part of me that has given up and decided to die is so much stronger than the fading part of me that has a glimmer of hope...I'm tired of fighting...can't find any self-satisfaction in my accomplishments...can't think of anything that would be satisfying...I've just given up.' Resisted reality testing. Identified 3 'parts' of her or sets of feelings as the strong part that wants to give up that has taken over and pushed out the 2nd 'part' the hopeful and the 3rd part or set of behavior, that of superficial, social, 'bubbly' used to 'put on a front of doing OK'...'but it doesn't work. People think I'm doing OK when I'm not. I'm empty.' Discussed feeling difficulty 'telling what's real and what isn't.. Like I'm in a dream-like state a lot...and like in a dream you can fall off a cliff and not feel pain, I can die and not feel pain...I'm not sure what's real...nothing means anything.' Reaffirmed suicidal intent, then stated 'I'm not going to talk anymore...not going to talk to anyone anymore...' Expression faded to blank, flat, posture fixed. No verbal or physical response to staff. Appeared non-responsive for about 10 minutes, respiration deep, normal eye blinks. Several repetitive motions then began rolling things in hands, etc. Dr.

notified of suicidal discussion and non responsive behavior. Decision made to transfer to quiet room for observation and safety. During seclude procedure, became tearful and combative. Folded and carried to quiet room actively struggling as in past. Full restraints for safety. Pounded bed and pulled restraints for about 15 minutes. Spoke to staff about feeling relieved of tension thru physical struggle and expressing anger.

The above entry sounds like they were talking to someone who was really crying out for help. Someone out of control. Rather than being responsive to my needs, the staff was reactive and fueling the fire. I had come to realize what relief I got from struggling with the staff, that to regain some sense of control of my feelings, I needed to be involved in a struggle. Through learned behavior, I would manipulate them into a struggle so I could regain control of myself. I felt a sense of peace and calm after the staff struggles.

Anyone with a good eye and sense of understanding of MPD would have seen my behavior and comments as someone inflicted with the illness. Because of the uncommonality of the illness at that time, they viewed my problem as behavioral and somewhat psychotic.

I didn't know what I was doing at the time. I was rapid-cycling with my moods, and alters were switching all over the place. I can clearly see that now through how I have come to understand my illness and Group.

OCTOBER 17, 1980
"Pt. cheerful and relational as if nothing has happened, even though she is in the quiet room. Superficial and utilizing denial as defense...Pt. is quite regressed now playing a 2 year-old game of 'make-me-I-won't' which she elaborates sado-masochistically. - Dr. W. -- Pt. in quiet room at beginning of shift. Pt. cooperative and a little child-like trying to please staff. On contact with staff pt. said she is trying to be good so that she can be discharged next week. Slept in quiet room with door open."

OCTOBER 18, 1980
"Awake since 5 a.m. Says not suicidal but has a gamy attitude. 'I don't know why staff thinks I'm suicidal.' Made contract. Affect was cheerful and socializing in day room. Had long phone call from mother and seemed calm afterward. -- Affect behavior labile. Visit with mother superficially pleasant, talking quiet and freely. During staff time became fearful at intervals during discussion of feelings of conflict, then retreated to room refusing to renew contract stating she was having increased difficulty controlling impulses. 'I'm letting it take over...(the part of me that wants to give up)...it won't leave me alone.' Requested additional meds to control agitation and anxiety. Given Vistaril at 11 p.m. Remained up in day room refusing to contract with some evasiveness. Escorted to quiet room with door open. Affect sad, quiet."

I was trying to open up more to staff, but really didn't know what I was saying. I was continuing to switch between alters, big time. Staff seemed to be pushing some buttons that got me reactive. The quiet room felt safe whether I went voluntarily or involuntarily.

I got attention from staff. Attention I had been lacking and in dire need of for some time. I didn't care what it took. I just needed for someone to notice me and that I was having trouble coping. I needed some TLC whether forceful or not. Anything to satisfy this need.

OCTOBER 19, 1980
"Continues to refuse to contract with staff. Affect sad, depressed, quiet, saying not wanting to talk. Difficulty explaining feelings; they are 'all mixed up.' Made firm contract to eat lunch out of quiet room. Mother phoned during lunch; pt. refused to talk to her. Appears depressed, continues to display sad expressions and walks with shoulders slumped. Returned to quiet room at 1 p.m. and

refused to contract for time out. Remained in bed in quiet room with eyes closed and door open. -- Affect somber, calm, guarded. Behavior organized, self-directed. Out on unit for dinner and duration of shift watching TV and crocheting. Occasional superficial interaction with peers and staff. Highlighted with staff ambivalence on making contracts and unpredictable nature of moods and behavior. 'I just don't know how it's going to go...sometimes I have some control over how it goes and sometimes I don't.' Denied any clear pattern. Ambivalent regarding options and continuation of therapy with fairly genuine affect and appears to be seriously considering options. Complained of persistent difficulty sleeping and by 'confusing' dreams...awakes confused and disoriented.

OCTOBER 20, 1980

"Pt. continues elaborate neurotic struggle with staff. Our dilemma is that if we transfer her involuntarily to Bethesda, will she simply persist in this struggle with no therapeutic benefit? Alternating, if we discharge her will it mean we don't care? Definite characteristic of childhood and adult relationships. - Dr. W. -- Pt. reviewed chart and noted that review helps her remember sequences and circumstances. Dr. came in to unit but didn't see pt. Pt. was very upset about this and refused to contract with staff because of this. Encouraged to call doctor to talk to him instead of indulging in this behavior. Remained indifferent to contracts until doctor calls. -- Continued to be upset that doctor had not called after placing 2 calls. Pt. would not contract. Staff said put in call to doctor and pt. contracted not to hurt self till 6:30 p.m. then would not contract any longer if doctor hadn't called. At 6:30 pt. refused to contract or stay in visible area. When staff contacted pt. in room she continued to escalate and at one point pulled a piece of broken glass from a light bulb from under her pillow and said to staff 'would you get a thrill from seeing me cut my wrist?' At this point, more staff was called and pt. carried to seclusion and put in full restraints due to pt. combative behavior. Pt. had crushed some of the glass in her hand and seemed to have superficial cuts from this. Pt. was put in restraints at 6:45 p.m. and at 7:30 pt. was seen cutting her wrist with a piece of glass in her mouth. The glass was removed and pt. had small superficial cuts on top of wrist and was treated. At 9:45 pt. calmed by PRN and placed in diagonals with a contract not to hurt self. At 10:30, pt. gave staff a rubber band, needle and bobby pin that she had hidden on her and said 'this should show you that I can continue to hurt myself here and the fact that I didn't shows that I'm no longer self-destructive tonight and should be let out of restraints.' Pt. was let out of restraints and searched and put in hospital pajamas. Pt. contracted not to hurt self while in seclusion and will spend night in locked seclusion. Out of full restraints by 10:30 p.m.

What got me agitated was that Dr. Whittington did not come in to see me and I had some very important issues to discuss with him. I had the staff call him and I called and left messages a couple times with his office and service. No response from him. I felt he was either testing my control or didn't care enough about me to return my calls. This angered me greatly. I felt like I was being punished, neglected and not important — some of the contributing factors that prompted this whole hospitalization in the first place. Being punished by someone else was not acceptable. I had to punish myself. At the same time I had to rid myself of the build-up of anger. If not, I would have really exploded and done something terribly destructive.

I took the way people related to me personally. Because of my experience with anger displayed in my family growing up, I decided I would not take my anger out on others like my mom did. Instead, I directed it inward. This was mainly because I felt people treated me the way they did because I was bad for some reason or another or had done something wrong to be neglected.

After the impulse of breaking the light bulb, I somehow knew my actions were not going to be taken lightly and hid some of the glass inside my bra. When they came to carry me to the quiet room, I would not release the broken glass from my hand. When they tried to take it away, I got some superficial cuts on my hand.

Once in the quiet room, Kim had another driving destructive impulse. She was able to position herself while in restraints to pull the glass out of my bra. She took the glass and somehow managed to cut my left hand by holding the glass in her mouth. The cuts drew blood, but were not deep enough to require any kind of stitches. In fact, when cleaned up looked just like scratches. It looked bad enough though to alarm the staff.

At this time in my life, I had no learned behavioral way of dealing with my anger. Kim was my anger. She acted out on it the only way she knew how; by being self-destructive. This cat and mouse game seemed to be endless, because there was so much anger built up inside of me that all this little stuff that was going on at the hospital was just grazing the surface.

My anger was also one of my ways of doing a reality check. If I didn't get angry and blow up somehow, meant that I no longer had feelings. If I no longer had feelings, then I felt like I didn't exist.

OCTOBER 21, 1980
"TEAM CONFERENCE: Pt. clearly of danger to herself. We will transfer short term treatment order to Bethesda. - Dr. W. -- Pt. attended conference with doctor and staff. Seemed to accept news of continued hospitalization well. Pt. reviewed chart. States that her intent in reviewing the chart has changed; she is no longer feeling that staff has been misinterpreting her, and that it is helpful to her to read what happened at the times when she has lost control because she does not remember these times. -- Affect stable, animated, relaxed. Behavior calm, organized, interactional, appropriate. Contracted easily with good eye contact. ('Let me put my glasses on so I can have eye contact with you.') Placed/received phone call regarding ranch job patient considering. (Talks a lot about ranching job.) Talks about control/lack of control of two 'parts.' Expressed apology for behavior when angry. Retreated to own room at approximately 11 p.m. appearing to be in good spirits and feeling in control without self-destructive impulses."

OCTOBER 22, 1980
"Pt. transferred to Bethesda Hospital by Ambo-Cab."

ADMISSION INTERVIEW, BETHESDA HOSPITAL: *"When I evaluated the pt., she surprised me by the degree of control she exhibited. She was able to relate appropriately, and clearly was an intelligent and appropriate woman, though the history of acting out behavior at Mt. Airy could not be discounted. However, after a lengthy interview it appeared to me that one of the difficulties at Mt. Airy was a power struggle for control that had developed between her, the ward, and possibly the physician. Therefore I will attempt to treat the patient in a much more open manner and give her considerably more freedom and not attempt to control her, and simply assume that she could function since she had functioned so well previously. Her mental status showed a neatly dressed female who related comfortably. Had only a mild depression with no evidence of delusions, hallucinations or looseness of associations."*

TRANSFER ORDERS: *Diagnosis at time of transfer: Depressive Neurosis and Schizophrenia with complex character disorder: borderline state; complex partial seizures; states post suicide attempt; states post mutilation with minor lacerations and abrasions. Behavior at times belligerent, noisy, suspicious."*

I had a big gap in my diary from the time the conflict arose at Mt. Airy until I was transferred to Bethesda. I had to count on the staff notes to be my memories.

Bethesda was quite different from Mt. Airy. The ward was a separate building on the hospital grounds. It had a cold, dark atmosphere to it. The other patients largely kept to themselves. Staff was not very interactive. I definitely wasn't going to stay there any longer than necessary.

I had a new doctor assigned to me. His name was Dr. Wirecki. (What is it with these doctors? Do all their names begin with a 'W'? Wanberg, Whittington, Wirecki?) I guess he is okay. He wanted to talk right away about a possible discharge plan. That was quite all right for me. I got a lot out of my system at Mt. Airy and was ready to try to get back into the mainstream of things.

I got a pass a couple days after my transfer to discuss going back to work with Linda and Nenad. It was an emotional experience, but I had to hold it together and retain a stiff upper lip. It was decided that when I did come back I would have just one responsibility; to finish setting up the map files. After that, we would re-negotiate my responsibilities. I told them that I thought I worked better independently and that maybe I wasn't cut out to be a Lead unless there was more structure to the position with clear guidelines.

A new air passed through me. I was still somewhat depressed but in more control and had clearer thoughts. I don't know whether it was the medication I was on or the new surroundings. I was ready to get out and on with my life. The good alters were back in control. I did have destructive thoughts pass through my mind but nothing obsessive.

I was so convincing in my new attitude toward life that Dr. Wirecki discharged me on November 2nd. I was going to be on probation and would have to be on my best behavior or they could reinstitutionalize me involuntarily because the court order would not expire until January. He also stipulated that I would have to continue with some kind of outpatient therapy. I elected to go back to Dr. Whittington and made an appointment for November 7.

One thing I did learn in the hospital was to make short term goals. I did take it to heart. Despite my depressed feelings and thoughts of ending things, I promised myself to hold on for at least another 6 months, or until the files were completed at work.

I went back to work for half days for two weeks after my discharge. Nenad was on vacation so the transition back to work went as well as could be expected.

THE SECOND WIND

My family and Gene suddenly wanted to spend a lot of time with me when I got out of the hospital. The hospital intimidated them; especially a psychiatric hospital. I had been exposed as someone weak and vulnerable and they must have felt like they had to protect me. Either that or they had a lot of guilt over possibly contributing to my problems. It is still hard to tell whether they were overprotective out of guilt or genuine concern. I'm sure it must have been a little of both.

I had snowed Dr. Wirecki into thinking I was doing much better; enough so to be back on the outside world. Actually it was the opposite. The turmoil continued on a daily basis. I was still quite depressed and fighting the will to live or die. I felt like a tennis ball in a game of doubles being batted back and forth among various alters.

I did manage to keep going through the short term goals I was setting for myself. I didn't want to leave this earth with any task incomplete. The secret was to stay busy and keep taking on new responsibilities. I have this thing for commitments. When I commit to doing something for someone or myself, it is extremely difficult to just let it slide.

The geologists at work were glad to have me back. One of them confided in me that I was the only one in the drafting department that they trusted with their work. That comment was a real ego and esteem builder. It gave me that little extra umph to make me feel that I was needed and life was worth hanging in there a little longer.

Life seemed to be a little more under control and not as rattled as it was in the hospital. That was greatly due to the fact that I was once again the controlling issue in my life; not the hospital staff. I did have lapses of time. In some cases it seemed like days. I would miss them all together and not have recall of what occurred. Sometimes I had a picture of what happened but no clue as to why or how things transpired.

When I was working half days after my discharge, I spent the mornings over at Mt. Airy thoroughly going through my chart. I was aghast to what really went on in there. I couldn't believe it was me that they were talking about. I was never that physical around people before. In fact, I'd consider myself quite sedate. Something had set me off. My actions are clear to me today, but back then just left a big question mark in my mind.

I was intrigued by the reports about the abnormal EEG so decided to pursue the idea of a physiological disorder further. I had made appointments with Dr. Quintero, the attending neurologist, after I got out of the hospital. He suggested a repeat EEG at Mercy Hospital to confirm if the first one was accurate. Maybe a confirmed diagnosis might explain why I had been having so many headaches. I would like to think it is something that can be treated, and not just due strictly to the tensions in my life.

The report of the EEG came back borderline, and Dr. Quintero decided to classify it as normal. He began to take me off the seizure medicine I was put on in the hospital. He said the temporal lobe seizures cause episodes of trances or daydreaming and lapses in memory. That seemed to describe my life. Was he so sure that I was not having seizures? I guess he must have felt that because I also was having psychological problems, my trances and lapses in time were due to those problems and not seizures.

Nenad was aware of the interest I had in computer drafting and told me that I could work with the committee to evaluate any CAD system that may be brought in. He even suggested that I may be put in charge of that part of the department. I thought, "great, now I really will have to work hard to stay alive if he thinks enough of me to give me this responsibility." One more commitment I wasn't sure I wanted to take on. Because I have a strong desire to succeed as long as I'm alive, I agreed to work on the project.

I had fasting tantrums when in the hospital, but began to eat all the time when I got out. I didn't know whether it was the medication or not. I had put on ten pounds within the month of my discharge. My depression was causing me to eat, feel lethargic and not be able to sleep much. When I did sleep, I had the same disturbing types of dreams that I had in the hospital.

Every day was a struggle, but some how or another I made it through to the next. I knew the energy to live must have been there or I would have done myself in as soon as I got out of the hospital. It was just so difficult having to fight the depression.

I knew Gene was dating a lot of women or one woman a lot. We saw each other maybe once a week, if that. I figured we were old news and he was just politely trying to break things off. He must have thought of me as extremely fragile, but I could see through him. I didn't really care for his leading me on.

I continued with my journal until the end of November that year. I had a variety of handwriting styles appear. Some were neat while others were scribbles. I just thought it was the mood I was in when I wrote it. It didn't occur to me at the time it may have been other people inside doing the writing.

I made it through Christmas okay. I was hoping Gene would spend the holiday with me, but he informed me he was going to Michigan for Christmas with a friend. He might be back to spend New Year's with me. He got back the 30th and called to see if I wanted to go out the next night. I told him I would really like to just have a quiet evening together.

New Year's Eve was our last big fling. He seemed to be real romantic, but his eyes told me the truth. I knew he had gone off to spend Christmas with his new girlfriend and her family. He tried denying it, but with these things you just kinda know. He finally admitted I saw through him and said that he thought it would be better off if we called it quits. He said I had a lot of turmoil and issues in my life that I am trying to work through, and he thought I didn't need the confusion of our relationship to contribute to my problems. I was heartbroken but agreed. At least I now knew where I stood and would no longer have to guess what was going on.

Losing Gene did not help my depression. I was obsessed with the man. We had a really fantastic relationship. Sally, Monique and Francie spent most of the time with him, and they loved him dearly. I would not get over this quickly. That was for sure.

I managed to survive through the winter. Spring was well under way and I was seeing Dr. Whittington weekly for therapy after the first of the year. I didn't seem to be making a lot of headway in the sessions. They seemed to be a broken record. I would just talk about how much I missed Gene, the problems at work, and how depressed I was feeling. He said he was not going to give up on me and let me die.

Things were building back up at work. Incidents caused me to lose what little self-esteem I had gained. Hopelessness was setting in again. I was becoming extremely depressed and the suicidal ideations were becoming overpowering. I was taking my anger out through self-destructive behavior as with the last time. I wound up in the hospital again in April. This time Dr. Whittington admitted me to St. Luke's Hospital psych ward.

APRIL 21, 1981
ADMISSION STATEMENT: "In outpatient therapy she has continued to deal with feelings of worthlessness, self-depreciation, depression and annihilistic thinking. Seemed to be making progress until recently when she experienced an increase in depressive symptoms and began to de-

scribe a great amount of mental confusion, indecisiveness and feelings of hopelessness. She was experiencing on 4/21/81 marked suicidal ideation and pressure, and hospitalization recommended to evaluate cause of worsening."

"Staff got impression that pt. was threatening suicide as a power-play against staff. Partially confirmed by Dr. W. who suggested that the pt. not be put on 15' checks, but should be watched closely unofficially. Pt. thought process seems intact, depressed affect, poor self-esteem. -- Pt. gamy w/staff challenging us to keep her here and verbalizing suicidal intent but did not act on this. Seems more like a power struggle/control issue where she seeks caring and then rebels against limits. Brief contact with mother who seems to be controlling and demanding and gives love when expectations are met. Sees pt. as perfectionist (as mother appears) who drives self and is never satisfied."

This hospital stay came off with minimal incidents. I was never confined in seclusion. On one day, I did get into a self-punishing ritual and ended up cutting on my arm and hand. I managed to cut myself one other time a few days later; again a self-punishing gesture and not suicidal intent. This probably resulted from the phone calls I got from my company in Alaska about a possible promotion and job transfer. I did not feel that I did a very good job on the telephone interviews. It was difficult trying to explain where I was.

I displayed a considerable amount of anger in group therapy when discussing the guilt feelings imposed by my mother and used feelings from my relationship with Gene.

Dr. Whittington placed me on Parnate, an MAO inhibitor antidepressant, to try and break the severe depression I was experiencing. This medication seemed to take hold and improve my affect by the end of the hospitalization.

Even though I was in a depressive swing, I did have a few light moments of mania as the records indicated my affect being cheerful and optimistic. Actually I believe alters were making appearances.

Katherine and Bobbie spent a considerable amount of time out during this hospital stay. Katherine wrote a number of poems reflecting my mood and relationships with self and men. Bobbie designed a cover for the patient information brochure the staff was putting together. She also did a lot of crocheting on a huge afghan she was making.

My interaction with staff was gamy and testing, but they didn't over-react as the staff did at Mt. Airy. They gave me a little more rope and talked me through my more difficult moments. They didn't punish me for my destructive behavior. Rather, they tried to help me try to understand why I had a need to deface my body. They wanted to understand me.

I did a lot of thinking and contemplating on whether or not I could change my behavior patterns. I also thought about whether or not I wanted to if I could. I had a life full of neglect and was in desperate need for attention to me and not what I did. No matter what I did, I could not achieve this appropriately. Acting out was the only way I knew to get attention. Attention for my accomplishments was not personally oriented but focused on the accomplishment; I was secondary to the attention.

MAY 19, 1981

DISCHARGE NOTES: "Initially aloof and uninvolved, testing and manipulative. Treated with Parnate, pt. became cooperative and increasingly insightful. On several occasions she inflicted superficial lacerations on her arms and hand, but without suicidal intent. Used assertiveness during group therapy and individual therapy quite effectively. Focus on resolving conflicts with mother, guilt, difficulty with sexuality, unmourned loss of father and conflict regarding career choices. Prognosis great." - Dr. W.

The new medication seemed to be working when I got out of St. Luke's. At least for awhile. The depression subsided considerably, and I didn't have as many suicidal-like ideations.

I was able to complete the files at work. They hired a file clerk to maintain the files which I had to train. A number of supervisory positions were opening up within the company, and I was applying for all of them. The only one that seemed promising was the one in Anchorage, because I had two telephone interviews. It was real hard to focus for those interviews and the fact that they were talking to me in the hospital had some affect on my responses to their questions. I think I seemed rather aloof, even though I really wanted the job.

I was spending part of my time evaluating computer aided drafting systems for the department. I would make my recommendation by late summer. We were planning another move into the new ARCO Tower that was going up next door. That move would come the following spring.

Therapy had kind of reached a stalemate by summer. I was not progressing well with any sort of recovery. Dr. Whittington thought I needed feedback and interaction from other people so suggested I join a therapy group that had been formed by his office. I still had a lot of anger built up that I would not let go of. I felt Dr. Whittington was giving up on me and found me to be an impossible patient who was narrowly focused. I really had little choice but to join the group.

I found it very difficult at first to contribute to the group. I was angry that Dr. Whittington had pushed me aside. Slowly I started to open up but in a guarded way. Most of the others' problems stemmed around social issues. Mine were personal and dealt with work. I didn't know how to communicate the tremendous build-up of anger that I had. I did resolve that my anger was my worst enemy. Somehow I didn't feel I fit in very well.

By mid-August, frustrations had once again built to an unbearable level. I was having more self-destructive thoughts resulting from the anger build-up and frustrations of life and work. On August 19, things reached a climax. I got the idea of playing Russian Roulette with my medication. With Parnate you had to maintain a strict diet. Well, I doubled my dosage that day and drank a lot of coffee and took a caffeine Dexatrim tablet. Just before I went into group therapy, I drank a third of a pint of straight bourbon.

Despite all I had done, I didn't start to feel anything until about halfway through group. I suddenly became very spacey and drowsy. When group was over, I didn't feel alert enough to drive home. I fell asleep in the doctor's office for about an hour. They tried to arouse me to get me to leave. I was very groggy and had trouble getting up. Dr. Whittington came in and threatened that if I didn't leave, he would put me in the hospital. He thought I was faking for attention. This made me very angry because I was really having trouble.

I staggered out of the office thinking that if I could just make it to my car, I would sleep it off there. I must have looked like an intensely intoxicated individual. I was hanging on to signposts and falling asleep. One of the building security saw me and went to get the group's psychologist. He came out and forced me into a wheelchair and took me over to ER at Mercy Medical Center.

I was angry that they were going to put me back in the hospital. While in ER, when no one was looking, I grabbed another 8-10 Parnate out of my purse and swallowed them. I came close to dying that night. Kim had done a real good job. At one point, I had stopped breathing on my own. The respirator was the only thing keeping me alive. I remember feeling a sense of calm at that time that was so wonderful and peaceful. All the anger was gone. I was floating on a cloud. I was in euphoria with no troubles or concerns.

AUGUST 18, 1981
ADMISSION REPORT: "Pt. brought into ER at Mercy for psychiatric evaluation and disposition by her staff psychologist, but brought to ER in a combative and hysterical state. Soon became stuporous and then lost consciousness. At initial evaluation at 6:45 p.m. she was unrousable with BP 145/100. Eyes in oculogyric crisis — deviated extremely superiorly." ASSESSMENT: "Pt. in evident drug overdose presumed secondary to Parnate. At present BP stable but decreased respiration since admission to ER are bothersome and underwent elective intubation by nurse and anesthesiologist at hospital. Now presently on IMD mode of respirator for control of respirations.

Did receive charcoal. Did vomit some." PLAN: "Pt. will be monitored and kept in ICU until she resumes her own respirations and is alert. She is under 72 hour mental health hold so will be restrained as necessary when she awakes.

AUGUST 22, 1981

DISCHARGE SUMMARY: "27 yr. old single female brought to ER for psychological evaluation when found wandering around parking lot outside Mercy in confused state. After brought to ER, progressively declined in awareness and became unconscious. At that time evaluated by Dr. Benedeth, the ER doctor, who obtained history of ingestion of uncertain quantity of Parnate. During ER evaluation she noted to have a respiratory rate of 16, BP of 145/100, HR of 106. Physical exam revealed BP of 124/84, pulse 110, resp. 8 and shallow. Temperature of 101.2. In general, she was a disheveled white female, lying in ER bed, unconscious and her only reaction to stimuli was to tighten up her eyes when her eyelashes were stroked. No response to deep pain, such as squeezing fingernails or rubbing knuckles on her chest. Deep tendon reflexes were intact. Head and neck exam; the fundi could not be examined as her eyes were in a deviated superiorly position. No gag present. Heart and lungs revealed clear breath sounds and no murmurs or gallops. The abdomen was soft w/o masses...Pt. transferred to ICU because she was unconscious and there she underwent elective intubation by the nurse and anesthetist, after multiple tries and vomiting and mild clonic contractions of her musculature, she was successfully, finally intubated and the proper ET tube placement verified with chest x-ray. Placed on 40% inspired oxygen concentration via a respirator and put in intermittent, mandatory ventilation mode, which satisfactorily controlled her respiration. Continued on respirator throughout the night, but did awaken in early morning hours and was observed to have some widespread, muscular contractions which were thought either to be myoclonic seizure etiology or hysterical seizures. Did respond to intravenous Valium while still on respirator. In a.m. when fully awake, was extubated and remained alert and transferred to room. Started on IV Penicillin for aspiration pneumonia. "

While unconscious, my mind was somewhat aware of what was going on. I could hear the respirator working, I could hear when my parents came into the room to see me. I faded in and out mentally, but the rest of my body would not respond or move.

I think this little incident alerted Kim to the fact that, yes indeed, I was vulnerable, and her behavior could hurt me and the rest of the Group. I also understand that when Kim gets extremely angry, she goes into a state of delirium where she has little thought of the repercussions resulting from her actions.

The attending physician at Mercy was Dr. Lee Anneberg. To show you what a small world it is, he also happened to be the attending physician during my OD the year before when I was at Presbyterian Hospital. He found me to be a very troubled individual and questioned whether I was happy with my therapist if he could provoke such a serious gesture. I explained that I was lost in my therapy and felt I was getting nowhere. He said that if I was interested, he knew a good psychiatrist that he would recommend to me.

A week after my discharge, I went back to Dr. Anneberg for a follow-up on the pneumonia. I had given it some thought and asked him for the name of the doctor he was talking about. The name he gave me was Dr. Greg Wilets. (Another "W")

I called Dr. Wilets and scheduled an interview. He was quite young and must have been starting out in his practice when I came to him. We hit it off from the start. I had a very good feeling about him and felt very comfortable around him. I decided I would not go back to Dr. Whittington or the group and began seeing Dr. Wilets on a regular basis.

I was just going through the motions of day to day life. I had plenty of vivid thoughts of things I wanted to do or say but had great difficulty with follow-through. I seemed to be losing control of what I was saying and doing. I was impulsive and sporadic. I was feeling like my life was a dream and having problems with reality.

Since Gene and I broke up, I had contemplated selling the condo so I could be free of any further commitments. I was looking at buying a house. I had decided on where it was going to be. I just had to find a buyer for my existing place.

That fall, I had started writing in my journal again. In my entry for October 1, 1981, I had a rude awakening. Someone other than myself was making comments in the journal. They were invading my privacy. I don't know who it was, and it was a big shock when I went back and found it. I suspect it was Kim or the Big Guy, because it was very negative. The handwriting was different. A lot of the final pages in this journal were filled with various kinds of handwriting.

I was experiencing a real identity crisis. I felt like an outcast that no one cared about. I would look in the mirror and question if what I saw was what other people saw of me. I was also having a lot more headaches again with a sort of "dissociative" dizziness. Someone kept telling me that I didn't matter, and if I died, would not be missed. It was real hard to fight back these negative thoughts and voices.

TUESDAY, OCTOBER 13, 1981

Dear Diary,

"Yes, I know it's been a week. It's just that I've found it difficult to talk. I've been absorbing any and all thoughts and experiences going on and not verbalizing them. Things have not gone so well lately, to say the least. Yesterday, was bad. If things had been any worse, I wouldn't be around today to talk to you. I was angry with myself and what was going on around me. No hard formed reasoning behind it. It was just there and I was experiencing it. My session with Dr. Wilets didn't help matters much. I remember hitting things that were difficult to discuss or face. I guess that's suppose to be good. But anyway, in my current state of mind it wasn't good. I dashed out in a fit of anger and got home as fast as I could. I had to do something fast to relieve the anger before it got so bad I'd do something that I'd regret if I could. I immediately got a razor blade and did a meat tenderizing job on my right wrist. For some reason, I can't ever cut deep enough to be fatal. Maybe that's why I do it. I don't know. Anyway, I proceeded to get carried away. I'll end up with a nice cross-hatch scar. You know, Diary, watching that blood seems to make things OK. After I relaxed from the mass of tension, I took 16mg. of Trilafon and went to bed. This morning I woke up feeling a little better. The biggest part of the anger had subsided...They keep telling me that things usually get worse before better. Well, I believe things are going to get so bad, things won't be able to get better. I've had this obsessive thought for a few weeks now. Tonight, I asked Mom if she thought she wanted to be buried with Dad or with Roy. I've had continued thoughts about joining Dad on the 11th anniversary of his death. That's just 2 weeks from now — the 26th. Mom said she'd probably be buried in Denver, so that leaves a spot next to my dad that won't be filled. It would just take a change in the gravestone. *I told you I would continue to keep my finger on you. I'm slowly taking control. Last night? That was me that made you do it. You sure did a good job and didn't bat an eye, did you? You didn't get sick like the last time. You enjoyed it — No, I enjoyed it. I've got you where I want you. Your tolerance level is getting low. Two weeks, that's not long. Believe me. It won't be painful. Talk to you later...* God, this can't be! I don't believe what is going on. I've got to regain control. I couldn't wait till I got off work today. That impulse is getting so strong. I need more time. I can't continue to have days where I go to work and then rush home to go to bed and avoid facing this nightmare! I need someone to pinch me so I can wake up. — Please!

By October 16, the impulse to take another overdose grew too great. I left work around lunch time. I got home and battled the urge to take the pills for a couple hours. Finally, the urge was out of control. I took 300mg of Vistaril and 44mg of Trilafon. After realizing what I had done, I placed a call to Dr. Wilets. I don't know what I was wanting from him when he called back. It should have occurred to me that he would certainly demand I go into the hospital. I became quite angry and hung up on him. He called back two more times and I again hung up on him. He then called 911. After hanging up with Dr. Wilets, I took another 1.5 gms. of Dilantin.

The fire department and an ambulance responded. I had forgotten to lock my door in the distress when I came home, so they were able to gain entrance to my condo without difficulty. I was laying on my bed very groggy when they arrived. They took vitals and escorted me to the ambulance. On the way to the hospital, they connected me to an IV. When I got to the hospital, they forced me to consume some ipecac to make me vomit the pills. They succeeded. After stabilizing me, I was transported to St. Joseph's Hospital that evening.

It was nearing the anniversary of my father's death. Eleven years since that event and I still was deeply affected by it. I cried a lot at his death, but somehow had not allowed myself to thoroughly mourn his loss nor come to final grips with it. My mother was also out of town, and Dr. Wilets thought I experienced a great deal of dismay over separations of prominent people in my life. He felt that I felt rage when other people leave me. I then punish myself by directing that rage inward.

During my other two previous hospitalizations, I was found to be healthy other than my suffering from depression. During my admittance examination this time, my heart demonstrated a II/VI systolic ejection murmur at the lower left sternal border with radiation to the apex, and a questionable click was heard at the left lower sternal border. I had also been experiencing some tachycardia. The tachycardia could have been due to the medication. After ultrasound, it was felt that I possibly was suffering from mitral valve prolapse.

Numerous future other hospitalizations and examinations would conflict with this diagnosis. It was almost as if sometimes it was there and sometimes it wasn't. After developing a better understanding of MPD, studies show that some alters can have physical defects that others do not experience. This is the only thing I can attribute to these conflicting diagnoses. I also attribute the sometimes abnormal vs. normal EEG's I have had to this same phenomenon. The only thing I haven't figured out is who has what problems.

OCTOBER 21, 1981
Dear Diary,
..."*It is now quiet time and time to make my entrance. Now that Michele is trying to relax, I think it's about time she and I conducted some more business. I don't need that stupid comb any more; besides the markings are too wide and obvious. I easily removed a knife from lunch. So what if it's plastic. It's serrated and that's all that's needed. I did a pretty good job on the back of your hand when you were at Mercy. At least that 'N' isn't as evident anymore. Michele is getting weaker and weaker all the time, and I have a way of making her forget our encounters. I know when to show up. I know how to get her to her room to keep from making a scene in front of staff. That way they don't see her and can't stop me. I'm not as dumb as some people take me for. In fact, I think I'm real smart. So smart that I'll get the two of us out of here in no time at all. They don't see her fits and fights and get the idea that she is on her way to recovery. Pam, her last roommate, was also a big help by pulling the curtain and shutting the door when she was fighting with me. Well, if I'm going to do anything today, I better quit this jabbering and get on with my business...*Yeah, Diary, it's me, Michele. By the looks of the writing above, I haven't said much to you. I make a habit of not reading that scratching above. Partly because I'm afraid and partly because I can't accept it's me that writes like that. I noticed another cut on my wrist. I think things are getting a little ridiculous. I also noticed a cut on my ankle when I was taking a shower. I felt a stinging when the water hit it...*"

This entry in my diary was too much for me to not become anxious. I got a little manic after my session with Dr. Wilets. I got some medication to calm me down. It worked for awhile and then things escalated again. What ensued was a power struggle with the staff. I ended up in restraints from about 4 p.m. until the next morning.

My mood swings were all over the charts. I was up, then down, then up again. I was experiencing mixed states and in a real confusion crisis. I didn't know which end was up. I had a lot of control issues I was fighting with the hospital staff. I wound up in restraints on numerous occasions during this hospitalization.

OCTOBER 18, 1981
"I just want to be left alone. I don't want anyone to care for me...I'm tired of feeling, of always giving and giving. I feel used...I do hear these voices; no they don't have any sex, I'm sexless...When I cut myself, I don't feel any pain. I know what I'm doing but don't feel it...I've been hearing these voices for 1 to 1-1/2 years. They've gotten stronger lately."

OCTOBER 21, 1981
"The voice I hear is my inner self. I've tried to fight it but it gets stronger...It's much stronger than last year and I'm afraid to relax because then it'll take over. The real me is a very weak person."

OCTOBER 22, 1981
"Depressed, clinging to bedspread. Isolating, tearful at times, later losing control attempting to bolt the unit. Increased acting out by threatening to harm self and regressed behavior to indicate how she feels. Pt. placed in restraints with 15 minute checks."

OCTOBER 26, 1981
"Pt. in restraints."

OCTOBER 29, 1981
"Pt. very gamy today walking off the unit and returning on her own in which her clothes were taken away from her. Pt. acting out the remainder of the day. Running off the unit having nursing staff pursue her and putting a big struggle in being returned to the unit. Pt. was placed in 4-point restraints for control."

OCTOBER 30, 1981
"Pt. talking about 'other' selves and being scared."

NOVEMBER 8, 1981
"Pt. remains very despondent and suicidal. Claims to have taken 8000mg of Tylenol yesterday. Called Dr. Kerchen in ER. Will get tests to see if mucomist is necessary."

NOVEMBER 9, 1981
Pt. rapidly regressed today after being exposed to the violence of male pt. She remembered her father's violence and her hitting him. She now feels she must hurt herself for relief. Pt. apparently must punish herself for her hitting her father years ago. She also appears depressed. Pt. placed in restraints at own request."

NOVEMBER 18, 1981
"In 4-point restraints. Angry with self that she can't keep control. She was progressively more depressed as the day went on."

NOVEMBER 30, 1981

"Pt. became angry and agitated about a broken light bulb — pieces found in wastebasket and were confiscated. Pt. still stating she had to hurt self. Had made superficial cut on wrist. Pt. placed in 4-point restraints. Pt. stated she had light bulb hidden on the unit. -- Pt. definitely regressing around discharge. She is getting involved in conflicts over sleeping medication (i.e. wanted pills early), along with broken light bulbs. She is having self-destructive thoughts making it hard for her to be discharged. These are incidents that represent her fear and panic about leaving hospital."

DECEMBER 2, 1981

"Pt. cut on self. Had three small lacerations on right wrist. No blood noted. Pt. stated glass was in her jeans pocket. Staff retrieved glass and disposed of it. Pt. does not appear suicidal — currently does cut on self 'to relieve pressures'."

DECEMBER 7, 1981

"Agreed to go into seclusion rather than restraints. Appears close to losing control. Placed in 4-point restraints for self-destructive behavior of beating on walls, window and floor with head and fists."

DECEMBER 8, 1981

"Speech is not pressured but her thought content is grandiose. Affect is manic and grandiose."

This was a long hospitalization. I did not get discharged until December 20. The only thing that saved me was that I was allowed to go to work during the day and return to the hospital at night. It subdued the fear of losing my job so I could work on other issues. Because of my work schedule, I got to see Dr. Wilets only on Mondays, Wednesdays and Fridays, either early in the morning or once I returned to the hospital.

I had to make a written contract each day with staff that I would not hurt myself while away from the hospital. One problem I have always had was with keeping my word. When I promise to do something, I will do anything and everything humanly possible to carry through with my word.

I had a tremendous amount of internal conflict that was not getting resolved in addition to the bipolar swings I was experiencing. Dr. Wilets gave me a depression test which came back positive. He started treating me with Ascendin. The depression was playing havoc with my body. I had a lot of gas and constipation. I was having numbing, void feelings. Then there were the "voices" that I couldn't seem to get rid of.

Staff was again reactionary to what was going on with me. I took every opportunity to try to convey to them that I was not responsible for the behavior I was exhibiting. No one seemed to piece it together. I wasn't sure of what was happening to me, either. All I knew was that it certainly could not be "normal" feelings and behavior.

The antidepressant seemed to be working. It was contributing to my tachycardia, but I could handle it if my body could. Anything was better than being depressed and out of control.

I had problems with the thought of discharge from the hospital, because, despite control issues, I was becoming comfortable with the staff relationship I had. I needed the staff interactions to relieve the pressure and anger I was experiencing from therapy and work. I knew how to push their buttons and get the needed resolutions, no matter how temporary. Somehow I knew I was going to have to find a better way to control my feelings. I could not act out at work. I needed the attention the interventions produced. I wanted to be recognized by someone no matter how or where. I was starving for attention with a release.

My life managed to get back to a tolerable state after discharge. I still had uncomfortable feelings and vast mood swings. The confusion and disorganization in my feelings seemed to subside. The voices became more subdued. I felt I was regaining some control in who I was.

My short term goal after discharge was to finally sell my condo and move into a new home I had contracted for. That was the main thing that kept me going in the hospital. I, in fact, became obsessed with that house and what it represented. By selling the condo, I would be through with Gene for once and all. I finally did sell it in January. I took a loss on it. It was difficult going to Gene to tell him he had lost his investment in the place, but I think he was finally glad to be out of that joint obligation. He could now get on with his life, also. My parents helped me to get approved for the loan on the house by loaning me some money to pay off some of my debts.

I was experiencing some loneliness, and knowing that I was going to have a house with a yard, decided to get a dog. I had done some thinking about what kind I wanted and was watching the paper. Before moving into my house, I bought a Yorkshire puppy and called her Nikki.

Preparing for the move and final separation from Gene generated stress and anxiety. My depression started to slip back into the picture. In February, I went back into the hospital for a very brief stay to try to get my medication readjusted and to resolve some of the anxiety I was experiencing. The stay picked me up, dusted me off, and did a reality check for me. It went off without a hitch or power struggles.

A NEW BEGINNING

I moved into my new house the first part of March 1982. A long-sustained dream had come true. I was as happy as I had ever been. I felt a real accomplishment and felt that my problems were a thing of the past. I became obsessed with that house. It consumed all my non-working and sleeping hours. I bought a 2-story, 3 bedroom house that was in a cul-de-sac and on one of the biggest lots.

On the day of the move, Bobbie was busy in the spare bedroom painting the walls. She and Bonnie had big plans for decorating the inside. They had gone to an art/decorating store and picked out wallpaper to hang. After the decorating that had been done at the condo, they were experts at wallpapering. I slept in the spare bedroom for the first few weeks, until the painting and wallpapering in the master bedroom was complete.

First big outdoor project on the agenda was to get a fence built. I couldn't let Nikki out in the yard to roam freely without a fence. My next door neighbor was getting ready to build his fence. We shared the cost of an auger and he drilled all our fence post holes at the same time. My dad helped me get started putting the fence posts up and showed me how to keep the fence even. Mike went into high gear and did 90% of the work. My mom came over and pounded a few nails, and when I was done, my dad came back with my brother-in-law to help me put up the gate.

Mike, Bobbie and Bonnie then sat down to plan out the landscaping for the yard. It was decided that I would have a large vegetable garden and plenty of flower garden in the back. I got a couple trees, evergreens and rock for the front yard. Mike got callouses on his hands from all the rock that was spread. It prepared him for what was to come in the back yard.

It was May before the grass was ordered. I had figured that 4400 square feet worth of sod would be needed to cover the areas not designated as garden. When it was done, I had little to spare.

It rained the first day I started to lay the sod, making the rolls just that much heavier. About an hour into the project, I lifted a heavy roll and put it down in such a way that I strained my back. The neighbor on the north side of me just happened to come over. His name was also Mike. He was living with his parents. He was about 2 years older than me. He offered to help when he learned what I had done. With his gracious help, I got the sod all laid in two days. Mike and I would soon become good friends. We helped each other with our new home projects.

By mid-June, the yard was complete and all but one room of the house had been painted or wallpapered. I was proud of my accomplishments. The only thing I had not done that I wished I could have afforded, was to put in a sprinkler system. The other work had taken more money than originally anticipated. I had to draw the line somewhere.

The soil around my yard was a very hard, sandy soil. Since the house was built during the winter months, the ground was hard. During spring and early summer, there was a lot of rain. The ground was starting to settle and I got some sink holes. One big one was in the middle of the front yard. My Mike had a plan to fix this. I had been to a number of home and garden shows that spring and he had the great idea of building a wishing well planter. He had fine-tuned his skills in carpentry and yard work, and now was going to try his hand at masonry. The base of the planter would have a cement and brick base. It went together well. I had problems with how the roof was going to go on, so my dad and Larry, my brother-in-law, came over one weekend to help get the roof on.

I kept busy that spring and summer. So much so, I didn't have any time to think about getting depressed. All that started to change when summer was winding down and the yard work was wrapping up. About mid-August I noticed I was starting to get depressed. Before I knew it, the depression was engulfing me.

Not helping my downward mood swing, was my finding out that Gene had gotten married that August. I was devastated and deeply hurt. He had led me to believe that it would be some time before he would make any kind of commitment to a woman. What hurt even more was that this woman was five years younger than I was, and I was seven years younger than Gene.

It appeared that the Ascendin I was on was losing its potency and effect. I was defenseless against this depression. Work was very stressful with the anticipation of taking on new and different job responsibilities. I began having suicidal ideations of overdosing again. I would threaten Dr. Wilets with these thoughts to the point he had no choice but to insist I go back into the hospital. The gain I had made that year meant too much to risk losing everything, so I agreed with some dissension.

Dr. Wilets had also gotten married that fall and I was feeling that all the men in my life had abandoned me. My father left me, Gene, and now Dr. Wilets. Dr. Wilets knew me better than my own mom. I felt the only person who could help me was now going to devote his time and energies to another woman. I seemed to be a failure with men. I could not relate to women, so men played an important role in my life. I thought of women as my mother, being hard and forceful and unloving. Men provided me with attention and caring and love.

Once again a predominant issue in my hospitalization was the upcoming anniversary of my father's death. I was obsessed with wanting to join him. I was feeling guilty that my life was going so well at the expense of my father's. This guilt was adding to my depression. I could not get in touch with the inner anger I was feeling over my father killing himself with booze. Instead, I made myself feel guilty and responsible for his death.

Early on during this hospitalization, I made two serious overdose gestures. I had also been on a binge of vomiting up my food after eating, and had lost 5 pounds in that first week. Dr. Wilets and the staff realized that I was bound and determined to pursue using a self-destructive course in the hospital. A Dr. John Lightburn was brought in on the case to evaluate whether electroconvulsive shock treatments would be of any help.

Dr. Lightburn and Dr. Wilets saw my behavior as rather characterologic in the borderline spectrum. At that time they did not feel I suffered from a major affective disorder. However, they did feel that my disorganization was significant and without some major intervention, I could become lethal to myself while in the hospital.

I was in a considerable amount of despair. The doctors caught me on a good day when I was not interested in pursuing any further confrontational behavior with staff. They convinced me that the only chance I had to come out of this hospitalization was through undergoing ECT. I agreed and signed the necessary paperwork.

I was given eight ECT treatments during this stay. I suffered the usual disorientation and memory lapses. The treatment kept me amnesic and disorganized that I did not act out during the course of the ECT. One day I woke up in my hospital bed wondering where I was. I had no clue as to how long I had been there or what transpired up to that time. I could not remember how I had put a big gash on my right wrist. I was extremely frustrated over the memory loss. As my thoughts began to reorganize after the conclusion of the treatments, my depression returned and I reinstated my compulsions to hurt myself.

It took me about a week to regain my full orientation. I had returned to my gamy struggle with staff as before the treatment. One day, I escaped the ward. I borrowed five dollars from another patient. I went to a local pharmacy and bought a big bottle of Tylenol. This occurred right after the anniversary of my father's death. I went to another nearby hospital to get a big cup of water to take the pills. When I returned to the hospital, I would not tell staff where I had been. A struggle ensued and I was put in restraints. I was transferred to another ward. They were suspicious and began to monitor my vitals. Finally, they were able to get me to tell them I had taken 100 extra strength Tylenol tablets. They immediately transported me to ER where they tried to get me to take ipecac and charcoal. I refused and they forced it down through a tube.

My drug levels were extremely high and I was started on mucomist therapy. I would not voluntarily take the medication. They placed an NG tube down my nose to facilitate the administration of the anecdote. I was taken back to the ward and kept in restraints for the next several days on strict suicide precautions.

SEPTEMBER 23, 1982
"OD of 50 aspirin and 50 extra strength Tylenol."

SEPTEMBER 25, 1982
"Cut a slice in right wrist while on patio."

SEPTEMBER 29, 1982
"Pt. returned to 4 South from pass and informed staff she had taken OD of meds which she had been hoarding (works during day and given meds by staff to take while out of hospital.) was given Ipecac on unit and became unresponsive after vomiting. Unresponsive upon arrival to ER. Eyelids fluttering with ammonia; no other response. Beginning of refusal to eat or drink."

SEPTEMBER 30, 1982
"Talks constantly about wanting to be with father. Wants to communicate with him, touch his fingers, experience him again. 'When I OD I don't want to die, but if I die, I die.' Obsessed with communicating with father. Pt. has lost 11 pounds in three days."

OCTOBER 3, 1982
"Pt. admitted to vomiting after eating. Way of acting out self-destructive behavior. 'I don't deserve to feel good.'"

OCTOBER 4, 1982
"Remains depressed. Shifting her battle to not eating or drinking. This is probably responsible for her decreased BP. Is consciously not eating to harm herself. Will run IV fluids in A.M. Don't trust her with IV needle in tonight."

OCTOBER 5, 1982
"Less depressed. Still hypotensive. Wants to still deprive herself of water and food. Will give IV fluids. Michele is somewhat giddy at this point. She appears somewhat amnesic and quiet. She spent much of the day in bed or isolated in room."

OCTOBER 6, 1982
"Pt. up and about mid morning after ECT. Seems increased amnesic, giddy, smiling, eating well. No evidence of vomiting. Pt. admitted to self-induced vomiting."

OCTOBER 7, 1982
"Still suffering from some dehydration, so will give another litre D5LR today."

OCTOBER 8, 1982
"Quite confused. At this time remembers little of what has gone on including self-destructive thoughts and actions. Not now self-destructive but this could change when the amnesia wears out. Will watch carefully."

OCTOBER 14, 1982
"ECT #8 today. This completes the series. The results thus far appear to be minimal therapeutic gain but with considerable confusion which may have decreased her ability to act out. Pt. remains very ill and a therapeutic challenge. Continued work on the issues of loss, anger and low self-esteem with role of father played and plays may eventually produce sufficient improvement. - Dr. Lightburn.

It seems shortly after this last treatment, I woke up from what seemed a long sleep. I had no memory of my hospitalization thus far. I felt what I did remember was just a bad dream. I remembered seeing myself down in a cold treatment room. The doctors tied me down, put something on my head and a stick in my mouth. The next thing I remember is waking up in a strange bed in the hospital. I have no memory of ever consenting to the treatment.

OCTOBER 20, 1982
"Frustration increased over memory loss and she is having the beginning of self-destructive thoughts again. In a masochistic way. She is punishing herself for not remembering event. Will watch. Pass this weekend if she is safe."

OCTOBER 25, 1982
"Pt. left unit at 8:45 p.m. threatening to hurt herself. Returned to unit at 9:10 p.m. with scratches on bilateral forearms and broken light bulb in both hands. When told of plans for seclusion made threatening gestures at staff. Pt. was combative making it necessary for 4-pt. restraints. Pt. seems to enjoy the physical contact with male staff while combative acting out. Due to difficulty of management, possible transfer to 5 South."

OCTOBER 26, 1982
"Today is the anniversary of her father's death. She sees me of depriving her of her job and ruining her life by not letting her go to work. She sets me up as the destroyer of her world as a displacement of her father. She has no comprehension of her setting me up. There is no doubt she will force a conflict with me or the staff whether she is secluded or not. She is definitely of high risk to herself. Multiple interpretations were made about her father's death. - Dr. Wilets -- Pt. depressed. 'I'm not going to stay here. You're doing this to me. What do you mean I'm not in control?' During early part of shift sarcastic and gamy. Dr. Wilets here. Pt. very angry that she was not going to be let out of restraints. Trying to get out of 2-points; placed in 4-points with a struggle. Screaming and writhing and trying to bite staff. Calmed down a bit after being in 4-points. Today is anniversary of father's death; pt. acting out. Continued with 4-point restraints to give patient some control."

OCTOBER 27, 1982
"Pt. depressed. 'Dr. Wilets is making himself to be like my dad so I can be angry with him. The only pleasure I get is when I hurt myself. I can understand how my father felt. (That drinking was his only pleasure.)' Pt. in 4-point leather restraints for out of control behavior. Wanting to get out of restraints. States that 'I was good for 4 hours so now you should be able to trust me.' Pt. shifting blame on others. Not accepting responsibility for her own actions. Continued with restraints until pt. able to show more control. -- 'I just don't think that what Greg is trying to get at has any

validity. I have to get back to work.' In later part of shift seems a bit less gamy. Taken out of restraints progressively. Shower taken. In seclusion. Manipulative and gamy. Pt. did contract not to hurt herself or act out. Still questionable whether pt. is in control. Maintain safe environment. Starting tomorrow 1 hr in seclusion, 1 hr. out. Any acting out, back in restraints."

OCTOBER 28, 1982

"Pt. depressed. 'Would you call Dr. Wilets? I need to talk to him about going back to work. Well, can I talk to Kathy? Why can't I talk to Kathy?' Flat effect. Remains very gamy and child like to include tone of voice. Has needed very little structure with time in and out of seclusion. Has been gamy and refused to eat, but continues to take medication. 'It's the best turn on. It's better than a climax. It's so much better than having sex with some bastard.' In 1:1 talked about the compulsion for the restraints and the Tylenol OD; States she wants to do it this weekend so she can go to work on Monday. Also says 'I can be a goody two shoes until Monday and do it then. I think I'm a pretty good actress, but I don't know when this compulsion will hit.' Also talked about possibly being discharged tomorrow for follow-through with plan. Followed through with limits set on her with some reservation. Affect during 1:1 difficult to describe. She was gamy but very certain of herself. Planning on OD and acting out. During 1:1 it was like talking to a different person. Need to have staff to determine direction to go now. Maintain strict suicide precautions.

The turn-on I was speaking of was a result from the struggles with staff in being placed in restraints. It was a safe way to get rid of my aggressions and feel good. I was not a frail woman during these struggles. It usually took 4-5 staff people to wrestle me into the bed and restraints. Dr. Wilets rightly thought that the confrontation set-up with the staff was to force staff to restrain and wrestle me in a highly sexualized manner. He thought it was reminiscent of the struggles I had with my brother while engaging in intercourse when I was in grade school. On the contrary, I believe it stems back further than that. I can't help but to think that a struggle resulted during that day in the basement over at Johnny's house when I was in first grade. It was after that incident that I discovered my sexuality.

OCTOBER 29, 1982

"Pt. depressed. 'What can I do to make you all (staff) feel better?' Pt. has been testy much of the day. Not demonstrating ability to contract on her behavior or to take responsibility for her feelings — relating to Mr. Wilson that it is not what her behavior means to her but to staff. Looks angry, smiling inappropriately. Left unit in a manipulative walk down the hall; then ran out of the unit. Security notified. Dr. Wilets answering service notified. Hospital searched by staff. Pts. roommate reports that pt. borrowed $5.00 from her this a.m. Pt. returned to unit. Hid in linen closet after being seen by staff. Resistive to going with staff. Transferred to 5 South room 524. She was angry and resistant. Refused to say what she had done off unit — 'I did what I did off the unit. I'm not dumb enough to bring it back here.' Pt. placed in 4-point restraints in 524. Continued resistive and self-destructive acting out of feelings. Pt. again requiring restraints for her behavior. Ipecac as ordered. Watch LOC and vital signs. Drug screen as overdose. To ER for more intensive Rx of OD for response to Ipecac. -- 'I don't need that tube. I don't like this.' Pt. remains in 4-point leather restraints. Seen by Dr. Wilets at 3 p.m. Shortly thereafter taken to ER for placement of Ewall tube and gastric lavage. Refused to take Mucomist orally. NG tube passed to facilitate Mucomist dosages. Pt. more complacent and cooperative later in evening. Got out of restraints to go to B.R. by contracting with staff to remain in control and return to restraints when finished. Vitals remain stable. 8:30 Acetominiphen level 135, down from 210 at 4:30. Severe Tylenol OD. Pt. still unpredictable, needing restraints. Mucomist protocol. Strict suicide precautions. Monitor vitals.

OCTOBER 30, 1982

"Pt. depressed. 'What you people don't understand is that when I get this compulsion, I have to follow it through no matter what. I wanted to do it sooner than I did so I could get back to work on Monday. Now I can't go till Tuesday, but that's OK, because someone called them at work. I'll drink the Rx (mucomist). How long do I have to keep it down so you won't have to repeat it? I'm nauseated, but I'm not trying to vomit.' Fairly compliant except around mucomist. Has been in 4-point restraints all day. Allowed only 3-pt. for meals. Eating ok to fair. Given bed bath and shampoo. Tampon changed by pt. having menses. Voided 1X very dark urine. Walked around unit 2X. Complained of nausea and dizziness. Pt. unpredictable and needs restraints to prevent self-destructive. -- Pt. states is all over and currently she feels in total control now. NG tube in place. Pt. took mucomist P.O. Appears much less gamy this evening. Restraints are reduced to diagonals. Pt. contracted not to hurt self or mess with NG tube."

OCTOBER 31, 1982

"'I've had diarrhea a couple times (loose, dark brown with foul odored stools). My stomach's more upset, This tube is irritating my throat.' In 2-pt. restraints in A.M. Vomited 2X after A.M. dose of mucomist, in P.M. told her I was putting her in 4-pt. restraints so it would be more inconvenient for her to vomit. Did not vomit afternoon dose of mucomist. Taking fluids only fair, eating lightly. Gotten up out of restraints in A.M. to walk around unit, shower, got up to B.R. Complained of feeling weak, nauseated, wobbly. Dozing on and off during day."

NOVEMBER 1, 1982

"Mood much improved and no self-destructive impulses. Pt. repeats that the obsession to hurt self has been fully relieved. Will quickly wear from restraints. Back to work Thursday is possible. May consider Wednesday. No severe liver toxicity. No imminent danger to self."

NOVEMBER 2, 1982

"'I feel that my wanting to hurt myself is over. I apologize for the problems I have caused the past few days.' Spoke of wanting to return to work by the end of week. Expressed some anxiety but felt she would be able to handle new job. Patient was able to tolerate being out of restraints one hour at a time, returned to restraints without difficulty. Affect is brighter and more sociable. Concerned about personal appearance. Contracted to visit with people from her job without restraints.

This hospitalization was a very trying ordeal. I was finally discharged on November 6. The trauma from that final overdose set me straight. I did not want to go through that again. It was real hard for me to take all those pills. I nearly got sick doing it, but that force inside of me kept driving me through the motions until every pill in the bottle had been taken. It wasn't until 1989 that I ever attempted another medication overdose. Hospitalizations since then were also kept to a minimum. It seemed that the longer I was in the hospital the more I regressed in my behavior.

When I returned to work, I was suppose to be placed in charge of the new computer aided drafting department. I told them that I didn't think it was a good idea that I spend all my days in a cold, dark room. I also didn't feel as strongly about the computer system that the company decided to buy. It was not the one I had recommended. I knew it was inferior to what we wanted to accomplish. I asked to remain out in the regular drafting department and be assigned to special projects. They obliged me with my wishes.

I tried to go back to work after these hospitalizations with the attitude that nothing had happened and I wasn't gone for great periods of time. I was allowed to go back to work on many occasions while still in the hospital. That helped a little. I'm sure, though, that their patience with my problem was wearing thin.

I tried to get on with my life and be as normal as possible. I still had recurring bouts with depression. Dr. Wilets would just bounce me from one drug to another to keep me stabilized and out of the hospital. I think I have tried every type of antidepressant that has ever been made.

I soon got back to a routine. Nikki had been staying with my mom during all my hospitalizations. She almost knew my mom better than me. I did miss her a lot when I was away. I was preparing for my first Christmas in my new home. I bought a nice artificial tree and had my presents all bought by mid-December. Karla and Larry and I were going to spend Christmas day at our folk's.

We got off work early on the 23rd because it was snowing real hard. Weather reports spoke of a severe blizzard and everyone was asked to stay at home till it was over. There were times when I looked outside to the back yard and could not see the back fence line. The snow just kept coming and didn't seem to want to let up. I lost my power for a few hours. By Christmas Eve, we had well over two feet of snow on the ground. The snow had drifted in the cul-de-sac such that it was waist deep. Needless to say, I did not get to my mom's for Christmas. The city was at a standstill. Only emergency vehicles were on the road. This was the first Christmas for me alone. My neighbors called me and asked if I wanted to come over to play some games. I grabbed some munchies and wine and headed for the house two doors away. It took me at least fifteen minutes to get there. I had to trudge my way through snow that was waist high most of the way and in some places almost up to my shoulders.

When the storm had subsided the snow plows did not come down my cul-de-sac. They concentrated their efforts on getting the main thoroughfares plowed. The only 4-wheel drive on the block was in Kansas. I was snowbound. Finally on the 27th, a front end loader came into the cul-de-sac. For twenty bucks from each neighbor, he would plow a path to the main street. I missed two days of work before being able to get out of my driveway. It was quite an experience, but I survived the Blizzard of '82.

I went into the new year with some stability and hope. I figured nothing could ever be as bad as the last. I had regular therapy sessions with Dr. Wilets and he kept me on antidepressants. When one would seem to fail and I started to slip into another depression, he would try another drug combination. One way or another, I managed to stay out of the hospital in 1983.

I allowed a new friend I had made from the CAP program talk me into joining the Association of Desk and Derrick Clubs. This was a professional organization for women in the petroleum industry. I got active right away. I joined the Speaker's Bureau.

In the spring, my sister made the announcement that she and Larry were expecting their first child. I was very excited about this. Roger's wife could not have children, so this was going to be my first chance to be an aunt.

I was once again invited to go out to Washington, D.C. for another annual CAP gathering. This time I took some vacation time and went out to see some sites. It kind of backfired on me. My baggage got misplaced and I was cooped up in the hotel room for two days. I did not even have a toothbrush. From that experience on, I learned to travel with daily essentials in a carry on bag.

In May, I got a brainy idea to start a side-line business to make maps. I was so frustrated with the poor quality of maps that we had at work, that I wanted to start my own base map company. I contacted a lawyer and had corporation papers drawn up. I was President and CEO. My dad agreed to be VP and my mom Secretary.

My first customers were a couple of landmen at work who were originally from Texas. They had done some research and found that all the major ski resorts in Colorado were once part of the Texas Republic. I designed the artwork for a major promotion they devised. It included T-shirts, posters and bumper stickers. This project lasted about a year before everything was done.

That summer I took a class at the community college on small business management. Word of my venture eventually worked its way to management. Corporate lawyers evaluated the intent of my business and felt it would be a conflict of interest to build base maps. I didn't let this stop me. I tried to just get the word out that I would do graphics.

That summer, Mike and Bonnie designed a deck to be built off my back patio. It was octagonal in shape to match the new hot tub that I had decided to purchase. I contacted one of the builders who was at a spring home and garden show to build it. The first attempt failed. I was very disappointed in the way that it turned out. It barely looked like how I had planned it. I made the owner of the company come out and look at it. I told him they were going to redo it correctly or I would see them in court. The guy I was working with on the project lost his job over it. They did rebuild it and looked a lot better the second time.

I managed to make it through the fall and the anniversary of my father's death with little incident. I did see Dr. Wilets twice a week during that time, but did not need hospitalization. I thought I had finally come to grips and resolved my anger and guilt from his death. He tried to assure me that women with mental problems seem to have the most difficult time in their late twenties and early thirties. I was really hopeful that the worst was behind me.

I was still seeing Dr. Quintero quarterly for my seizure activity. He had me taking anticonvulsants to hopefully sideline the spacey feelings and lapses in memory and trouble with coordination that I was having. He would not fully admit that I had epilepsy, but wanted to remain cautious.

By Thanksgiving, Karla was as big as ever and reaching the term of her pregnancy. She was due in early December. After the first of December, everyone was on alert to getting a phone call. On December 10, my mom called and said my sister had gone into labor. I dashed up to Westminster to see if I could be any help. She woke up sick that morning and was vomiting. My mom drove Karla and Larry into Boulder to the hospital. I followed in my car.

We waited around the hospital for something to happen. The labor was not progressing very quickly. The labor was hard. She said she just wanted to have it over with. Karla said she didn't care if she gave birth to a frog. She just wanted the baby to be born. Finally, about 4 p.m. my mom said it could be awhile and said there was no reason for me to stay. She said she would call me when the baby was born. I left the hospital to get something to eat. I went to a shopping center to do some Christmas shopping. I was too excited to just go home and wait.

I got home about 7 p.m. Around eight, I got a call from my mom. She was excited and said that Karla had finally given birth to a perfect little baby boy. They decided to name him Daniel. I was so overjoyed that I was in tears. I couldn't wait for tomorrow to come so I could go see the baby.

Christmas was especially joyous this year with my new little nephew in the picture. I was also on a bit of a high. I had no depression but was, instead, in a bit of a hypomanic swing. I was going into the new year very upbeat.

The previous year had brought about major shake-ups in my department at work. Jim had retired. We had moved into the ARCO Tower. With the installation of the new CADD department, a new department director, also named Jim, was hired to manage all aspects of the drafting department. Nenad was put in charge of just the manual drafting, so I still had to answer to him. Another guy, Larry, was brought in to manage the computer drafting.

Work had more than doubled, but we had no room to bring in additional drafters. Overtime had been implemented. By January, I was working overtime three to four nights a week. I had over 40 hours of overtime that month. The only way for me to wind down and relax when I got home was to take a nice dip in my spa.

One of the other guys in my department was manic-depressive. He had snapped in December. He was in a manic episode. It was cold and snowing outside and he went out to run some errands without a coat on. Where he went was four blocks away. When he returned, he was out of control, talking a mile a minute and doing bizarre things. I recognized this from my own illness and knew we needed to get him some help. It was one night during overtime. I got him to give me his home phone number and called his wife. She couldn't get there for at least a half hour. I called security downstairs. They in turn called an ambulance. I just hope I have never been that out of control.

I was so manic myself in January that I was going to bed early in the morning. Toward the end of the month, on top of my overtime, I had to work on a poster for the two landmen I was doing the Ski Texas art for. I got up that Sunday at 9:30 in the morning. I worked early in the day on laundry and housework, then started on the poster. I worked all night on it without any chance to go to bed. I did not go to bed until 11:15 that Monday night.

Dr. Wilets didn't like the level my mood was at. He was sure I was going to come crashing down big time if we didn't get control of it. I was on Lithium at the time and he had me increase my dosage to 1500 mg. a day. It sure did the trick. My mood level remained strong, but I was experiencing some real bad, uncontrollable grogginess during the day. I scared myself driving home from work on a few occasions.

My physical and mental state started to deteriorate. I was starting to have more episodes of losing momentary consciousness, my vision blanking out, or going into hypnotic like trances. I was losing track of what I was doing and the things around me. Dr. Wilets had me stop the Lithium. He thought I may have reached a toxic level. The blood level came back well within therapeutic range.

I was also experiencing a lot of abdominal cramping. My stools had signs of blood in them. I went to Dr. Anneberg to have it checked out. He thought I may have developed a spastic colon or functional bowel syndrome.

By mid-February, all hell was seeming to break loose. I was out of control. I didn't know whether I was coming or going. Dr. Wilets suggested the hospital to run some tests and possibly get me stabilized. I said, "Absolutely not!" I was bound and determined to get through this thing without having to go into the hospital. I was losing a lot of time and feeling real spacey.

Dr. Anneberg had me go in for a lower GI test. It took two separate tries over two days before the test was successfully performed. As suspected, it came back normal. I was really beginning to think I was going crazy. Nothing was making sense, but all the tests were coming back normal. Dr. Anneberg and Wilets suggested I see my neurologist, Dr. Quintero. Dr. Wilets started me on Tegretol and was still talking about me going into the hospital. I still refused.

Early in March I was plagued with regular symptoms. I was having a lot of dizziness, confusion, and would get "zaps" in my brain that would disorient me further. My moods were swinging wildly and would sometimes feel like I was crawling out of my skin. I had trouble recognizing who I was or where I was throughout the day. I was running into things and literally bouncing off the walls. My coordination was completely shot. I had real trouble trying to stay alert. It may have been caused from the Tegretol I was on.

My performance at work had really deteriorated. So much so, that my supervisors called me in to talk to me about it. I told them I didn't know what was causing my problems. They asked if I needed a medical leave. I told them "not if I could help it." They backed off and gave me some simpler tasks and projects to work on.

I had another EEG with NP leads the second half of March. The results came back with an abnormal reading because of bilateral temporal-occipital spike discharges with poly spike discharge of the right, and left frontal spike discharge with phase reversal across the left frontotemporal area. The abnormalities did suggest a seizure disorder with two possible independent epileptogenic foci.

I was falling asleep a lot when I got home from work. When I would get up to go to bed, I would have to have something to eat and drink. I was needing a boost to get me through the days. I started taking Dexatrim, a caffeine diet pill. Not long after taking it, it would wear down before the 12 hours was up. Soon I started taking two a day. They worked only for a couple days, so went back to taking one a day. All my doctors suggested I cut back on it to every other day. Reluctantly, I agreed. I eventually phased out of the Dexatrim, because it wasn't curbing my appetite. I started taking No-Doz tablets.

I got on a spending frenzy in the spring. Had no control over my impulses. I didn't remember buying the stuff, just seeing it around. Dr. Wilets was concerned about all the spending I was doing. He made me contract with him to put on the brakes or he was going to put me back on Lithium and call my mom. After about a week I lost control and sometime bought two camera lenses for $540. Dr. Wilets told me to go back on the Lithium that I was getting too manic. I asked him how I could be manic and then have so much trouble with all the drowsiness I was experiencing.

May of 1984 was quite a month. It was the time that I had the reunion with my Group. I started out the month with a lot of abdominal cramping and diarrhea. I missed a few days of work. I was taking antacids like candy to help me get by. The doctors could not find anything wrong or causing it.

I was not staying up nearly as late in the months previous, because I had slipped into a mild depression. I was still on a spending spree. I charged most of everything. I had three or four major credit cards with large limits on them. I didn't know how to control things. I tried to make myself stay at the office during lunch, so I wouldn't be tempted. Dr. Wilets was real concerned and still threatening me with the hospital.

I left for Sheridan, Wyoming on May 16. I was headed for a Desk and Derrick meeting in Billings, Montana. I wanted to stop and visit with Roger and Linda. I pretty much drove straight through. I got to Sheridan before they got off work, so went to the high school for a visit. I walked the halls to regain a few memories. My real purpose was to see if they still had my painting. If it wasn't hanging in the halls, I was going to ask them for it. However, when I got to the second floor, I found it hanging in the main hall. It had been fourteen years and was still hanging in the school. That gave me a real feeling of pride.

Roger, Linda and I went out to dinner. We visited for about three or four hours when it got to be time to go to bed. Linda had to get up early to be in to work out at the mine. I got up early to say goodbye. Roger was working a late shift out at the mine. They both worked at the Decker coal mine just north of the Wyoming border.

Roger checked my coolant level in the car and found it to be low. I had lost my air conditioning outside of Casper the day before. I wasn't sure if that caused some damage to the radiator. He also replaced my wiper blades for me, because it was almost certain that I would hit some rain along my trip.

I got to Billings just long enough to take about a half hour nap before having to go on a field trip to the Exxon refinery. I was gone for about two hours. When I got back, I noticed that a lot of coolant had drained out of my car. I decided that I would have to miss a field trip the next day and take it into a garage to have it checked.

I waited for two and a half hours to have a thermostat replaced in my car. I wasn't convinced that that was the only problem. They said they could not find any leaks in the radiator. I don't know a lot about car mechanics, but that coolant had to be leaking from somewhere. I bought some extra coolant and oil just in case to take with me.

The meeting went well on Friday and Saturday. Friday night I stayed at the party they had scheduled until I and a few others closed down the bar. I hadn't partied like that for a long time. I drank a lot and had a real good time. On Saturday, we learned that next year's meeting was going to be in Regina, Saskatchewan. I knew right then that I was going to plan to attend.

Sunday, I left for my real vacation. I was going to drive to the Pacific Northwest, then down to Corvallis, Oregon to visit with Ken and Carol, my best friends from college.

I made it to Anacortes, Washington in two days from Billings. I had a number of stops along the way to take pictures. I had to stop in Osburn, Idaho. They had a shop there with all kinds of wood carvings and furniture. I couldn't get out of there without spending about $500. I bought a rocking ram for Daniel and had it shipped to them. I bought myself a wood sculpture of a buffalo and took it with me.

It was late when I got to Anacortes. I drove around the entire town to find a motel room. I had not made any reservations for this trip because I didn't want to feel pressured into having to be some place at a certain time. I finally found a real dump of a motel. It was fairly run down. I felt like the room might be infested with bugs or lice or something. I was tired, though and ended up sleeping well once I finally got to sleep.

I worked my way across Puget Sound and down around the Olympic Peninsula. The weather was not cooperating very well. It was cloudy and drizzly or rainy most of the time. On my way out of Washington state, I took a detour to where the Mt. St. Helens volcano had erupted. The land was all barren and covered with ash and dirt. They had helicopter rides up around the crater. I decided to take the ride. I had to wait for a couple hours until someone else came that would fill the helicopter. It was going to cost too much for me to go up by myself. The people I ended going up with were from Sheridan. I didn't know them. They had moved there after I left. We did know some of the same people, though.

I got to Carol and Ken's on the 24th. After dinner, Carol talked me into going to her jazzer-cize class. Boy, was I out of shape. I could not last through the whole class. I stayed with them for a day and a half. Carol took me into town to do some shopping. I think I got away spending less than $100. We had some real good talks and shared a lot of memories. They had four kids by then. I couldn't believe how big Matthew was. I knew him when he was born. He was born when they were still living in Phoenix and I was in school.

The rest of the trip took me down the Oregon coast and into northern California. I then trekked across to Reno, Nevada. From there, on to Salt Lake and back home.

THE SECRET'S OUT

I couldn't believe I had been gone for sixteen days. I felt so rushed that I couldn't see all I wanted or have a chance to really enjoy it. The whole trip seemed very hazy to me. I was hoping that all the pictures that were taken turned out so I could remember where I had gone.

I had what seemed like a lot of chatter going on inside my head the whole trip. Voices were telling me to pull off here, go there, and I was listening to them. Sometimes this noise seemed to be so great that I felt I was losing touch with reality. My body was exhausted from all the driving and I felt I ended the trip in a daze. I lost all track of time the last few days because I was not wearing my watch. I did make it home safely and a day early.

When I got back the trip must have caught up with me. I felt some excitement when I was gone, but was now feeling depressed and confused. I saw Dr. Wilets on June 7. He was going to put me back on Vivactil to hopefully take the edge off the depression. He suggested the possibility of consulting with a depression specialist to see if there was a way to get a grip on the massive swings I was having. I told him I had no recall of my trip between Kellogg, Idaho and Spokane. I also told him that I had discovered a sore area on my forehead that felt like a bruise after that day. Things really went crazy towards the end of the session. I thought I must have climbed into high gear. I was acting real unpredictable and didn't know who I was. This must have been when I began talking to him about the trip in third person. He called me on the carpet for it and asked me if there was a reason for me using "we" in the conversation. He thought I had gone alone on the trip. I didn't know what to say.

Things that Greg was saying to me didn't seem to register. At least I didn't include any of it in my diary. Somebody heard what he was saying. I saw him again the following Thursday. Things were real messed up. The entry in my diary says it all:

"Things are getting bad again. I'm so confused. I'm being swallowed by something — I don't know what. I don't have much true control over who or what I am. My body is an observation post or movie theater in which I'm strapped to my seat. I'm scared. It feels like a time warp. I can't move forward or back. I can recall past memories but everything else is suspended. My mood and personality changes so fast I can't keep up with it. I felt so odd at the RMED luncheon. I don't remember a lot about my session with Dr. Wilets. He said to increase the Vivactil. We talked a little about separation, but the rest is a blur. I just recall bits and pieces...Things were screwy when I left Greg's office. I felt so weird when I got to my car. I don't know how I got to D&D at the Ramada, but I did. Like someone else drove me. I felt that way several times on vacation."

JUNE 17, 1984
"Today was real strange. I didn't seem like myself at all...I put the lawn mower away without trimming the front. I didn't even dump grass from mower. Said hell with back yard. I just seemed to wander around the rest of the afternoon. In the garden taking pics, talking and wandering. No real sense of time or purpose. Just a lost soul. I had no motivation...After movie I watered garden and moped around again. Got in shower, walked into bedroom to see I had,not made my bed. So

what? I put pillow cases on, grabbed my robe and slept on top of the mattress pad. What am I doing? This is not my nature but I can't control myself.

JUNE 18, 1984

"Well, at least I've been consistent. Consistently confused with my moods and behavior. Today I found myself primarily low. Had a morning appointment with Dr. Wilets. He could be very right in saying the thought of separation is bringing on my strange behavior and feelings. He hypnotized me to see if I could remember the part of my vacation I couldn't consciously recall. I got to Osburn, Idaho...No Cour D'Alene tho. I had a couple dizzy spells later in the afternoon and partial blackouts. Felt part of me left my body."

JUNE 19, 1984

"What a change!!! I feel good for a change. Like an entirely different person. Not a gradual improvement as usual, but BINGO! Now, if it just keeps moving upwards. Just kind of bouncy, bubbly. And this is despite a runny nose and sore throat. Good for this, cuz I got my annual performance review...Was going to mow lawn, but blew it off. Instead, spent all night on my files and trying to empty my briefcase. Finally got it all put together. Out of the blue, at midnight, I remember the lake and where I stopped in Cour D'Alene, Idaho! Eureka!!"

JUNE 20, 1984

Gotta keep going while the goin's great. This mood came on so fast I don't know how long it can last. It has already slacked off a bit. Yesterday was great. God, please don't let that depressed self come back too soon. I've got to stay "up" until I get the verdict on those 2 job applications. I know I'd say yes to either one without batting an eye. I wouldn't need any doctors if I could just continue to have "yesterday's child" permanently. What does it take to keep you inside me? It's getting to be too difficult to predict who I'll be from day to day, hour to hour. I don't think I can live through another episode of this again."

JUNE 21, 1984

"The day started well. I was in a good mood and had a very positive attitude. Some confusion and occasional absence of sense of self. Nothing I couldn't deal with. Got my performance review comments written, and given to Bill. Now, for Dr. Wilets. I went into the session up, but I slipped. My deepest, darkest secret became exposed. I fessed up to having more than one Michele sharing my body. I said 5 or 6. That's the dominant ones for the last 8-10 years. Boy, is everybody mad. I'm being pulled apart. I don't feel together. Things don't feel right. Got home, changed clothes, grabbed Nikki and headed for Lookout Mountain. Only, I ended up on Havana north of I-70. Saw smoke and headed for it. Wound up at 56th and Chambers, hypnotized to the worst lightening storm I'd ever experienced. It was all over and around me setting fires and killing people. Got home around 10:30. Watched myself take a new x-acto knife to the top of my right foot. Took a Dalmane at 11 p.m. but was restless until after 12:30 a.m."

JUNE 22, 1984

"What a nightmare! I don't need this. Today, what's going on? SHIT! Dr. Wilets wanted me to come back in this morning at 11 a.m. I hate this. They're starting to show signs of irritation at me always going to the doctor. I always make up my time. I don't know why, but Dr. Wilets wanted me to come back in at 5:30 p.m. or tomorrow. They didn't like that at work at all cuz I was scheduled for 2 hours O.T. Things got real crazy after that. Dr. Wilets tricked me and called the cops and made me go into the hospital. I can't be here. It's not fair. I didn't do anything. I'm just a bit confused is all. That's no reason. I have too much to do."

STAFF REPORT: *"Admitted ambulatory to 523 a 29 y.o. female accompanied by Dr. Wilets, 2 security guards, 2 Denver policemen and staff from 4 South who met others at tunnel from Midtown Medical Building. Dr. Wilets asked for help bringing pt. to unit because he felt she might attempt to leave when he told her he wanted her to be admitted. Michele appeared quite tense and anxious regarding admission, angry although not physically aggressive. Did attempt to run X1 on way to unit. Spent a long period of time talking with Dr. Wilets. Afterward, made phone call -- tearful on phone. Quiet on approach other than to say she is upset about being in the hospital. 'I'm only confused.' According to Dr. Wilets, pt. has been sharing new information about herself with him and appeared quite overwhelmed, anxious after doing so. Pt. appears oriented x3. No evidence of delusions, hallucinations. Affect sad at times; increased anxious at times with increased symptoms of anxiety and depression when sharing new experiences and feelings with doctor. Pt. to be encouraged to talk about feelings. Watch closely for increased acting out, escape, self destructive behavior. Continue to evaluate."*

JUNE 23, 1984

"I had a real restless night to say the least. It took me awhile to orient myself this morning. I panicked a bit thinking I'd lost several days here like the last time. What threw me off was the gray, dreary clouds I saw out the window. It was suppose to be a nice day in the high 80's. I had a lot of confusion. This has to be a real bad dream. I took a real long hot shower trying to set things straight. Dr. Wilets came in this morning for a long time. He was never like this before. He decided not to have another doctor see me. Almost got out today, but wanted some more observation time. Promised tomorrow at 8 a.m. Slept a lot in hopes of keeping it together. Stayed secluded in room most of time so things would stay cool. Can't spoil things. We all have to team up and work together."

STAFF REPORT: *"Regressed and tearful on approach and then angry and controlled. Upset over staying in hospital until tomorrow but seemed more resigned to it as we talked. Pt. has not acted out or attempted to leave unit. She at times is regressed and tearful, other times very much in control. 'I was lying there just trying to stay in control telling everyone if we can only keep it together, we could go home. It's just too hard to stay in control here -- at home I have lots I can do.' Pt. in room most of evening. When out at times is angry then seemed regressed and anxious. Came out later seemed less anxious, calm. Then in room working. No acting out or attempts to leave. Seems to be having difficulty with confinement and the increased stimuli on the unit. Trying very hard to control her anger. Possibly discharge in a.m."*

JUNE 25, 1984

Real tired. The weekend was a bit exhausting. Tried to get Dr. Wilets to fill me in on the weekend cuz it's just one big blur. Asked what may have caused bruises on my arms. Said I tried to slip out and down the stairs at the hospital and got tackled. Asked what his therapy plans were for me now. Said it was for us to jointly work out. I don't think anything was really decided upon. Maybe we'll decide on Thursday. Not feeling all together with it. I'm cranking out my work, tho, but as if I'm running on automatic..."

I don't know who it was that told Dr. Wilets that there was more than one of me inside. I had the awareness that there were voices inside my head that kept me company, but was not really consciously aware that they surfaced and actually did things without me knowing it. All I knew was that strange things had been happening and from time to time, I exhibited behavior that was not at all like me. I didn't have a clue as to when, where or how things shifted. All I knew was that I felt things suddenly really got out of control. If I had an identity problem before, it just now kicked into fifth gear. I was really kind of scared of all the possibilities of what may have happened or was going to happen.

I tried to go on with my daily routine, but with a guarded perspective. If my alters were able to do things without my knowledge when they were a secret, I had to try and think about what they might do now that the secret was out. Deep down I felt there was a lot of turmoil and anger that was about to be released.

I began seeing Dr. Wilets twice a week when I got out of the hospital. I know he used some hypnosis during some of the sessions to coerce some of the alters to show themselves. I didn't remember a lot of what went on in many of these sessions. I was just hoping that Dr. Wilets was keeping track of things so he could inform me at a later time.

At first my alters did not have names. When they first appeared they identified themselves to Dr. Wilets with descriptions of their Group task or specialty. Soon, when they knew it was all right to have a name and they were someone of value, they started to slowly identify themselves with a name they wanted to be called. I'm sure some of their names evolved from people I had known in my life that they identified with. Some of the names made no sense and I had no clue as to where they came from. Regardless, I honored them for who they were.

I was more aware of periods of dissociation after the diagnosis. I didn't necessarily have more control over things, but allowed me to comfort myself when I would discover some surprises. My moods were still out of control and all over the chart. Dr. Wilets felt that my dissociation and conflict within the system may be intensified by the quick cycling and mixed states I experienced.

JULY 5, 1984

"Today, yeh, right. Things were on top when I started. I thought I felt good when I got up, so put a dress on. Seemed to do ok at work till the end of the day. Then my mind couldn't get thoughts to piece together. Had a number of errands to do and go to RMED bd. mtg. at lunch. Was not altogether when I went to Dr. Wilets. Used hypnosis. Don't think that was a good idea. Got Shell to discuss some real personal things. Has put everyone in real turmoil. The anger is pulling me apart. I can't control or fight everyone. They don't like each other. They'll never unify themselves. I'm afraid they'll destroy me and them first. I'm scared. Barely made it home. Took couple of Dalmane to sleep it off and get it out of my mind."

JULY 6, 1984

"Things are not going to work. I woke up this morning with the back hose going, front and back doors open and several small scratches on my feet. I was in my underwear and big t-shirt. I'm having lots of difficulty keeping things under control. The Big Guy is showing anger and fighting his way through. I'm so confused. They are very hostile to the idea of joining forces and working together. Things need to be left alone. I feel impending disaster and doom if not. Talked to Dr. Wilets for some time on the phone. Wanted to call therapy quits. Just disrupting things too much. Canceled 2 hr. O.T. then left early for 4 p.m. appt. with Dr. Wilets...Took 2 Dalmane and went to bed real early. Feeling real low and confused and angry and unpredictable."

I was doing things just out of the blue. Nothing was making sense. There was no reason to my madness. I set an agenda to do one thing, and end up doing really crazy things. One example is that I was going to a hardware store to buy some wood for a display booth. On the way there, I pull into a car dealership and come away with papers signed to buy a truck. My car was having problems ever since I took my vacation. I just couldn't figure out how or why I settled on buying a new truck.

JULY 31, 1984

"I feel I'm dreaming this whole truck thing, but I've already become so attached to it. I can do and go more than with Bessie. I personally feel good about what I've done, but am scared about explaining to Mom, Roy and Greg. Time — I can't keep track of time. I was so messed up during my session with Greg. I can't keep track of myself or the group. I don't have any control of them; they have control of me, and without warning. They say things I'd never say...Just in a daze bouncing from place to place. Am very tired today. Somewhat on the more depressed side. On an eating binge, too. I'm getting strong urges to just take this life and shove it — it's too screwed up to set straight..."

Around September I swung into a manic episode. I also started to have regular blanking out spells. They didn't seem like dissociative spells. Dr. Wilets observed some of them in my sessions and thought they may have been some mini seizures and had me call Dr. Quintero. He had me increase my dosage of Tegretol.

I took another long trip the end of September. Another chance to get to know some of my alters a little better. I went to the annual Desk and Derrick Convention that was being held that year in San Antonio, Texas. My club had an energy puppet show we had inherited and were scheduled to present at the meeting. I volunteered to take the stage, puppets and sound equipment to the convention.

Mike drove the truck and did an excellent job. He packed the back so well that none of the show shifted during the trip. The second day out, Elizabeth had Mike stop a number of times for pictures. She took a lot of pictures on the field trips and the way home. She ran out of film when I got to a small rural town in New Mexico. She made me promise to come back on my next three day weekend to take some more pictures.

I was still having some seizure activity when I returned from my trip. Dr. Wilets said he would call Dr. Quintero and explain what he observed during my sessions. My mind would be racing then suddenly I would get "hit like a power surge on a computer. Everything pops up blank, then scrambled and I have to start all over putting things in order again."

It seemed that by November things were not letting up. I would have days when I had the most difficult time trying to carry on a conversation. I would black out in the middle of a sentence and not remember what I was trying to say. I was beginning to have more frequent headaches, too. I was more tired than before and found myself going to bed one, two or four hours earlier than I had all year long. My muscles were also aching. My arms, legs and body would sometimes become jerky and uncontrollable at times. I didn't know what was happening to me. All I know is that this problem was distressing me and had the doctors concerned.

Dr. Quintero decided to change my medication. He added Mysoline to the regiment of drugs I was taking. The first dose I took was way too strong. My vision got way out of whack and I staggered around my house running into things and found that I could barely stand up. I felt real intoxicated. He cut back my medication to a level that was less affecting.

Over Thanksgiving weekend, I promised Elizabeth a trip back to New Mexico to take pictures of the old adobe communities I had passed on my way home from Texas. I went down on Friday. Along the way, I got a real void feeling as I was driving. I had numbing and tingling in my arms and hands. There were times I felt that if I went fast enough, I could fly with my truck. On my way back into Las Vegas from Dallas, I became very drowsy and had a terrible headache. I also felt very spacey. I ended driving back to town about 25 MPH. I wasn't sure I would make it. I had never been so scared with my driving as I was that day.

By the end of November, things started to get a little messed up. Alters were no longer afraid to speak out to me. They even started to make notes in my diary. All the spending was also catching up with me and I was getting hit hard with the reality that I may be in big trouble.

NOVEMBER 28, 1984

"Work as usual. Went to bank to cash in some savings bonds which hadn't matured. Yes, things have gotten that bad. Got $300 worth. Have about $300 left and that's it on our reserves. Need to get loan application to credit union. We're sure they won't grant any kind of loan. Hit the jackpot and got $60 from 1st Interstate mini bank. Have enough to pay bills due before next pay day. Don't know where I will get money for Dec. mortgage payment. If we can just hold on till March — 4 months is a long time. — Quit worrying...things have a way of working out. Don't bother yourselves with such petty things. Let the others do some typing and book work."

NOVEMBER 29, 1984

"We've got to get rid of that damn masochist. She's going to hurt us permanently sooner or later. Couple people from drafting went to Walt's funeral. I finally got to talk to Greg. He's a real neat guy. I kinda like him. I told him we heard about MP's on Phil Donahue Wednesday — thanks to Marsha. It was very informative. Shelley took good notes, but I couldn't quite follow them. He said there's such a thing as MPD's which know about one another. I didn't think our club counted, but guess it does. Why do the other members dislike me so? Is it cuz I'm so carefree and don't let hurt or pain disrupt things? I do want to be accepted and have more time. I'm not going to take anything away."

NOVEMBER 30, 1984

"Today was a real tough day. So many of us were out today that things have been a real turmoil or headache. I don't care if it is Michele's club. She's going to screw things up for all of us. That damn ball baby. She's so emotional. No wonder we can't convince anyone at work how totally competent we are. Everybody's fighting for time. Things are going to burst! God, please help us all. It's so hard to keep it together. I don't know who I am. It's so hard to think. Where's our unity and sisterly love for one another's individualism? Greg, please help!! I'm being smothered. I'm getting so tired. We have to get organized. Please, let's all set back and discuss things as adults who generally care for one another. We've done it many times before and things have been running well for the most part. Let's not end up back in the hospital. We can't afford it, the time, or the opportunity to allow the less desireables to screw up all we've worked for these last couple years. I'm scared, too, but we've got to be strong. We've got lots — so very much — opportunity ahead of us. We can't let everything crumble. The Big Guy is getting our losers together. You can all see it with the lack of control we have against that masochist. We've got to prove to everyone, but mostly ourselves, that we can maintain that stamina and highly controlled environment which can be shared fairly by all. Please!!!"

From the best that I can tell, it was mainly Shelley and Francie that made these entries. On the 30th, it seems like there were others who were also crying out wanting their concerns to be heard. They must have been talking about Kim's threat to the Group.

I made it through the holidays despite a very domineering mother. She has this problem with co-dependency. Even at thirty years of age, I was her little girl. I had health problems and she didn't think I knew how to take care of myself. I finally conceded and decided to let her do what she wanted. Anything to avoid an argument with her. Arguments were real nasty and I didn't want to relive the arguments of my childhood. I let her clean my house and do my laundry. When she wanted to buy groceries or clothes or other things for me, I didn't fight it. Besides, I was having money problems and I could use all the help she was offering at the time. In repayment, I would call her during the week and visit with her when she came out on weekends. My house was about 15 miles one way from hers and that was a long way for my mom to drive.

Her deed of all deeds that Christmas was to buy all my family Christmas presents for me. I took great pride in buying my own presents since I could remember. It gave me a warm feeling inside. This Christmas had a cold touch to it, because it wasn't a part of me. I was weak, confused and numb. I really wasn't in a position to say no.

Dr. Wilets knew I was having a great deal of difficulty dealing with my mom. He began to schedule some joint sessions which both my mom and I attended. I saw him by myself the following day to discuss that session and try to work through things. This helped him to understand just what I had to live with all my life. He agreed that she was a very demanding and overpowering woman. He also knew where I got my perfectionistic behavior from. We concluded that she had no ill-intent and that her actions were not deliberate or premeditated. It was just her nature, and I was going to have to learn to live with it, yet be able to take some control.

By the end of the year, I wasn't writing in my journal any more. I was having an increase in seizure activity and doing whatever I could to hold on. My Group was not communicating with me. They did write in my journal before I stopped, but they were all going off in their own direction. I was scared that things would get out of control.

After the holidays, I began having greater difficulty in my daily functions. I was literally bouncing off walls and unable to concentrate. My reflexes were not spontaneous, they were labored. I was confused and disoriented with what was going on around me.

I stayed home from work on January 25, 1985. I could not pull myself together. I had a migraine and my eyes were extremely sensitive to the light. I slept all day with shades and drapes drawn. My mom finally came over late in the afternoon and saw that I was not doing very well. I was having episodes where my body would begin to jerk uncontrollably. My mom had me call Dr. Quintero. He suggested she take me to the Mercy Hospital ER for evaluation. I was admitted that evening.

JANUARY 25, 1985
ADMISSION REPORT: "Pt. experienced 5-6 days of confusion, disorientation and disconnection from what has been going on around her. Problem progressively worsened 2 days ago. Developed a recurrent sharp headache over left frontal head region. Felt so disconnected from environment that she was unable to go to work and spent most of the day in bed. Did not take any of her anticonvulsants with very limited fluid and caloric intake. Mysoline and Tegretol drug levels done in ER were both very low and sub-therapeutic."

NEUROLOGICAL EXAM: "Very functional with pt. having intermittent total body jerks each time deep tendon reflexes were tested. She had irregular give to all muscle testing and had fluttering eye movements. Pt. responded slowly to questions and appeared to have difficulty understanding questions posed to her. Was oriented to self and time. Did not know name of hospital. Able to name mayor, governor, president but was very slow. Had difficulty performing simple arithmetic problems and unable to interpret proverbs." MOTOR: "pt. cooperated poorly for formal motor exam. However moved all 4 extremities equally well. Did have an irregular give to all muscle testing but no weakness was found."

JANUARY 26, 1985
"Hand grip very weak. Leg strength very weak. Moves slowly with difficulty. Pupils dilated and non-reactive. Jerky movements of extremities continue at intervals. Movement jerky and weak. Pupils remain dilated; react very slowly. Twitching arm and legs. Respiration shallow. 5 p.m. - Pt. remains unresponsive. Unable to open eyes. 5:30 p.m. - Remains unresponsive. Dr. Quintero notified. Here at 5:45. Pt. does not acknowledge presence. 6 p.m. - Pt. beginning to respond. BP 160/100, pulse 104, resp. reg. 16."

JANUARY 28, 1985
EEG: "This is an abnormal EEG due to the presence of frontotemporal dysrhythmic activity. The cause of this activity cannot be determined electrically. These findings could be consistent with a seizure disorder or migraine disorder. Clinical correlation is recommended." Dr. Marc Treihaft

DISCHARGE SUMMARY: "History of suspected Partial Complex Seizures and long complicated psychiatric history presented with an approximate week history of feeling of losing touch with reality and what was going on around her and comcomittant severe left frontal headache and anorexia. An EEG as outpatient this past week revealed paroxysmal slowing. Physical exam on admission normal. Neuro exam reveled lethargic female who is slow to respond to questions and appeared to have difficulty understanding questions. Exam was quite functional in that she'd demonstrate an intermittent total body jerk when her reflexes were tested. Had an irregular all muscle testing and had constant fluttering eye movements. EEG on 1-28 abnormal due to frontal temporal dysrhythmic activity. CT scan normal. On day following admission the pt. became unresponsive. When examined at that time she appeared to be quite hysterical. When lifting her extremities they would drop limply, but when lifted above her face or other parts of her body where the drop would cause injury to herself, she would avoid hitting herself. This spell cleared spontaneously. Meds at discharge were Mysoline and Tegretol." FINAL DIAGNOSIS: "Mixed seizure disorder, complex partial seizures and functional seizures."

I did not feel like myself during this hospitalization. I felt I had no control over my bodily functions. I had great difficulty, walking, talking and eating. I felt someone else was in control. Someone I could not reach. To this day, I am uncertain of who it really is that experienced these neurological disabilities. My guess is that it may be more than one alter, but no one has really come forward. At least I do not believe it is any of my dominant alters.

I wasn't out of the hospital two weeks when I had another episode similar to the first. This time I went to work. I fell ill after lunch and went up to the medical clinic at work. They tried to reach Dr. Quintero. He suggested they bring me back to the Mercy ER. Jim and Larry, my supervisors got a company car and drove me to the hospital. This time they kept me in the hospital for a week running tests and trying to regulate my medication.

FEBRUARY 8, 1985
"Neuro exam normal except for periodic blinking eye movements, head and neck jerking forward and jerking of arms. During these episodes pt. unable to converse. Continued to experience intermittent jerking movements. However, when not aware people observing these would stop. Movements would start immediately when I or nurse entered room. Dr. Marc Treihaft felt this was a difficult picture to sort out but did feel that the pt. had complex partial seizures as well as functional seizures."

COMMENT: "The problem is one of differentiating complex partial seizures from hysterical disorder. This is a difficult problem and may not be resolved easily. As discussed by prior observers, the pt. may have one or both disorders concurrently. Would agree with treatment with anticonvulsants and would attempt to maintain Tegretol level in therapeutic range to see if any change in behavior. 3 months trial on meds would be appropriate. Secondly to differentiate real from hysterical episodes, might be worthwhile considering video monitoring with running EEG record."

FEBRUARY 10, 1985
"Pt. lethargic and oriented. Grips weak equally. Leg strength weak. Oriented to place but not time."

FEBRUARY 11, 1985
"Seizure activity noted. Episode lasted approximately 12 minutes. 2 p.m. Observed seizure lasting approximately 3 min. Pt. in fetal position jerking of head and both extremities. Did not respond to name during episode. Eyes rotated upward. Hand grips are weak. Appetite poor."
FEBRUARY 13, 1985
"Chrissy came out and placed her on the floor." -- Dr. Wilets

It seems as though I had finally lost total control of my body. It was simple when I was younger. The spells I had were quite predictable. They usually happened when I got up after sitting or lying down. My hearing would become muffled and my vision would narrow then go black. I would see stars. If I did not grab onto anything, I would lose my balance and fall. I adapted to these episodes and did very well at covering them up to observers.

Suddenly everything was different. Nothing was predictable. I could not draw any similarities to what was happening. At times I felt someone was zapping my head with an electrical shock. I would be reading and my eyes would cross then roll back into my head. My eyes would become extremely sensitive to any and all light. I would have a tingle run down the back of my neck and then get hot flashes. At the same time my hands would become ice cold. I would forget where I was in the middle of involved conversations. The jerking would happen when I seemed the most relaxed. One by one all my muscles would seem to tense up. Sometimes I felt that I was in an ice house and began shivering uncontrollably. I could hear people talking to me, but found myself unable to respond in any way.

My alters must have felt the staff and doctors were not doing enough to figure out what was happening. After waking from a seizure one night in the hospital, one of the alters, identifying herself as Chrissy, made me fall to the floor and stay there until the next morning when someone came into the room. This did not set well with Dr. Quintero or the staff. Dr. Quintero no longer felt he could objectively treat me with the interference of alters.

Dr. Wilets helped me to find a new neurologist that could be objective to the seizure activity I had and, yet, work with the MPD diagnosis. In March I began seeing a Dr. Bernstein at Colorado Neurological. After several visits and examinations he and Dr. Wilets conferred that they felt the tensions and stress from work and my financial situation were contributing to the increased seizure activity I had been experiencing. By April, both doctors were in concurrence that I take a leave of absence from work to try to get my health under control.

The day before I left on sick leave, I got a written warning regarding my increased absenteeism. I was away from work from April 19 until May 8. My supervisor was on vacation when I returned, so a suspension was on hold. Larry called me into his office with the employee relations representative a week later. I was informed that I was being suspended without pay for 10 days. Because my excessive absenteeism was recently due to the increased seizure activity I was having, I felt I was being discriminated against for a disabling health reason. I went to the Civil Rights Commission and filed a complaint.

The suspension came at kind of an opportune time. I was scheduled to leave for another Desk and Derrick Regional Meeting the following week. Despite objections by Dr. Wilets, I was going to drive by myself to Regina, Saskatchewan. I felt safe enough to drive, because the seizure activity seemed to have let up from the time I had away from the stress of work. I did OK on the trip and found someone to ride back with me.

I returned to work from my suspension on May 31. Before leaving, the office had been informed that the company was scaling down its staff in the Denver office. It was not known as to whether or not union represented employees would be allowed to take the early retirement/severance option. I was informed the day I returned that represented employees could participate. Because of the problems I had been having and the bad taste I had from the suspension after all I had done for that department, I decided to take the offer from the company to leave. In fact, the 31st was my last day. They expedited the paperwork and I was processed. I ended my career with them on May 31, 1985.

Suddenly I had a lot of time on my hands. I had new stresses to deal with. I thought about trying to get another job, then decided I would try to make a go of my business. I would build a client base doing contract drafting and mapping for small oil companies. I had a lot of contacts through Desk and Derrick and kept abreast to what was going on in the industry. I began a concentrated marketing plan. I had joined the Chamber of Commerce back in April and was going to try to make contacts through their activities.

It was slow trying to build a business with little business experience. I had a couple chance connections and picked up my first real clients. I also went to work on a contract basis for another drafting company owned by a guy I had met through Rocky Mountain Energy Drafters. I managed to make a smidly living through the summer. In the fall I got some more profitable contracts. I spent a couple months solid doing work for SOHIO in their office.

In November, I got a big contract with a mining company that was trying to market itself to investors. After a few weeks on the job, I realized I had bit off more than I could chew. I needed help if I was going to meet the deadlines. I asked Randy, who I was doing contract work for if he knew of some drafters that could help. He allowed me to use his facilities since I did not have an office of my own.

Despite these strong contracts, my financial situation had reached a serious level. I was experiencing extreme anxiety from it. The pressures of carrying out the contract to the expectations of my client became overwhelming. By December, I was at a level of desperation. I was expressing a lot suicidal ideation in my sessions with Dr. Wilets. It was decided that I needed to be hospitalized. Dr. Wilets agreed to allow me to continue work on the project but enforced strict precautions. Once again, Kim, who was posing as Chrissy, was antagonizing the staff and acting out.

HISTORY OF PRESENT ILLNESS: "*Current illness seems to have evolved from the fact that a number of the personalities were unaware of what others were doing, and many of them had procured credit cards accounting to a debt of over $40K. It was my hope that the crisis would reemphasize the need for her to integrate the various personalities. I had stated that one goal of the hospitalization was for there to be unified decisions as some of the personalities wanted admission to the hospital, and at least one wanted to leave, that is, Chrissy. She was told that this was her treatment and I told her that she was responsible for her treatment. She is now admitted with suicidal thoughts. She also has a history of MPD and the personality, Chrissy, was presenting. She was suicidal over her identification of having serious debt. She is quite frightened, sees no recourse to eminent bankruptcy, and says there is only one solution, and she sees suicide as a real possibility. The other personalities are not sure of her suicidal intent.*" -- Dr. Wilets

HOSPITAL COURSE: "*Upon admission to the hospital it was important for her to maintain her work. She basically said that if she could not maintain her job and her various projects that she definitely would be suicidal. This posed a number of difficulties, because the more she works, the more she is stressed; the more she is stressed the less she sleeps, and the less she sleeps the fear was the greater her disorganization would be, and the possibility that seizures would erupt or that negative personalities would take over. It was confronted early in the hospital that each of the personalities were very selfish, each wanting to take their own course, and not working in any kind of integrated fashion for the well-being of the total being. In fact, by 12-13-85 "Chrissy" had cut herself with a pencil sharpener blade, because she didn't feel understood by the staff. This borderline acting out behavior was heavily confronted. Suicidal thoughts persisted, and she made some attempt to have herself discharged from the hospital. She was informed that she needed the hospitalization to reorganize, and by 12-18-85 we were talking about integrating the personalities. She is afraid of dealing with issues of sexuality, and also uses the personalities to defend her-*

self from loneliness and loss. It needs to be understood that her initial multiple personality organization occurred around her feeling of being very neglected as a child, and needing to have imaginary companions to make her feel better. Some general acceptance of her sexuality was felt by her on 12-19-85. Another personality was identified in the hospital called "Whispering Owl." This personality, she claims, was responsible for starting the multiple personalities earlier in her life when she was feeling quite neglected. The patient continued to make some progress it appeared towards unification, and on 12-26-85 four of the artistic personalities were unified successfully for a brief 15-minute period. This initially seemed quite successful, but shortly thereafter it appeared that she decompensated and was not able to maintain the personalities intact. This was actually on 12-27-85 that the fusion took place, on a more intensive effort, but this did not persist. It was around this time that the patient stated that she was having increased seizure activity. This was exemplified by her having greater difficulty in being able to talk and remember. It was thought that we could fuse other personality constellations, but it was not thought timely, in view of the fact that she was feeling increasingly depressed, and this may have been secondary to the earlier fusion.

By 1-1-86 it was clear that the patient was going to have to file bankruptcy, and then she started feeling extremely suicidal. She started talking about having a gun so that she could shoot herself in the head. The personality 'Chrissy' appeared to be sabotaging the progress of the rest of the group. The intrapersonal dynamics of this patient became quite complicated with various personalities forming factions and siding with one another. Unfortunately, a pervasive belief of mine was that she was quite potentially lethal in the eminent future, and I had suggested that I meet with her and her family.

On 1-4-86 she was found to have a tight band wrapped around her neck, and this was thought to represent a suicidal acting out, and my concern about her lethality warranted. At the family meeting she felt supported both by her parents and a plan to file bankruptcy worked out. With this decision her suicidal ideation appeared to be much less. She also was receiving Paxipam for anxiety. The reality of her hospital insurance running out was also addressed, and it was clear that she did not want to be transferred to Fort Logan Hospital. She made a commitment not to be eminently suicidal and her privileges were increased. We continued to talk about bankruptcy. Around the discharge the patient was less than frank in the information she was giving her mother. I had asked her not to be driving at a time when she felt she was having increasing difficulty with her alertness. It was unclear as to whether or not she was getting toxic from the Tegretol, or whether or not the seizure activity was increasing. As her insurance was expiring, a plan was made for her to be discharged from the hospital. I did discuss her neurologic difficulty with Dr. Levisohn, who was now seeing her, and suggested checking a peak and trough with the Tegretol. Both these seemed to be reasonable.

By the time of her discharge she did seem much improved with less anxiety and depression. She was not eminently suicidal at the time of discharge, but certainly posed a long-term suicidal risk. This was explained to her parents that I thought the patient had a definite possibility of a lethal suicidal attempt in the past secondary to any number of problems, including her multiple personality disorder, her depression, her anxiety, or the continuation of uncontrolled complex partial seizures. She was discharged, to be followed in my office the following day."

DECEMBER 20, 1985
"Back from pass. Was smiling. Said she worked today and last night but had no complaints. Watched movie on VCR with pt. group. Later appeared child-like in her behavior, a little flirty with male staff. Asked what her name was. Responded 'I don't have a name.' Pt. appeared to have

a different personality tonight. An easy-going, cheerful, child-like one compared to the workaholic of the past nights."

DECEMBER 27, 1985
"Dr. Wilets used hypnotic suggestion to try to fuse some personalities."

This attempt at fusion was quite an experience. I was a bit apprehensive about it at first, but then accepted that it should be tried in hopes of gaining more control in my life. I was successfully placed into a hypnotic trance. What transpired from the point of the fusion suggestion was remarkable. After the suggestion, I remember getting very heavy in the chair. Things all around me began spinning profusely. I was afraid I would fall out of the chair. From that point on I felt a sense of vibrance and clarity with my thoughts. I felt that the suggestion was successful.

Within the hour after Dr. Wilets left the hospital, I felt a struggle ensue. I'm not sure whether alters getting wind of this fusion became disgruntled or what. I began to get very agitated and hypomanic. My mood level was all over the place. I told the staff they had to do something, because I could not handle the intense pressure I was experiencing. They put in a call to Dr. Wilets. He called and over the phone, he initiated a suggestion that would break the previous fusion. A deep calm overcame me and I was back in control. I vowed never to do that again.

DECEMBER 29, 1985
"During midnight rounds found pt. asleep with belt from bathrobe tied around her neck 3xs. No redness noted and moved pt. to seclusion. Pt. calling out for help from 2-4 a.m. Door locked for safety. Remained awake and agitated."

JANUARY 1, 1986
"'I just don't know what to do. I can't go on like this anymore. I just want to go to sleep and never wake up again. I just don't know if I can go on like this anymore. I just think it would be better if Michele wasn't around any more.' Asked to have 1 to 1. At beginning part of 1 to 1 was hyperventilating and talking sadly about her situation. Upset because she slept all day and didn't get any work done. Talking about not being able to think clearly at present. Talked about wanting to die, but wasn't very clear about this -- or if she was planning on hurting herself. When this writer confronted about this, Michele wouldn't answer the question about hurting herself. Another personality came out which was angry. This writer told this personality she would only talk with Michele. This other personality said it was in charge and wouldn't let Michele talk.

JANUARY 2, 1986
"Pt. at desk at 12 a.m. requesting Paxipam and repeat sleeper. Affect depressed. Pt. then went to B/R for 20 min. and went to bed. She went to the B/R again at 1:45 and 2:15 a.m. Complained of nausea and vomiting. Pt. given 7-up to drink. Skin warm and dry. Pt. stated she had ingested 25 Comtrex. Poison Control notified and Dr. Wilets notified. -- 'I'm angry with Chrissy about last night. I'm just feeling depressed today.' Slept most of the afternoon as she did most of the day. Joined pt. group in cafeteria for dinner accompanied by staff. Spoke on phone and had 1 to 1. Still expressed feeling depressed. Quiet in evening group, appeared preoccupied. At end of group volunteered to bring some movies in for the VCR. Appeared brighter after group. Socializing a bit. Signed out at 8:25 for a walk and was back at 9 p.m. At 9:15 wanted to leave unit again and was asked if she was walking within the hospital. Said she's walking outside the hospital. Given feedback that it's dark and probably unsafe. Pt. responded 'I'll get security.' Told to sign out but later noted that she didn't. Brought back to unit with handcuffs on by 3 security guards. Security guard said pt. asked to be escorted to her truck and there asked if his gun was loaded. Then wanted to borrow his stick. He said pt. asked him if he'd use his gun if somebody tried to get it. When guard

responded 'no' pt. said she needed to use it (gun). Was handcuffed and brought to the unit. Pt. claimed she didn't know what happened and she wouldn't do anything. Just wants her sleeping pills and other meds. Refused to change to gown for awhile. Refused to walk to seclusion by herself and had to be escorted by 2 staff holding her arms. Pt. provided with paper gowns as she was playing with the ties of her gown. Talked in a child-like manner with staff. Said she was 'being punished for somebody else's behavior.' Informed she's in seclusion for her safety until Dr. Wilets sees her at 6:30 p.m. tomorrow. Given Paxipam and sleeping pills as requested. Placed on 15 min. checks. -- ADD: Security also stated pt. asked 2x what someone had to do before he shot them. Prior to handcuffing, she reached for the gun."

JANUARY 4, 1986

"Pt. found on 15 min. check with rope apparently made from gown tapes tied together and wrapped around her neck. Pt. coughing with air cut off. Redness around neck. Dr. Wilets notified and he ordered 4 pt. restraints and 30 mg Restoril given to be repeated in 1 hr. Pt. banging on door and wanting to get out thinking it unsafe in room. Placed in restraints with 4 males and female supervisor present. Offered bedpan but unable to void. Took Restoril 30 mg with difficulty. Pt. very suicidal (afraid other personality will kill her). 6 pt. restraints necessary because of agitated behavior at 4 a.m. and reduced to 4 pt. as pt. calmed down. Frank Beck came down to look at pt. and ordered Haldol injection 3mg x2 given at 4:15 and 5:30 a.m. Pt. calm at 6 a.m. "

I don't know where Chrissy (Kim) got the ideas for her behavior. She was real cunning and gamy and knew what buttons would get her restrained. It seemed like a real trip for her. When she got the staff involved, she appeared to gain additional strength. It took several men to restrain her. This fueled her fight. Her behavior was impermeable by the tranquilizers. She was the "Hyde" in the Group. In most instances, the struggles would end almost as abruptly as they began. Kim got her anger and frustrations out of her system and then would disappear until the next time. Things finally got back under control and I was discharged on January 9, 1986.

I seemed to have stabilized enough to get that big work contract completed. I was still experiencing a great deal of confusion and mixed states. It was very difficult to function during the day. I would get done only what absolutely needed attention. The stress over performance issues was swallowing me up. Between the mixed states and seizures, I was having identity problems, and my Group was in an extreme state of chaos.

By early February I was exhausted. I didn't have the energy to go on. I was out of control of my mind and body. It got to be so bad that I just wanted to sleep the bad dream away. One evening I felt that if I could just sleep for a day or two things would straighten themselves out. I took a large dosage of the Halcion I was using for sleep. My mom called me and somehow got me to tell her what I had done. She had me call my neurologist, who at that time was Dr. Paul Levisohn. I told him I was having difficulty with my seizures and just wanted some peace. He suggested that my mom bring me right to Porter Hospital.

The staff in ER made me take some charcoal. It had been long enough since I took the pills that they didn't think they could get me to throw them up. My vital signs concerned them so they transferred me to ICU for the night for observation. Dr. Wilets came by the next morning to talk with me and my parents. He and Dr. Levisohn thought it would be a good idea to admit me to the neurology ward and have some tests done to try and shed some light on my increased seizure activity. I was very weak and incoherent.

I agreed to the admission because I wanted to find out what was causing my problems. I did have some hesitation to the hospitalization because Karla was pregnant and expecting her second child in February. I didn't want to be in the hospital when the baby was born.

The doctors certainly ran the full gamut of tests on me. I had physiological and psychological testing done. The seizures were causing my brain to shut down. They did repeated EEG's and blood work-ups. They even scheduled me for an MRI. I was having problems at night and during sleep so they scheduled me for a 24-hour monitoring EEG in their sleep lab. I had some Neuro psychological tests done. I was so shut down that my IQ rating was a 70. I had extreme difficulty concentrating and recalling what I had learned throughout life and in school.

I was pretty much confined to my bed during this hospitalization. For my own protection, I was to stay in bed with the rails up. When I did get up to walk around, my legs felt like rubber. I could not walk without holding onto something. I had trouble just getting up and going to the bathroom. I slept a lot and had a very small appetite.

Dr. Wilets visited me fairly regularly to give me moral support and to see that none of the alters would sabotage my stay like they did the year before. He conveyed the importance of not acting out while in the hospital. I was too weak to act out even if I wanted to. I was very lethargic and my brain was numb. They tried a number of different drug combinations to try and stabilize me and bring me back to a functional level. I was able to maintain control and be as helpful as possible to the hospital staff.

Fortunately, none of my alters acted out. That's not to say that none of them showed themselves in the hospital. I'm almost certain that some of them were present, but we were all so weak that nothing happened to jeopardize my relationship with staff and doctors.

The doctors were baffled by what was happening to me. They didn't know what to test for next. After conferring and making some calls, they decided to discharge me the first week of March to prepare for a trip to Boston for some additional testing and to be seen by some stronger experts. I had regained enough strength to get out of bed and take care of my basic needs. My mom and dad did insisted that I stay with them the week before going to Boston.

While at Porter Hospital, though, Karla did have her baby. However, it was not without complications. The doctors had to do an emergency C-Section. As she was in the delivery room, one of the nurses noted the size of the baby's head as it was trying to pass through the birth canal. There was something very wrong. They did some tests and decided to move Karla immediately to surgery. Stephanie was born on February 22, but was diagnosed with hydrocephalis. They rushed her to Children's Hospital for stabilization and to prepare for surgery to place a shunt to remove the fluid from her brain. The doctors had not detected any problems with the pregnancy to that point. Karla had gone to the hospital the week before with labor pains, but was told to go home because it was false labor. It was not. I couldn't help but think how much more damage was done during that additional week before her birth.

I was so devastated when my mom called me to give me the good and bad news. I was in tears and very scared for Karla, Larry and Stephanie. I wanted so much to be with them. I got very religious and asked the nurse if I could go down to the chapel in the hospital to pray and meditate. They got an orderly and wheelchair and let me go down for a little while. I needed to be with my sister and felt so guilty about being cooped up in the hospital in the shape I was in.

My mom flew with me to Boston. This was my first trip there. I was going to be admitted to Beth Israel Hospital and the neurology ward. When I got there, they had no beds in the neurology ward so I was admitted to the cardiac ward. My mom stayed overnight at a local hotel and flew back to Denver the next morning.

My first night there was a real doozy. I don't remember all that happened. I did not review my charts or records so can only go on what I remember and what the staff told me happened.

Evidently that first night I experienced a number of seizure episodes that lasted for several hours. My body was out of control. I remember the staff coming in and trying to get a response from me. I sensed their presence but did not have the ability to respond. I forgot where I was. The night seemed like a big dream. My vital signs were all over the chart. Finally, early in the morning, with medication, they were able to get the seizures under control.

Because of the disturbance that ensued from the previous night, they moved me the next day to a private room in the cardiac ward that was closer to the nurses station. I began what was going to be two and a half weeks of intense testing. They took me for blood tests and a CT scan first.

By the third day, a private room had opened up in the neurology ward and I was moved there. It was in an older wing in the hospital.

The testing involved several EEGs. I remember having a seizure during one of the EEGs. I wanted to be still for the test but could not help myself. I also had some additional neuro psychological testing.

The CT scan that I had early on showed something faintly so they decided to inject me with something and do it again. The results from the second scan were strong enough that they wanted to schedule me for an angiography. I was not aware of what I was getting into with that test. All I knew was that they had me sign all kinds of releases and told me there was some risk to the test.

The angiography was scheduled for one afternoon. I was allowed only fluids for breakfast and not allowed to eat lunch. They came in around noon and started an IV with Valium. I was alert when I went down for the test but certainly not feeling much of anything. They took me into a cold surgical room and prepped me. The test involved sticking a big needle and small tube into the vein that was in my groin. It went up through my heart then to the base of my brain. This was not so bad. The test really got uncomfortable when they started injecting the dye into my brain. It was very difficult to lie still for the x-rays. The dye had an intense burning sensation and was somewhat painful. They increased the amount of Valium they were giving me. I was sure glad when that test was over, but the worst was yet to come.

After the test, they wheeled me out on the gurney to a small recovery area. I was told to lay perfectly flat and not bend my leg. I did as I was told, but when they came out to check me before taking me back to the room, they noticed that I was hemorrhaging where they inserted the needle. They jumped into third gear to get it stopped. I was in recovery about 2 hours. This was one of the risks they warned me about when I signed the release for the test.

I got back to my room around 6 p.m. They put weights on my leg to keep me from raising it or moving it around. They gave me some juice and jello for dinner. They catheterized me so I would not get up out of bet to go to the bathroom. I developed a real bad migraine and felt my head was going to explode. They finally came in and gave me some Valium for that. Sometime shortly after, I started seizing. They could not keep my leg still with the jerking I was doing. They tried more Valium and couldn't get things to stop. They used leather restraints to try to keep me as still as possible so I would not rehemorrhage. Not much was working. Finally they gave me a suppository with some medication (anti-convulsant) in it and were able to get me to relax and stop seizing.

I guess my mom tried to call to see how I came through the test during all this. The doctor answered the phone and said I was having some difficulties. This was not too reassuring. I'm sure my mom was fit to be tied.

I was sore all over the next morning. I felt as though a steam roller had run over me. The last thing I remembered was the headache and some doctors or staff working around me with the light on. The rest was a big blur. I found out about what happened after I got up and went to the bathroom the next morning. My bowel movement was loose and orange and I questioned them as to what they gave me. That was when they explained what happened.

From the angiogram they discovered a small venous angioma in my brain. It was only about the size of a pea, but to me seemed significant. They said that I probably had it for some time if not most of my life. Maybe this is what caused the blackout spells I had been experiencing through a major portion of my life.

After I recovered from the angiogram and succeeding trauma, they decided to put me on 24-hour EEG monitoring with video. I had gone through quite an ordeal to this point and wasn't sure of what was going to happen next. Evidently, one night Samantha got very scared. She came out and cried and said she wanted to go home. She is a little girl alter that doesn't like hospitals. They ended up bringing in a staff psychiatrist to talk to me. Things calmed back down until after the 24-hour monitoring was concluded.

Over the next few days, Kim made an appearance and threatened the staff. I don't remember what transpired but somehow or another I ended up in restraints and with a staff on guard outside my door around the clock. They were wondering if some of my behavior was not related to the seizures. After a couple or three days I felt back in control and reassured them there would be no more acting out.

I was discharged on April 1, 1986. My mom flew back out to take me home. We did half a day of site seeing around downtown Boston. I did have to take a couple prn's to make it through the night and the trip home, but made it without incident.

Dr. Schomer tried to explain to my mom and me some of the findings they had made over my hospitalization. He explained that if I could get my alters and their behavior under control and be able to avoid any outbursts like I had this time, he would like me to come back for a possible depth electrode study in December. I didn't know much about what it involved and told him I would think about it.

APRIL 2, 1986
"Dear Dr. Levisohn:
...My clinical examination of Michele suggested that she had some left frontotemporal dysfunction, probably congenital or early acquired, with some growth asymmetry particularly of the face and thumb on the right. The EEG reports that I had from you all suggested bursts of generalized abnormalities with left hemisphere predominance. Our EEGs here showed primary generalized abnormalities, some more epileptiform than others. Initially, no left-sided predominance was found to our EEGs. Then, she underwent a CT scan with infusion. A suggestion of either an AVM or an aneurysmal dilation of the middle cerebral artery on the left was noted. Angiography then revealed a small venous angioma in the left anterior temporal region.

We continued to perform EEG monitoring on a long-term basis, including video monitoring. We found that she had frequent clinical events which were no different than as described in your notes. With about half of her clinical events, there did appear to be some subtle suggestion of left inferior mesial temporal potential epileptiform activity of a sustained nature, but an equal percentage of events with no electographic markers. She was then started on Clonopin and watched for several days. During that time, she had a spinal tap which was unremarkable. Her neuro psychological testing, which had been started by Dr. Powers in Denver, was completed by Dr. Spiers here and confirmed the presence of predominantly left temporal and posterior frontal abnormalities.

Putting all this together strongly suggests that this patient has left hemisphere cognitive abnormality associated with behavioral abnormalities, i.e., cognitive testing abnormalities, and the past electroencephalographic evidence of left-sided predominant abnormality. Therefore, I suspect that she has bursts of secondarily generalized potential epileptic activity. During the remainder of her hospitalization here, she was seen intensively by our Psychiatry Department which became quite concerned about the suicidal issue. Late in her hospitalization, following her last 24-hour session of EEG monitoring which showed essentially normal EEG throughout with the exception of one epileptic spike from the left temporal region and a couple bursts of semi-rhythmic slowing from the left temporal area, no correlation between behavioral events and EEG events was noted. She then developed a marked change in her affect, becoming violent for a period of about 45 minutes. She required four-point restraints and injections of Haldol prior to resolution. Over the ensuing 36 hours, she did quite well with no further outbursts and then was scheduled for release. Her mother flew out from Denver to accompany her home and she did quite well during the over-night stay in a Boston hotel...

I have scheduled Ms. Newman to come back to Beth Israel in about nine months for consideration of stereotactic depth electrode placement. The issue is whether or not sustained electrical activity can be correlated with her behavioral events with a degree of regularity. If not, then a surgical for control would not be entertained. If such a relationship can be shown, she may very well become a candidate for surgery, barring worsening of her behavioral state. Much of this has been discussed at great length with Dr. Wilets, who will continue to follow her closely for her psychiatric issues."
-- Dr. Donald L. Schomer, MD Director, Clinical Neurophysiology

This report suggests that some alters are afflicted with temporal lobe seizures while others are not. Some may have followed the attention that resulted from having a seizure and decided to mimic such events to gain attention from hospital personnel. This might explain why some seizure events were recorded without electrical activity.

When I got home from Boston, I had to try to get myself together enough to finish pulling all the paperwork together for filing my bankruptcy. Everyone agreed that that was the only solution that would allow me to get a fresh start and take away a lot of the stress I was dealing with on my financial issues.

I couldn't believe how far in debt I had gotten. It made me extremely depressed to face how alters had spent everything I had and a lot more. Being in the hospital didn't help matters much. I was self employed and had no income while in the hospital. Thank God I had insurance to cover some of these expenses. My previous employment insurance converted to a Cobra policy the first of June.

The lawyer that was helping me with my bankruptcy and Dr. Wilets suggested that I go to Social Services and see if I couldn't get some benefits to help me buy groceries. It was a long and trying process but I was able to receive food stamps and some additional monetary benefits from the state Social Services department. The money I had gotten from my separation from the oil company had pretty well run out. I only had some stock that I had not cashed in.

After six months of gathering records, I was able to file the paperwork for my bankruptcy. With my unpredictable health and the emotional stress this caused, I reached a breaking point by mid-June. I had become extremely depressed and very confused about my future. The depression had almost incapacitated me. I wasn't feeling overly suicidal, but Dr. Wilets decided to take some precautionary measures and suggested I go back into the hospital until he could get a grip on the depression and adjust my medication. I had little strength and resistance in me to refuse.

I was in the hospital for a little over a week. During that time, he did some checking within the medical profession to see if he could not get me some help. Among the seizures, depression and multiple personality and not having a regular job, I was overwhelmed and losing my wits. I was getting desperate. I needed answers and solutions.

For the previous year I had been experiencing bouts of constipation and blood in my stools. One day in July, I lost my appetite. I had some intense cramping in my abdomen. At first I was constipated, but by late afternoon all hell broke loose. I was running to the bathroom every ten or fifteen minutes. After awhile there was nothing to come out but I still had the need to go to the bathroom. By then, my movements consisted of blood and mucous. I was having hot and cold flashes. My mom had talked to me earlier and came out to see if she could help. When things turned to blood, she thought it was time I called my doctor. I called Dr. Anneberg and he told me to go to the emergency room at Presbyterian.

My mom took me to the hospital. They kept me in the ER for tests and observation all night. Dr. Platt was on call the next morning and came in to examine me. He did a rectal exam and said it was a bloody mess. He had me admitted to a room for more tests. They put me on IV's because

I was so dehydrated. I was in the hospital for three days, but the doctors could not find any reason for this episode. The problem disappeared almost as abruptly as it began.

Dr. Wilets learned in July that a study was being done at the National Institute of Health on individuals suffering from MPD and seizures. He sent a letter to Dr. Frank Putnam at NIMH to review my case and consider me as a possible candidate for the case study for his program. He received a response from Dr. Putnam in the early fall saying that they were interested in using me in their case study. I was to make a trip back to Bethesda, Maryland in early October to be evaluated.

I was honored that my situation was complex enough to warrant review by some of the foremost authorities dealing with the problems I was experiencing. I was excited about the trip but cautious at the same time. I was almost scared to think about what they might find. Were my problems really serious and complex and offered a bleak outlook for my future? Or, was everything that was happening to me something I had dreamed up and gotten out of control. I didn't know what to think any more. I didn't know who I was or what I was about.

I was really concerned about my inability to support myself. I found it very difficult to do what little work I had coming in, and was too afraid to look for more work because I might be unable to perform. Dr. Wilets suggested that I go talk to Social Security. He felt I was definitely qualified to be considered for disability compensation. I made an appointment and went with my mother. They told me about the paperwork I needed to present them and fill out. There would be a review process once everything was filed. It could take several weeks or a few months.

It seemed like October was never going to come. I somehow managed to get through each day as it came, doing my best to take care of my basic needs. My mom seemed to be supportive and sympathetic, but I sensed that she was really trying to get sympathy from her friends for my misfortunes. Mike, my neighbor, was understanding and tried to give me some companionship. He was one of the few people I told that I had MPD. He didn't think less of me but was there for reassurance.

October finally came. My mom asked if I didn't want her to come with me. I told her I really needed to go by myself and did everything to make her believe that I would be okay. Besides, my parents had spent a lot of money on me when I went to Boston. They bought plane tickets for my mother and me. I couldn't see them spending money on two round trip tickets back to D.C. It was a long flight, but I had made it before and had medication with me. I just hoped that I would not be too stressed and have a seizure on the plane.

I was admitted to the neurology department at the National Institute of Health. The testing and my stay would take place there rather than at NIMH. Dr. Putnam would consult and contribute to the evaluation. The admission was a long process and the admission interview very thorough.

Dr. Putnam came by to introduce himself the next afternoon. They were doing admission tests and blood work-ups in the morning. I found him to be a very friendly gentleman and one who seemed to understand what I had been going through.

Late in my session with him, Kim came out identifying herself as Chrissy. She was very agitated and became very threatening. I'm not sure if it was Dr. Putnam that seemed threatening or made her angry by something he had said. Regardless, her threats made the staff concerned enough that they decided to give me some Haldol to calm me down.

Part of the evaluation process was to take me off all the medication I was on. I was not sure about this. I felt I was being stripped of all my precautionary support. They finally made me realize that I was in safe hands and they needed to evaluate how and what was happening to me without the aid of drugs.

Dr. Orrin Devinsky was assigned as my staff neurologist. He came in and explained the process of the evaluation they were conducting. I was informed that I would have an initial EEG to use as a baseline test. I would then have sphenoidal leads placed in my cheeks and I would be placed on 24-hour video EEG monitoring. This was to capture any seizures I may have on tape and check the electrical activity during these episodes.

During the baseline EEG I experienced an intense dizzying sensation. It was as strong as that which I felt when Dr. Wilets hypnotized me and tried to fuse some of my alters. I felt I was spinning profusely around the table. Then I felt like I was vibrating up and down. I thought I'd surely fall off the bed I was on. I told the tester what was going on, but nothing seemed to show up on the chart.

My alters were cautious about showing themselves but did manage to appear during some of the testing. Most of it happened during the neuro psychological testing, because the evaluator encouraged them to show themselves. Everyone knew they had to be on their best behavior, because it was important to get answers from this testing and evaluation that was going on. For the most part, this hospital stay went off without any major incidents.

During the course of the monitoring, I did experience seizure-like activity. I developed a real keen awareness to a whole series of sensations my body was going through. I had a lot of time to do nothing. I was pretty much confined to my bed for ten days.

The doctors all came in to talk to me toward the end of my stay to tell me what they had found. What they had to say was both disturbing and a relief. They informed me that there was minimal to no abnormal brain activity during my seizure-like episodes. They came to the conclusion that my seizures were psychogenic in nature. They also said that the seizure activity was probably due in large part to the stress I had been under the past few years. I felt I took the news fairly well, however, I was not too sure how my mom was going to take the news. She had told all her friends that I had epilepsy. How was she going to explain that my seizures were all in my head and caused from stress?

I still wasn't 100% convinced that every seizure I had was all fabricated. Besides, the seizure I had at Beth Israel during an EEG did come back with abnormal electrical activity. My theory is that other alters learned about the extreme relief and calm that comes after a seizure and decided to imitate it for a stress reliever and as some kind of a controller and attention-getter.

I made it back to Denver without incident. I did have to take one of the Haldol they gave me for a prn. because of some anxiety. Other than that, I was off all medication and seemed pretty much under control.

SEPTEMBER 29, 1986 -- DISCHARGE SUMMARY
"Following admission, the patient had an electroencephalogram on October 14, 1986...During one period of the EEG, there is a notation that the patient complains of sudden onset of dizziness, however no change occurs in the EEG at this time...Impression is that this is a normal EEG. No focal abnormalities, no epileptiform discharges are seen. Of note, the patient complained of dizziness during the recording and had no change visible during this period. It should be noted that this EEG was obtained with simultaneous anterior, temporal and sphenoidal montages.

Laboratory Data: The patient, during admission also had routine blood work, including SMAC, CBC and differential; these were completely within normal limits.

The patient had consultations with Dr. Frank Putnam from the Psychiatry Service. His evaluation was that 'from a psychiatric evaluation perspective,' Michele Newman was interviewed on three occasions by Dr. Frank Putnam from the National Institute of Mental Health Inframural Research program. She fulfills DSM-III criteria and National Institutes of Mental Health research criteria for multiple personality disorder (MPD). She has an altered personality system of approximately 15 personalities, who represent the type of alters most commonly reported in MPD. These include: A depressed and depleted host personality, Michele, who loses time when other alters are active, and who suffers the consequences of this behavior; a persecutor/protective alter, Chrissy, who is responsible for self-mutilation and other self-punishment, or self-destructive behavior; a child alter, Peggy; a masculine-like, Mike; and a series of creative and occupational alters. Two alters who are responsible for different styles of sexual behavior, Sally and Monique, who are also identified.

There is evidence of significant alter personality conflict, and many of these seizure-like episodes are probably dissociative in origin, and represent the emergence of unidentified alters or the abreaction of tests or dramatic experiences. Michele has a childhood history of incest with a brother, but denies other childhood trauma.

During one psychiatric interview when she regressed to a child-like state, and briefly abreacted, being tied into a chair and beaten, suggesting that there is a more extensive history of childhood abuse that has been acknowledged. The results of her psychiatric evaluation have been discussed with her primary therapist, Dr. Greg Wilets; that is the end of Dr. Putman's evaluation.

In addition, the patient was seen by Dr. Jordan Grafman for neuro psychological evaluation. His report reads as follows: Michele was generally cooperative during the evaluation and demonstrated good effort on the testing procedures. She also showed a good grasp of test instructions and it is felt that her performances were both reliable and consistent indicators of her cognitive abilities (with a few exceptions). Parts of the evaluation were completed when an alternate identity of Ms. Newman's multiple personality was present. I will note these occurrences.
Michele was first administered the Wechler's Adult Intelligence revised form. She achieved a verbal scale score of 107 and a performance scale score of 104. Her subtest scatter was minimal, but she had particular difficulty on the digit symbol subtest, with a scale score of 6. Clinically, I felt that this performance still underestimates her intellectual capacities. Michele's auditory comprehension and naming abilities were excellent. Michele and Bonnie (an alternate identity) completed accurate and detailed drawings of objects for memory, as well as copies of objects already drawn. Michele's Wechler's Memory Scale, memory quotient of 113 was actually slightly higher than her WISC-RIQ score, reinforcing the suggestion that her I.Q. scores underestimate her true ability. On the Wechler's Memory Scale, she was well-oriented to time, place and current events. She had good retrieval of digits, geometric figures and stories. Michele's performance on the Peabody Picture Vocabulary Test was at the 60th percentile, which was quite acceptable for her age and education.

An alternate identity, Francie, completed several self-rating forms. Francie perceived a Beck Depression Inventory score of 24, which places her at high risk for depression. She complains of verbal and temporal memory loss, which are partly attributable to difficulty in remembering actions performed when different alternate identities are present.

Michele had several alternate identities perform a variety of memory tests to assess the amount and kind of information that transferred between or remain within identities. Given tests of autobiographical memory, each identity primary drew memories from its own perceived experience. Some slippage did occur. For example, Peggy (an alternate with a 12-year-old identity) included in her memory productions the same exact memory that Michele had offered earlier for this same stimulus probe. While this rarely occurred, it did indicate that there is a common 'pool' of somatic knowledge from which each identity draws its own 'character and moods.'
The slippage across identities indicates that all identities potentially have access to this pool. Several tests designed to assess proactive interference across identities were attempted. Interestingly, we found no category interference crossing identities from Bonnie to Michele. Typically, in control subjects who receive two lists of words drawn from the same category to remember, recall of

words from the second list usually finds intrusion of words from the first list; this phenomena was not found in Michele. Several attempts at priming were also made. Recognition of words presented in fragment form in one identity were primed by prior presentation of the same words in complete form in another identity. Priming of dictorial information was not successful. Several comparisons in cognitive performance were made between Peggy (12-year-old identity) and Michele. Findings indicated that across tasks, Peggy retained and processed information in age and intellectual level more consistent with Michele than a 12-year-old girl. The one exception was in the autobiographical memory recall task.

Michele's mood state was remarkably stable during most of our testing. We did not have a problem with her more disruptive alternate identities. In several instances, we had to delay the testing because of what appeared to be 'seizure-like' activity; the testing was never halted by such activity. She often would discuss her difficulty in day-to-day functioning with the test examiner, and worried about the effects of being told that she did not have epilepsy. The difference in mood state across identities appears profound, and may contribute to some of her amnesic experience through the mechanism of mood induced stated dependent learning and retrieval.

In summary, this generally cooperative female presents as a bright and curious test subject, whose major cognitive difficulties appear secondary to her diagnosis of multiple personality, i.e., amnesic episodes, state-dependent learning and retrieval, and swings in mood regulation. The slippage of information across identities in conjunction with her above-average intelligence level suggests that she would be amenable to therapeutic efforts that probe episodes that were primarily experienced by an alternate personality. That is the end of the neuro psychological evaluations by Dr. Jordan Grafman, Ph.D.

In addition, the patient had more than 110 hours of simultaneous EEG and CCTV video recording of her behavior. During this monitoring period, at least 12 episodes of what she describes as her 'minor seizures,' which are characterized by the sudden onset of tingling in the left hand or both hands which may migrate up to the left elbow, were observed. During none of these episodes was there any change in the baseline EEG, including paroxysmal flowing of either theta or delta activity; neither was there any evidence of epileptiform sharp wave or spike activity. In addition, the patient had approximately six to eight episodes during which she had jerking movements, usually starting in the upper extremities, but eventually spreading to include all four extremities, and often associated with tonic deviation of the head which could occur in either direction. During these episodes in which all four extremities were jerking, and the head was deviated, the patient also often had associated trunk flexion. However, during these episodes, the patient was fully responsive, could answer questions. She was able to name the president during these 'seizures.' In addition, during these minor and major episodes of which she refers to as seizures, the patient was able to move to command, so if instructed to move towards the middle of the bed she would do so without hesitation. These episodes could last between 5 and 30 minutes, and would often subside only to begin again shortly afterwards. These episodes never began when the patient was involved in discussion with other patients, with examiners or during testing sessions. These episodes never occurred during sleep.

On review of the electroencephalogram obtained simultaneously with the episodes, it was felt by all reviewers that there was no evidence of any change in background rhythm during these episodes. Because of the dramatic changes in her behavior, i.e., jerking movements of all four extremities with tonic deviation of the head and preserved consciousness and no changes in the baseline electroencephalogram, it was felt by the Epilepsy group that these most likely represented psychogenic seizures.

This diagnosis was discussed slowly, and in a gradual way with the patient, so that shortly before discharge the full diagnosis was disclosed to her that the available evidence based on extensive recordings and visualization of approximately 20 seizures revealed no clear evidence of epilepsy. At first the patient was quite disturbed by this information, and she said, mostly because 'my mother will be very upset that I do not have epilepsy.' This was discussed with the patient by Dr. Jordan Grafman, Dr. Frank Putnam, and Dr. Orrin Devinsky, and after a long discussion, the patient seemed to be accepting that seizures do not appear to be her primary problem. It was also mentioned that the possibility of simple partial seizures, with electrical discharge limited to limbic structures or deep structures within the brain could not be entirely excluded based on the information available. However, it is clear that the prolonged episodes of confusion and four extremity jerking movements which the patient referred to as severe seizures were probably not epileptic in nature."

This hospitalization was a major shift in where I was earlier in the year. I think the Group felt that this was an important study and there could be no screw ups. That's not to say what was going on earlier at Porter Hospital and at Beth Israel were screw ups. The way I was feeling was very real at the time.

I had no control over my mental alertness at Porter. I was very incapacitated. My true weakness showed through. I did not have the help and support of my alters at this time. I felt I was very much alone and they were not there to get me through it. I had to do it by myself. There was no acting out. They all stayed in the background. Maybe they were trying to prove to me just how much I needed them. That maybe I was a weak and frail individual without them.

My stay at Beth Israel started out in the same way, but soon changed. I admitted that I did need their help. The help was disorganized, but nonetheless there. I didn't approve of everyone's behavior, but it was not out of control like it was known to be in the past.

During these two hospitalizations I was not stressed. I was looking for answers. There was more pressure on me at NIH. These doctors were important and I didn't want to waste their time and the government's money. I was tired of hospitals by this time. I just wanted some answers. At this point I really didn't care what they were. I wanted to get on with my life and needed direction. The thought of epilepsy was something I could not control and scared me. At least with my mental illness I felt I had some sense of control.

When the doctors told me they didn't believe me to have epilepsy, I was quite frankly, relieved. As mentioned in the discharge summary, I had a great deal of concern about how my mother would take this new diagnosis. She ate up the attention she was getting from her friends when she talked about my problems. How could she tell them that her daughter was mentally ill or crazy? She was too proud.

My alters were not intimidated by the staff at NIH and felt comfortable in showing themselves. It wasn't like this at the other two hospitals. I'm sure the stress from a good performance and good behavior had a lot to do with the onset of the seizures I experienced there. The conditions were a bit tense. I know I was not fully functional, but everyone tried to cooperate. I was confused by all this interest in my alters. They did not know quite how to take all the attention they were getting. For a change, they were welcome to show themselves if they could maintain a sense of control. They were encouraged to come out of the closet and be recognized for who they were. They were welcomed to participate in the testing.

I came home with no medication. I felt cleansed to a degree. I also felt unprotected but no longer scared about having seizures. I knew that if I could control the stressors in my life that I would have some control over my seizures.

When I got home, I had a letter from the Social Security Administration saying that they were granting me disability status and I would be able to receive monthly benefits. Because of the bankruptcy, I stood to lose everything. I had no or very minimal income coming in. It was inevitable that I would lose my house. The only thing I said I wanted to continue to pay on after the bankruptcy was my truck. I needed transportation, even though I wasn't driving that much lately. It was my only sense of independence and was very important to me. I talked things over with my parents. They agreed to let me move back home with them.

I had put my house on the market earlier in the year but had few lookers. I did not have a very aggressive realtor and know this was part of the problem. I quit making mortgage payments in August. When I got back from Bethesda, I started gathering things up and deciding what I was going to sell. Nothing seemed of value. I was tired and didn't care about material possessions any more. I had a garage and moving sale every weekend in November. I ran ads in the paper for my furniture. By the middle of December, just about everything was gone. I boxed up what I was going to keep and rented a storage locker for what I could not store at my folks.

I wanted to put 1986 behind me. My parents gave me the two bedrooms in the basement for my things. I moved my drafting studio into the larger bedroom. That was about the only furniture I kept. I used the bedroom furniture they had in the other room. By the first of the year, I said goodbye to my house. The move was fairly uneventful for Nikki because my parents had taken care of her throughout the previous year. She knew their house well and felt quite at home.

I got a notice to appear in bankruptcy court the latter part of January 1987 to finalize my Chapter 7. The first half of the year was fairly uneventful. I tried to do some drafting but didn't market myself much. I just did what came along with the clients I had the early part of the year. I decided to start work on this autobiography. I thought it would give me some insight into my therapy and problems and possibly would help me grow. I did manage to stay out of the hospital. My moods were manageable and I was starting to feel more productive.

I was feeling good enough to start looking for a regular job. I went through the want ads weekly and sent out numerous resumes. I went to job fairs and on interviews but no luck in landing a job. Finally, the grocery store workers were threatening a strike. King Soopers was the retailer they decided to strike. I went to the local store and applied for a job. I got hired to work the strike as a cashier. I worked at the store for six weeks until the strike was settled. Shelley and Francie took the responsibility for the job. Shelley was good with numbers and the register and Francie had the people skills necessary to deal with the public.

I joined the National Association of Women Business Owners the previous December and tried to get involved with that. I bought a Macintosh computer after I got back from NIH. I wanted to improve my skills so took over as Communications Chairman and did the monthly newsletters. I did work that year to help bring the World Congress to Denver. There were women entrepreneurs from 21 other countries in attendance. Being in NAWBO and around all those women business owners got me motivated.

My job interviews did not go to waste. I got a call that fall from one of the companies I had interviewed with. They were looking for someone to do some contract work for them on a major project they were awarded through a government contract. I had decided to try to build my business because I was getting nowhere with my regular employment search and took the assignment. It was a project that would last at least through the following March.

In November I got the wild idea of finding an office for my business. I was not having a lot of luck motivating myself toward work in the basement at my folks. I found an old parking garage across from the ARCO Tower that had been converted into an office building. With the big contract with this company, I needed more room. There was a strong chance that I would have to have some other people working for me to complete the project on time.

I worked on the maps for this project until my office was ready the first part of February 1988. I bought a couple additional tables and equipment. It was a nice new office with one whole wall that was glass and overlooked an atrium. It became a joy to get up and have some place to go to work. I began putting in long hours. By the end of February, I was looking for help. None of the people I knew that drafted was able to help. They were busy with their own clients. I resorted to calling the drafting schools.

I ended up with three students or recent graduates to help me. They weren't the caliper of person I was hoping to get, but did help me get the work done. Two continued to help me through most of March because one had gotten another job. As I was reviewing the maps for their completeness and accuracy the day before they were due, I found some that were below my standards. I proceeded to redo them entirely. I worked 30 hours straight to get them presentable the next day. That week, I put in over 100 hours. With sheer luck, I made my deadline but decided to let the two students go after that.

I was in a manic swing that spring and was easily working twelve to eighteen hours a day at the office. In addition to the big project, I had work to do for my other clients and some other new ones I had acquired. That manic swing lasted from February to June.

In May, I landed a six week contract with a company in southeast Denver. I was working at their office during the day, and my own in the evenings. I usually worked eight hours without a lunch onsite, then get a bite to eat on the way to my office.

I made enough money from these jobs to meet expenses. I had enough to obtain a lease on a laser printer for my computer. I decided to ad desktop publishing to the list of services I offered. Through my membership in the Chamber of Commerce, I was able to get a contract to work on their Leadership Denver yearbook. This was a program for community leaders to learn about the local community and government. I did all the typesetting and layout for this project. It ended up being my first quality published piece.

Even though my business was doing well and I was lucky with getting work, I was still trying to locate a regular job. I was still receiving disability payments, because I was unable to clear enough money with the business to pay me a salary. That year, I paid myself only $500 and some medical expenses. I did not have health insurance until I became eligible for Medicare that fall.

I answered an ad during the summer for a job as a cartographic manager. It was for the Michelin Tire Corp. They were wanting to bring a mapping department to the states to create digitized atlases of the United States. I was contacted and interviewed by phone with the headhunter that was conducting the search for them. I was selected as a finalist candidate for the job and got a trip to Greenville, South Carolina for an interview with the company.

The flight went well, but I was nervous. Was I really ready to move away from my doctor and family? I hit it off big with the headhunter. The test was going to be the next day with company management.

I drove around the area looking for possible places to live should I get an offer. When I got to the company for my interview, I had to wait about half an hour. My nervousness had a chance to escalate. When I finally got into the interview, one of the gentlemen was from France and didn't speak real clear English. He was one of the main interviewers and I had trouble understanding his questions.

I felt some of my alters were having second thoughts about wanting this job and moving. In some respects, I think they did some sabotaging with the answers they gave. Needless to say, I was not offered the job.

I think not getting the job contributed, but more than anything, the coming of fall started to pull me into a depression. I had been high too long that spring and summer. I got back to the office and found myself lost. The work had slowed way down and I was wondering how I was going to pay the bills. I did not have any prospective projects on the horizon. I did go to the office from 7:30 a.m. to 4:30 p.m. every day; however, on numerous occasions found myself locking the doors and going to an inner room to lay down.

When I returned from South Carolina, I learned that my office building was being sold to the Post Office. The company that was selling the building offered to pay moving expenses for all the tenants. Bonnie and Shelley wanted to keep the business going. Dr. Wilets and some of the others thought differently. My depression was getting seemingly worse. I was confused. Bonnie had found a new office. My parents, Dr. Wilets and Chrissy decided that it would be best if I moved my office back to the house. There was no telling how much damage the depression was going to do this time. I had not been in the hospital since NIH in 1986. The discouragement of not being able to find a job was surely contributing to my depression and negative thoughts.

I ended up selling more than half of my furniture and listened to the direction my family and alters were giving me. I couldn't deny the past. With the unpredictability of my moods, I had to play it safe. I moved what I had left back home the end of October.

My depression did get worse. One difference this time was that I was not feeling suicidal. Kim was not angry at this time and that helped with not partaking in destructive behavior. It seemed that I was just going to have to ride this depression out on my own.

November and December were the pits. I spent nearly all my days in bed or laying on top of it. I rarely went outside or even out of the basement. I did not solicit any work. I only worked when the client called me, and was minimally productive at that. On the days I spent in bed, I barely ate or drank fluids. When I felt good enough to get up and dressed, I would have eating binges and couldn't drink enough fluids. That amounted to only about eight or ten days in December, but I ate enough to gain ten pounds that month.

Despite all the hours I was sleeping I did not have a whole lot of trouble sleeping at night. What I had trouble with was the dreams I was having. As with what happened during past depressive episodes, I would dream things that appeared very real; however, made very little sense. I was not in a deep sleep, just enough to feel confused about what was going on. My alters were also very shut down.

During many of my earlier depressive mood swings, I had small manic swings. I feel that not all my alters have the depressive tendencies I do and would kick into gear and try to pull me out. This time, it seemed that they had either gone on vacation (except for the days I would binge out) or had also succumbed to the depression. Needless to say, I made it through this cycle without having to be hospitalized.

During this depression, I was taking Depakote and Centrax. I also took Halcion every night for sleep. I'm sure the Depakote was what caused me to lose a lot of my hair. I almost felt I was going through radiation therapy. It was so bad that my mom bought me a wig for my birthday. I'm almost certain that it was also causing me to binge out on food from time to time.

The depression began to lift right after Christmas almost as quickly as it had come on. By the first of January, I was spending much of my time out of bed. Not knowing where my depression was going to take me, I decided to close my business the end of 1988. I would work for clients as a freelance contractor and not a company.

Dr. Wilets had started me on a new drug that had recently been released. It was called Prozac. He weaned me off the Depakote and other drugs. After stopping the Depakote, I continued with eating binges. Over the course of the following four or five months, I gained another 25 pounds.

I got called by a company I had sent some literature to back in 1987. They wanted to know if I could work on a project for a government hearing. Because I was feeling much better, I accepted and went to work in their office from the middle of January through much of March.

While working on that project, I continued to read the ads and apply for other positions. One day while reading the ads, I noticed an ad for an entrepreneurial program at one of the business colleges in town. I checked into it. I was still discouraged by my not having been able to get a regular job. I thought that if I had better training on how to run a business of my own, I could succeed at it. I ran my other business by the seat of my pants. I really had no clue as to what I should be doing. I just knew I had to do something to maintain some level of sanity and purpose as a human.

I checked out the program at Barnes Business College. It seemed like something I really needed. I checked into getting a loan and gaining admission. I was successful on both parts.

Mania began setting in again about February; about the time I registered for school. I immediately began dreaming up my new company. I came up with a name and logo. I had a note pad next to my work where I was drafting to jot down ideas as they rushed into my head. The floodgates seemed to just burst open. I put in some long hours to finish the project in time to start school. I was getting only three to six hours of sleep at night.

By late February I was experiencing some anxiety about the work I was doing and the thought of a new business. It was not clear as to whether the Prozac was causing this anxiety or not. Dr. Wilets prescribed some Haldol and Ativan to alleviate some of the distress I was feeling and to hopefully curb some of the mania.

School started around mid-March. About that time the mania also started to subside a bit. I was not feeling so grandiose. I was real excited about school and impressed with the instructor, Ike. He used to own a ski resort and had a strong business background. The class consisted of only five students so there was a lot of time to ask questions and have personal attention.

I studied for this class like I had never studied before. I turned in all my assignments on time and did well on all my tests. I got a 100% on one test that had about 100 true/false, multiple choice and essay questions. The final project for the class was to write a business plan for our venture.

I had purchased a software program that helped entrepreneurs prepare a business plan. I researched the market extensively and developed a dream company I had always wanted. I was optimistic but kept my plans to something that could have been manageable should I be able to get proper financing. By the time I finished my business plan, it was over 100 pages in length. Enough for a doctorate thesis but overkill for a bank or financial institution to look at. Ike thought it was great and wanted a copy of it to use as a sample for future classes to review.

Toward the end of the program, I had to make a presentation to the other members of the class. I took an hour and a half to present my business and plan to them. I was more thorough than anyone had ever been in the classes that Ike taught. When graduation came, this effort produced a Certificate of Excellence from Barnes for the program. Only the second one they had presented in the couple years the program had been in existence.

I was proud of my accomplishment and ready to build on my business. I wanted to succeed this time and was going to work hard at it.

I knew my chances of getting financed would be slim but I was going to try, regardless. I took my business plan to the bank where I had my business account. Nancy was impressed with the work but came back to me that without a strong track record showing that the projections were attainable, she was not in a position to take a risk on me. I had not made a lot of money in the past. The main thing she commented on was that even though I didn't plan on paying myself wages for awhile, that was unrealistic for a business. Employees needed to be paid.

Banks were also not very comfortable with using computer equipment for collateral. It didn't hold much value.

When the class was over, I continued to work diligently on building my business. I joined the Chamber of Commerce to try to advance my networking. They had a New Business Breakfast Club that I joined. In the class I met a man who had an oil company. I gave him my brochure and said if he ever needed help, he could certainly call me. He didn't say he had anyone in particular that he had been using in the past. This club met weekly and had some good presentations and programs for new businesses.

I was hungry for all the help I could get to become successful. I had to prove to myself and my family that I was recovering, and was coming back strong. It was so important to me to succeed. It seemed that in the past, just before I could attain success, I would do something to sabotage it. This was especially true with my career at the oil company. I had to show everyone that I was past that and a new person. At least that was what I kept telling myself to keep on going.

John, the oilman, eventually dropped out of the Breakfast Club, but shortly after the program had concluded, he called me to do some work for him. It seemed as though he had held off on putting together presentation quality proposals on some of his prospects. He had a number of projects for me to work on. I also got a call from a contractor that worked for him that had other projects and wanted me to do some work for him.

Things were beginning to look up. I tried to contact the guy I had worked for a few years back. It seems that another company had bought the Denver research and environmental division. Most of the people I had worked for had gone with the new company. I finally made contact with them and a few months later, they had some projects for me to work on. I kept busy through the summer.

I had gone to a local venture club for a couple of meetings. I submitted my business plan to them for review for a possible presentation at one of their meetings. I was accepted and scheduled to make my presentation the first Tuesday of October.

ROCKY ROADS AGAIN

By early September a change was coming over me. My antidepressant was losing its battle with my depression. Dr. Wilets said the FDA had finally approved a drug that he had been talking to me about for several months. He was thinking about starting me on it.

That time did not come soon enough. The latter part of September I got hit with a rolling pin. I woke up one morning and was hopeless. My mom had gone to the hospital to be with my father who had had surgery on Monday. By mid-morning, my depression became overwhelming and unbearable. All I could think of was dying. I became infatuated with the thought. I took off for the mountains, thinking that I would find some beautiful place and do myself in.

I drove to Summit County and found myself parked along the banks of Lake Dillon. I was parked in the sun and observed the people in the area; all the while thinking how happy they must be. Those pleasant thoughts were repeatedly interrupted with how I was going to kill myself. I could never really form any solid thoughts. I just kept hearing over and over in my head how I wanted to die; how I had to die. That this was the time for it to happen. Finally, I gave up and realized I was not going to succeed with this attempt. I started back to Denver at dusk, still thinking to myself that I had to die.

I got home and called my friend, Cheryl, whom I had become close to in my bipolar group that met at a local psychiatric hospital. Her doctor was also Dr. Wilets. She sensed how hopeless I was. I told her I would not call Dr. Wilets, because I didn't think he could help me. I got fickled and frustrated with the conversation and told her not to call Dr. Wilets. I broke off the conversation with her and just fell back on my bed. About twenty minutes later, I got a call from Dr. Wilets. Cheryl had called him regardless of my demands. I told him I was hopeless and could not talk. I didn't know what I was thinking or planning. I was very confused and frustrated and desperate. He suggested going to the hospital. I informed him that there was no way that I would go back into the hospital and hung up on him.

Shortly after that, my mom came home. She came down to see what I was up to. Moments later, the phone rang again. I told her to answer it and I didn't want to talk with anyone, knowing all the well that it was probably Dr. Wilets. It was Dr. Wilets. She asked him what was going on. He must have told her I was talking of hopelessness and sounded suicidal. He suggested to her that she get me to go to the hospital. He would call ahead and prepare them for my arrival.

When she got off the phone, I broke down. I could not put into words what I was feeling. I was choking on my words and must have sounded in great despair. I did not want to go the hospital, but in my heart, I knew that was what I needed to get me through this. My emotions were unpredictable and I was capable of doing just about anything. Deep down I know I didn't really want to die but it seemed like it was just about the only way I could get out of this stuck feeling I was in.

I was so frustrated that I began sobbing uncontrollably. I did not want my mom to see me that way and ran outside and sat on the swing. She took a moment to get a grip on the situation then came out to the swing with me. In a very calm and motherly voice she tried to sound encouraging but wanted to respect where I was at. This was the first time she experienced the pain I was feeling when I was in the middle of it.

After a half hour she convinced me the hospital was what I needed and assured me she would stick by my decision and support me. We both went inside and she helped me put together a suitcase of things.

Dr. Wilets had changed his hospital affiliation and instructed me to go to Presbyterian Denver Hospital. My mother drove me and stayed through the admissions processing. By this time it was about 10:30 p.m. on Friday, September 29, 1989. All the other patients were already in their rooms.

This was the first time I had ever been in the psych ward in this hospital. I had hoped that Dr. Wilets gave them directions for medication to help me sleep. I assured the admitting nurse and my mom that I had not taken any pills. Prior to just about all my other psych admissions, I had taken some kind of overdose. I just wanted to go to bed and sleep in hopes of waking the next morning to find that this nightmare was over.

The next day arrived too soon. I woke early as I usually did in the hospital. I was still feeling very depressed and hopeless. Thankfully, though the feeling and desire to die had subsided. I just wanted help and support to get me through this trough in my mood. Wanting to take a proactive approach to my therapy and to know what brought all this on, I immediately got active in the program on the ward. I attended group and Occupational Therapy. As usual, my inactive periods were hardest to get through. Keeping busy put the depression in the background.

Dr. Wilets came in the next day and said he was not going to wait any longer to get me started on the new medication he had been telling me about. It was just a few days before the Wellbutrin he prescribed was at the maximum recommended dosage. He had also prescribed an antipsychotic, Loxitane, to hopefully take the edge off until the Wellbutrin began to kick in.

The day after my admission, one of my long-time clients called with a job he wanted me to do. I convinced Dr. Wilets I was in control enough to go on pass to pick up the work and bring it back to the hospital to work on. He also let me out to go to Barnes Business College on Monday to make a trial presentation of what I was planning to give at the Rockies Venture Club meeting Tuesday night.

Tuesday was the big day. Things seemed to be going better. I was up for the presentation I was going to make. When I was out on Monday, I brought back a suit and make-up I needed to get ready for the meeting. I even brought in my curlers. Everyone in the hospital commented on how nice I looked and gave me strong words of encouragement as I went out Tuesday evening to the meeting. I was feeling good when I got back that evening and hopeful that things might be on the verge of changing for me. It was about time I got some kind of break.

The next day, I asked for another pass, because there was some stuff I had to do on the maps for my client that I needed to do at home. Each time I went out on pass, I had to contract with Dr. Wilets and the staff that I would not do anything destructive.

I took my suit and make-up and curlers home with me and got the work done that I needed within a couple hours. As I was getting ready to leave to go back to the hospital, I decided to get a few of my sleeping pills to take back with me. I was not getting much sleep in the hospital and was embarrassed by making a couple trips during the night to the nurses station for additional medication. I could not find my pills. I figured my mom must have taken them and hidden them. My father had come home from the hospital on Saturday and was upstairs in the TV room. My mom had taken my pills once before and put them in her bedroom. I went upstairs but my dad was awake and I couldn't get past him into the bedroom. I started to become very angry with my mother for doing this to me. I went back downstairs and started going through all my drawers in the bedroom and cupboards in the bathroom. It's very difficult to say just how angry I was. If my mom was home I would have fought with her and was angry enough that I could have hurt her with my abusive language.

I found a bottle with some Fiorcet tablets in it that I had gotten from Dr. Levisohn earlier in the year for some of my migraines. I also found about a dozen Vivactil pills from an old prescription. I gathered them with some more clothes and went back to the hospital. The staff was checking whatever I brought back so hid the tablets in one of my pair of socks. I contracted with everyone that I would not do anything while out on pass that would hurt me. I abided by this promise and brought the pills back to take at the hospital.

The anger towards my mom was still very intense. I loved my mom very much and didn't really like confronting her because she always would make me feel guilty when I was through. It was much easier to turn this anger inward, against myself. That way I could not hurt the ones I loved, because I really didn't love myself.

I got back to the hospital after lunch but before OT. I went into my room and pulled out the pills. I thought the pills would deaden the pain. I remember looking at the pills and thinking that this is not what I want to do. I don't remember actually taking the pills. I later found out it was Kim, my destructive alter. I was not suicidal. I just wanted to relieve the anger and I ended up taking 20 Fiorcet tablets and 12 Vivactil pills. Shortly afterwards, it was time for OT. I went as usual and began working on the project I had started as if nothing had happened.

About 3:30, I was beginning to feel something. The sounds around me began to get muffled and I felt like I was becoming distanced and detached from my body and feelings. I tried to act as if nothing was wrong, but all the while was feeling very strange. After OT, I went back to my room, put on my headphones and cranked up my music.

The next thing I remembered was one of the nurses in my room shaking me and telling me to get up for dinner. It was very difficult to respond. I was very groggy. She got me to sit up and was asking if anything was wrong. I said I wasn't sure, but that I was very tired and numb. She asked me if I took anything. I didn't know what to say. Even if I did, I couldn't have said it because I couldn't get my vocal cords to work. I just kept collapsing back on the bed. She called for help. I heard them searching through my things. One of the nurses found the pill bottle stuffed in my socks. They tried to get me to tell them how many I had taken. I don't remember whether I told them or not.

They took this very seriously and called the ER. My vitals were dangerously low. They immediately transported me to ICU on the bed from my room. Because I was so unresponsive they could not get me to take any medication orally. They proceeded to put a tube down my nose. Dr. Anneberg was still at his office a couple blocks away and rushed over. He said it was imperative that they intubate me because what I had taken could cause my air passages to become swollen shut, cutting off my air. It took them several tries before they were successful with the intubation and getting me on the respirator. All the while, I faded in and out of consciousness. One or two nurses and doctors worked on me throughout the night. They came in and took blood gases on several occasions. The nurse was trying to pump charcoal down the tube in my nose to absorb the pills I had taken. It did not stay down. I vomited back up every dose they put down. I was a mess with black vomit all down my neck, gown and chest.

I am very thankful they got me connected to the respirator when they did, because my breathing became very labored. At one point, I felt like I had lost all reflexes to breath on my own. My whole body was numb and shut down. Never in a million years did I think I would come so close to really killing myself. To top it off, I was not deliberately trying to kill myself. I had a lot of promising things going for me at the time with my business. It was an act of rage that made me take the pills.

I survived the night, thanks to the quick and effective care of the hospital. I was humbled and completely helpless. The next morning, all I could think of was being disconnected from the respirator. I was breathing on my own just fine, but had to wait for Dr. Anneberg to see me. My level of alertness was causing me to fight the respirator and put strain on the tube in my throat. They finally removed the respirator about 9:30 the next morning. They kept me in ICU most of the day for observation and to administer some potassium IV's. I had done so much vomiting the night before from the charcoal that my potassium level had dropped very low. I believe they gave me three bags of IV's.

That evening, they wheeled me back for readmission to the psych ward. I was immediately placed in isolation and locked up. I was angry and didn't understand why they did that to me. I now know that they were extremely angry with me because shortly before I came into the hospital, they lost a patient who had died while on the ward. They took my act very seriously.

My gesture had released the anger I was feeling, and I was ready to get on with my therapy and to try and work through it. They wanted a cooling off period and wanted me to give serious thoughts about what I had done.

OCTOBER 2, 1989
"Went on pass. Affect bright. At 8:10 said she felt 'wound up.' Pass went well and contributed to increased energy."

OCTOBER 3, 1989
"Fluctuation of feelings. Up and down. Required two doses of Loxitane. On pass to give presentation (Rockies Venture Club). 'I feel like I'm dissociating.' Affect flat w/sad facial expression.

OCTOBER 4, 1989
"Pt. appears depressed and states so. 3-3:30 pm - Pt. Lacks concentration; unable to do repetitive tasks. Pt. participating in OT group at beginning of shift. Pt. did not attend community meeting as she was on bed asleep with radio headset on at 4:45. OT therapist stating pt. was having a hard time in OT group and was unable to follow direction with project of repetitive nature. Pt. was aroused at 5:15 for supper and was lethargic at that time with slurred, slow speech. Stating 'I'm not hungry.' Pt. BP 136/94 lying, 134/100 sitting, p-68 apical and was regular, resp. 14. Pupils dilated. Staff searched room at 5:30 and found empty bottles of pills with Fiorcet label found in pts. drawer wrapped in stockings. Pt. questioned about pill bottle found, the amount of pills that were in the bottle and at what time pills were taken. Pt. verbal response, 'I don't know, a bunch, I don't know what time, it was when I got back from pass.' BP 110/100 at 5:45 pm. Pt. sitting at bedside remains lethargic with slow speech. Dr. Wilets called at 5:30. Dr. Spatt here on unit at 5:45 to assess pt. BP 138/100, p-32, R-16 at 6:00 pm. Pt. remains sitting at bedside stating 'I'm sleepy and numb.' Staff encouraging pt. to stay awake and to respond to questions. Dr. Spatt notified Dr. Platt and Dr. Anneberg at 6:10. BP 134/94 at 6:15. Dr. Wilets returned call at 6:20. Pt. lying down in bed at 6:25 and not responsive verbally but able to open eyes to verbal stimuli. Pt. gowned and clothes removed. Pt. transferred per bed to ICU rm. 108. Dr. Wilets called at 6:20 and shared information that over past 9 years, pt. has OD'd several times and usually in the hospital. When I was talking with pt. at 5:30, she kept saying 'I don't know, I don't know' to questions as to where she took pills, when, number, etc. Then later said pills were Vivactil and Fiorcet. When I asked her about the contract she had made with Dr. Wilets and staff, she said 'while on pass.' Stated she was angry with her mother. When asked why – 'She took all my medicine out of the medicine cabinet.' Mother was called at 7:00 pm to inform her of incident and transfer to ICU. She shared with me that on Sunday she had taken several bottles of pills from pt. medicine cabinet which included Advil, ASA, Ascendin 50mg, Tenormin 50mg, Haldol 5mg, Benztropine Misylate 2mg, Loxitane 5mg, and Temazepam 15mg."

OCTOBER 5, 1989
"Pt. returned to 3N rm. 367 in locked seclusion per MD order for potential harm to self. Pt. stating 'I won't be able to sleep. I've slept all day. Why do I have to be in here?' Explained to pt.

about OD last night. She needs close supervision and will be in this room till able to be assessed by MD tomorrow. Pt. lying down in bed resting quietly."

OCTOBER 6, 1989

"2:30 am - In seclusion. Pt. easily arousable. Voice loud, strident. Complained of throat being sore, bleeding spulum with small specks of red viscous liquid. 5:30 am - Somewhat restless. Poor eye contact. Loud tone of voice and angry manner. Seems to calm when talked to. 7:30 am - Lethargic, sad affect, but voice angry sounding. 2:10 pm - Pt. presents as severely depressed, impression is that pt. could be unpredictable as far as suicidal impulses. Pt. reported feeling 'compelled' to overdose. 3:30-11:30 pm - Pt. spoke of incest with brother only lasting a couple of years but was attention from someone in the family. Flat affect, tearful at times during interaction."

OCTOBER 7, 1989

"2:15 pm - Affect sad, appears depressed. Voice hoarse, volume low. Little appetite. Met with staff and mother at 1:15. Pt. angry and unwilling to believe mother's pain. Both talked with neither listening. 6:00 pm - Out of seclusion with staff. Behavior appropriate while on unit making eye contact, smiling and speaking to peers. Watched movie with other pt. Seemed to enjoy – laughing and joking w/peers and staff. Said difficult to acknowledge she came from an abusive family. 'Parents had to work hard with their business. They didn't have much time for us and now my mother tells me she loves me. I don't know how to respond because she didn't do that when I was growing up and now I don't feel that I need it.'"

OCTOBER 8, 1989

"'My parents had a 24-hr. business and we were left with baby-sitters or alone. My mother says she loves me but it's too late. She wasn't there when I needed her. I feel so...cold when it comes to her. If I act like I really feel, I feel guilty afterward.' Affect sad and depressed, appearing more animated than yesterday. Ate in dining room. Carried on lively conversation with peers and began coughing. When asked what the problem was by peers she eluded question. Asked permission to watch Harry and the Hendersons with peers. Eating popcorn and enjoying movie. Approached nurses station at 12 pm, 'I need a Loxitane.' Appeared shaky, eyes wide, winding gown string around her finger. In response to how she felt, 'I'm confused.' Pt. returned to room and laid down. Did not want doors closed, said able to contract for safety. Later observed in fetal position with blankets wrapped around her. Unable to ID any precipitant. Dr. W. called, prn of Loxitane obtained. Unpredictable inability to cope. Amiable most of shift. Ongoing depression. 2:30 pm - Given Loxitane upon entering floor. 'I don't know what brought it on; it's so unpredictable. I usually don't catch it in time.' Gave pt. positive feedback for asking for Loxitane and taking time out. Avoided eye contact, eyes downcast and having difficulty accepting positive comments. Pt. is 'other' oriented. Relies on the reactions of other people to define herself. Takes little responsibility for own feelings."

OCTOBER 10, 1989

"Anxious for Dr. to call or visit. Becoming angry. Watch closely. Given Loxitane prn at 4:15 pm for extreme agitation. Pt. agitated and becoming out of control. Demanding to leave unit. Encouraged to write list of concerns and complaints. Pt. called Dr. W. office. He called back, talked briefly with pt. and agreed to come see her. Pt. extremely hesitant and angry when asked to contract for safety. Tray checked for missing silverware; none missing at that point. Pt. later revealed she had slid a plastic knife from tray into bootie but returned it. Dr. W. saw pt. and both were able to verbalize anger with one another and are looking at possibility of 'burn-out' in relationship."

OCTOBER 11, 1989

"Pt. engaging staff in power struggles, splitting behavior which allows her to focus energy on other than goals set."

OCTOBER 12, 1989

"Began Biofeedback today. Muscle tension 8-10X normal level. Peripheral temperature within 1° of normal range. EDR readings 2X normal level. Participated in games during recreation group. Seemed easily excited and highly competitive with peers."

OCTOBER 13, 1989

"Anxious about case conference. Voice loud, more giggly. Able to chase more difficult questions. Able to accept compliments from another pt. and staff. Pt. had case conference with Dr. and staff. Able to make safety contract with staff for duration of hospitalization. Taken off 15 minute checks and has accompanied privileges. Affect bright. Contracted with Dr. for hospital outing. She went out and followed staff directions. She became quiet for awhile at park but then became more social. Participated in group and appeared to have good evening until 9 pm. Affect dulled and pt. seemed depressed."

OCTOBER 14, 1989

"Early affect was bright. Highly competitive w/peers and with activities. Also, very compulsive with many recreation activities, puzzles, cards, but pt. feels this is positive for her. 8 pm - 'I'm feeling really depressed. The last time I felt like this I OD'd.' Pt. asked what could be done if she felt really bad and was told she could be moved to safe room and she could contract to be safe again. Refused both and said, 'I'll be O.K.' Almost immediately she decided to contract for safety again. Pt. said she didn't know what caused her 'wave of heaviness' that overcame her. Pt. watched TV and movie with peers wrapped in her blanket. 'It makes me feel safe.' Pt. also stated that she knew she had to stay out of her room and being by herself as that makes her depression worse. Pt. displayed flat affect, slow movements, tired speech and depressed mood."

OCTOBER 15, 1989

"Flat, depressed affect. Has remained in her room in bed with her blinds drawn and wrapped in her blanket, knees drawn up. 2:00 pm - Affect brighter. 'I feel better. My depression is lifting.'"

OCTOBER 16, 1989

"Affect vacillates between sullen to superficially polite. Unwilling to accept responsibility for self happiness and actions. Superficial compliance. Lonely but unwilling to work on people skills; resorts to blaming and excuses. 7:30 pm - Affect bright at community meeting. Later found in room sitting on floor in the dark. Refused to talk about what was upsetting her. Remained that way for approximately 45 minutes. Came out of room and watched movie. Later talked about feelings of frustration around feeling like she has no control over her mood swings and cycling."

OCTOBER 17, 1989

"Affect seems depressed and flat. Stated she did not feel impulsive and was able to contract for safety on pass. Given nurse's station number if she needed to call. Went on a pass to work on project for client and to attend support group at Centennial Peaks. Appears depressed, anxious about discharge on Friday. Unsure if she's ready. Evaluated pass upon return. Checked pt's. belongings immediately upon return."

OCTOBER 20, 1989

"Went horseback riding. Preparing for discharge tomorrow. Flat affect. Seems more depressed, expressing anxiety regarding discharge."

OCTOBER 21, 1989

"Pt. manifesting increased depressed affect, but no suicidal material expressed. Plan around discharge changed by Dr. Wilets; not D/C today. Pt. experiencing feelings of depression and sadness, but is currently managing them more appropriately. Monitor for subtle change in mood suggesting a return to suicidal thought. Words expressing helpless, hopelessness. Stated light therapy 'not doing anything. I don't feel any different.' Lights removed from room per Dr. W. Removed plastic bags from room during routine room check. Sat outside nurses station after movie complaining of numbness and tingling in hands and arms and spasms in legs. Didn't want staff to call Dr. W. but did. Ordered to continue Wellbutrin 'seizures or not.' Dr. W. concerned with pt. behavior and will discuss assignment with pt. on Monday. Attempted to split staff and Dr. Questioned motive. Possibly angry over removal of plastic bags from room."

OCTOBER 22, 1989

"Complained of feeling extremely anxious and doesn't know why. Given Loxitane at 9 am and pt. agreed to listen to relaxation tape to help decrease anxiety. Pt. able to relax and fell asleep for hour. When staff approached she reported feeling anxious again. Having difficulty accepting responsibility for last night. Staff requested pt. to write a written contract for safety due to unpredictable behavior and she was unable to commit to that and began to write that she'd 'do her best.' Staff informed she would need to contract for safety without reservation. Pt. informed she needed to be out of her room, in the day room or in front of the nurses station until she is able to do that. Dr. W. called and 15 minute checks ordered. Pt. is to stay in public view until she can contract for safety in written contract."

OCTOBER 23, 1989

"Continued 15 minute checks. Affect sad, depressed at beginning of afternoon/evening shift. Isolated in room, lying on bed with covers on. 'I'm confused, I'm so down.' Repeating some statement of helpless and hopelessness. Stopped conversation since pt. feeling sorry for herself. Gave assignment to ride exercise bicycle. Call placed to Dr. W. regarding conference on Wednesday. Mood changed after dinner. 'I feel so much better now.' Dr. W. called again. He will have to call back in a.m. since he didn't have his book with him. Child-like need for attention and praise. Needing maximum encouragement to get out of bed."

OCTOBER 24, 1989

"Still on 15 minute checks until pass. Affect bright and cheerful and interactive. Looking forward to evening pass (D&D IAN). Pt. talks of tomorrow's D/C and appears ready."

I was discharged the next day. I had had 4 biofeedback sessions which helped me learn to control my levels of anxiety. I learned when it was time to take a time out and do my relaxation exercises.

My moods still fluctuated for a few weeks after my discharge. The uncontrollable swings and dissociation that ensues is very discouraging and frustrating. It made my behavior very erratic and unpredictable. Finally, after about six weeks on the maximum recommended dosage of Wellbutrin, my depression seemed to almost all but disappear.

I continued to see Dr. Wilets weekly for a month. In that time, he explained the anger he felt about me because of the overdose in the hospital. The doctors and nursing staff really came down on him pretty hard for allowing me out on pass in the unstable mood I was in. He said he was angry that I took advantage of his trust and decided to split hairs on the contract I had. He came close to dismissing me as his patient until we both had a chance to vent our anger towards one another. We came to an agreement that I would never let things go that far again.

During the last week of my hospitalization, I took the comments and suggestions from staff very seriously. I also talked with a social worker on how I might be able to better fit into society and build my people skills. She gave me a list of singles networks and support groups in the Denver area. I made a list that I promised to check out. Despite my rocky final days in the hospital, I was ready to get on with my life and had a lot of opportunity to think about how I would go about it.

THE LONG TRAIL BACK

Somewhere during or after my overdose, I had a feeling that if I got through the ordeal, I would renew my faith in God. That very next Sunday after my discharge, I mustered enough courage and determination that I went to Trinity United Methodist Church for Sunday School and church. I picked this church because I was somewhat familiar with it, having worked downtown near it for several years. The singles program was also on the list the social worker had given me. I wanted to start to meet other singles and develop a social life and felt a program sponsored by a church had to be a safe place to try.

I was very cautious in my connections with the people. They welcomed me warmly and made me feel like I fit in. Most of them in the class were a little older than me. They told me there were two other single's Sunday School classes that had a younger following. I decided to give them a try on the following Sundays. Not long afterwards, I felt myself comfortable and starting to fit in. I began attending church every Sunday. I even started coming down to the church on Wednesday evenings for their dinner and program. This program tended to have a more secular theme and was a nice change from Sunday. I also continued with my Bipolar support group at Centennial Peaks Hospital.

Once again, I began to claim my own friends rather than friends of my mother or boyfriends. I did not attend these activities with the thought of finding a companion. I was looking for acceptance from others and myself. By getting it from others, it was a little easier to obtain self-acceptance. This was something I had very little of.

I became a committed regular to the church. I enjoyed studying the topics covered in class. It brought back some memories of childhood Sunday School. I even got a lot out of the sermon in church. Never had I attended a church where the minister was as dynamic a speaker as Jim Barnes. No falling asleep here. I also really enjoyed the music and loved to sing the hymns. Church gave me an inner renewal that made it a joy to be alive.

Before long, I was getting active in the leadership of the single's program. First, I made a commitment and renewed my faith by joining the church. For the first time in my life, I had a home church I could call my own. No longer was I recognized as Harriet's daughter.

I volunteered information on my talents and hobbies and they immediately took me up on my offer to do the singles newsletter. I had time on my hands and had the equipment. I felt that any real world experiences I could get would only help me. Besides, I liked the singles minister, Dale Wood, and all the people. They were now my friends and I was happy to do anything to help my new friends.

Business had slowed up and I had a lot of time on my hands. It seemed that all I was doing was going to meetings. I was at church two to three times a week, Desk and Derrick, Bipolar Group, Dr. Wilets, NAWBO and the New Business Breakfast Club once a week. Even if the medication I was on wasn't working, I had too much interaction with people and things to think about other than being depressed.

My new church put out a call for interested individuals to be the Stewardship Secretary for the 1990-91 pledge campaign. Since work was almost nonexistent for me at the beginning of the year, I submitted my name. It paid enough to help with my expenses and rent. They must have been impressed with me because I got the job.

I spent three months, January thru March, working in the church office. I took minutes at all the committee meetings, coordinated all the correspondence and mailings and supervised the volunteers. I learned how to use an IBM compatible PC. I definitely came to the conclusion that I'd take my Macintosh computer any day over a PC.

I got caught up on some of my reading, because all I did on some days was babysit the printer when we did a merged letter. Some days were long when I had mailings to do. I would come in at 6:30 a.m. and start the printer so I wouldn't tie it up when the ministers and other staff were there. On other days of mailings, I had to start late and wouldn't get out of the church till 8:30-9:00 p.m.

I really enjoyed working with the ministers and volunteers at the church. I was always made welcome and considered a member of the team. They would invite me to share lunch with them and valued my opinions. This was a real switch from past work experiences. It almost made me think about considering a job somewhere in the church. I realized quickly, though, that paychecks are contingent upon pledges being kept and can be real stressful from payday to payday. I didn't need that. I decided I would continue to volunteer my talents and abilities when this job was over and plan on other things for a living.

Since work was slow, I also took on the added responsibility of doing my Desk and Derrick Club's monthly newsletter. This publication was quite a bit different than the church newsletter. With the church, Dale collected all the material and did most of the writing. Desk and Derrick, on the other hand, required me to do everything. I had a committee that helped to proof the newsletter and print and prepare the mailing. I did everything else from writing, collecting articles from members, to designing and laying out and typesetting each issue. This newsletter was not a piddly 4-pager, either. It was never less than 16 pages and usually ranged between 20 and 24 pages.

My committee would come over to my house on an evening or Sunday to proof. As they found things that needed to be changed, I would change them on my computer on the spot. One of our members worked at Petroleum Information. They had a complete print shop and copy equipment. We had an arrangement with them to do the reproduction of the newsletter. The gal that worked for them was on my committee and would take it to work the next day.

Along about April, things began to turn. I started getting calls from out of the blue based on contacts made a year or two earlier to do work. I took anything that came my way with open arms. Before long, I began to outgrow the small 12x15 bedroom I had all my equipment in. The small drafting table I had was not adequate for some of the projects I was getting.

In July, I began looking for office space. I definitely decided against space downtown because it was fairly expensive and I would have to pay for parking. I checked with some of the office buildings just down the street from where my folks lived. They didn't have the kind of space I needed. I ended up calling a fellow NAWBO member and asked her about the complex she was in. She thought they might have something that would suit my needs. I went and took a look. After looking at four spaces, I found one that I thought would definitely accommodate me. I made a deposit and filled out the paperwork. They would have to pull out the old carpet and repaint the walls before I could move in. I also had them put in some shelves. The space was about 750 sq. ft. and in the lower garden level of one of three buildings in the complex.

The complex was about three miles from my home. They had beautiful landscaping in the plaza. Lots of trees and flowers, a fountain and bridge across the water. My suite was in the same building and just below the office of my NAWBO friend. I negotiated a three year lease. I was almost tempted to go five, but pulled back at the last moment, because I could outgrow the space in three years or be out of business. After my bankruptcy, I was a bit more cautious about signing personal guarantees that had lengthy commitments.

Move-in was the first of September. In August I went to a local auction and got some good deals on chairs and a desk. Right after the auction, I went to find a storage place close by that I could store my newly acquired furniture for a month. I also read the ads to find a larger used drafting table. A good used table was in great demand. If you didn't call right after 8 in the morning on an ad, it was usually gone.

I got a local moving company to move me. I had some big and heavy equipment. I had acquired, in previous years, a diazo (blueprint) machine and copier. I also had a lot of books and some computer equipment. I was real disappointed in the way the move went. The movers were suppose to be there at 8 a.m. the day of the move. They didn't show by nine and I called, only to find out that I was not on the schedule for that day. They ended up calling a sister moving company that came late that afternoon. The move was not finished until 9 p.m. that evening. This put a real dent into my schedule because I had to be back up and operating within a day or two. I had some big projects on the board that needed to get done.

Getting a place with about five times the space I had at the house made a tremendous amount of difference in my motivation factor and enthusiasm about working. It also made me feel like I was really in business. The atmosphere also made me truly believe I could succeed this time. Elbow room and good overhead lighting brightened my mood and made me want to work and succeed.

I finished my project on time despite the problems with the move. Right afterwards, I began putting together a marketing plan towards getting more work. I was always reading the want ads looking for part time or temporary work. I read the *Denver Business Journal* looking for new companies in the area or stories about prominent businesses that could possibly need some additional help. I also read the Denver Chamber newsletter that would list new members and the type of companies.

I put together a brochure that had some samples of my work in it and began calling energy companies listed in the *Rocky Mountain Petroleum Directory*. I set aside one to two hours a day to make calls. I then sent out personalized letters and brochures to those who voiced an interest in getting some information.

I rejoined the local NAWBO (National Association of Women Business Owners) Chapter and began attending the monthly meetings. The local management office for the association was stepping down from the responsibility and they began to search for another Director and manager. I submitted a proposal to the Board of Directors for the position. I was interviewed by the Board. Another woman owned business with experience in association management got the job.

I did continue to attend the meetings and network and joined a Round Table of other women business owners. The theme of the group was to discuss problems and help one another develop their businesses. We took turns meeting at each other's offices or homes once a month. The focus of the meetings was to try to give the hostess ideas to improve her business or solve problems she may have been having with employees or the such.

I also joined a similar program with the Greater Denver Chamber. These round tables included men and women owned businesses. We also met once a month rotating to one another's offices.

When it was my turn to host the meeting, I had to put together an Executive Summary that explained the objective and position of my business and just what kind of business I was in. I made an agenda of what I wanted to discuss over the course of the 1-1/2 to 2 hour meeting. We discussed what my successes were and what I needed advice on. I got some very beneficial recommendations for trying to build my business. Everyone was always impressed with my operation. Little did they know I was not even making enough money to pay myself a salary. We never got into the financials of the business. Everything was held in confidentiality, though.

These round tables were very helpful in making friends in the business community. I developed a keener awareness of what owning a business was about. I no longer felt I was flying by the seat of my pants. I had developed goals and plans.

I was at meetings or in my office every day by 7:30 a.m. I stayed at the office till at least five, but when working on a deadline project, would stay till 9:30 or 10 p.m.

My mom felt sorry for me when I did this and would sometimes pick me up dinner. It was very quiet working in a place for that length of time with little or no outside contact. I had a little portable black and white TV and radio that generated noise throughout the day. I also had a small refrigerator, microwave and coffee pot in my supply room just for days that I could not get away. It was very homey and I enjoyed being at the office.

Shortly after moving to my new office, I was contacted by the Colorado High School Activities Association. I had given them my name that spring at a trade show. I told them I would be interested in judging speech meets. After years of thinking about doing this, I was finally faced with the opportunity.

I attended the judges training one Saturday in October at Golden High School. I took the training for individual events and debate. I also took the test for both and was certified. Forensics had changed a bit since I was in high school, but I was excited about going to meets and seeing the caliber of young people that were in the schools now.

I began attending speech meets almost weekly from the end of October thru April the next spring. Douglas, Arapahoe, Adams and Jefferson counties seemed to host most of the meets. That year, I only attended one meet held in Denver.

Because they were always short on certified judges or judges interested in debate, I spent almost all of my time judging this event. I judged both cross examination debate with teams and the new Lincoln Douglas debate. This was something that had been started since I was in school. I never did do debate when I was on the forensics team.

I got to know and converse with other judges that attended meets regularly. I made a few new friends, but no one that I got together with outside of the meets. Judging was not only a service to the schools and a way for me to get out in the community, but also brought in a few extra dollars. I got paid from four to seven dollars for each round I judged. I would judge from four to six per meet day.

On a few occasions when I judged interpretive events, I heard cuttings from what was done when I was in high school. Things had not changed all that much. There were some new pieces that I had never heard, too. I still think that the deliveries that were presented in rounds when I was competing were a bit more professional, though.

I tried to be thorough in my critiques, because I felt the judges that judged me did not offer enough suggestions and comments that would help me understand why I ranked poorly in a round, or why I did well in one. I would almost write a short story on the debate critiques I gave. I guess that was because debate was more structured and disciplined. There are more rules to follow.

This extracurricular activity was very enjoyable. It was easier to give fully of myself, because many of the meets began on Friday afternoon. Being in business for myself, I could leave work and help out with the earlier rounds.

THE REJUVENATED WHIRLWIND

Nineteen Ninety became a year of self-discovery. I tried to reacquaint myself with myself and just what I was about. It seemed like I was reborn and given a second chance after my hospitalization in 1989. Finding a church home I felt comfortable with gave me the courage to rediscover my inner faith and helped me to do some self-discovery.

My inner Group reaffirmed their promise to cooperate as long as my moods remained stable. When that is the case, there is harmony, not chaos and pushing and shoving. There is a sense of order to what I try to accomplish. I am able to remain focused.

As 1990 was winding down, I felt healthier than I could remember about the last ten years. I was happy about what I was doing and fairly enthusiastic about life and what it had to offer. I know pushing myself to be out and around people had a lot to do with this. My alters were all given tasks and assignments to drive me in a new direction. They readily accepted the challenge.

I received a mailer in December about a new networking group that was forming early in January. I decided to RSVP and check it out. This was a nation-wide networking organization. I felt very comfortable at the meeting and decided to join. I thought it could add quite a boost to my bottom line.

The group met every Tuesday morning from 7-8:30 a.m. at a local restaurant for breakfast. The object of the group was to generate leads for other members through the course of their daily dealings and contacts. Because I did not get out regularly in the business community, I found I was having difficulty creating leads for the members. I would generate leads that consisted of myself, family and church friends. I wasn't alone. Many of the leads from the other members were the same. As it turned out, most of us would work for each other. The ones with a higher rate of leads were those who met numerous people every day in their business. Sometimes, that Tuesday meeting and church were my only contact with outsiders.

I struggled with my affiliation with this group. I felt guilty that I could not generate the leads they stressed. I did make myself attend the Chamber functions in hopes of generating leads. I was not going to be beaten with this. My drive was strong. The leads I received did generate about $5000 worth of work in 1991.

I caught wind that a couple of the guys from the group were trying to develop a similar program with the Denver Chamber. I dropped out of the national leads group in early fall to sign up for the Chamber program. It didn't sound like it was going to be quite as competitive and cut throat as the other group. This program started one year later in January. I was much more comfortable with this group. There was not near the pressure to have large numbers of leads each week.

I was extremely active in anything I partook during 1991. Church and my faith played an important role in this revitalization. I missed maybe six Sundays of church and Sunday School all told that year. I became a real leader on the Single Adult Council and volunteered to be the single's rep to the Administrative Board. I continued to put together the singles newsletter every month on a very tight deadline. I even found myself teaching a Sunday School series on anger.

Thank God for my alter, Carol. I could not have done it without her. I only wish I could have given her more time to prepare. I know she could have done a superb job.

Shelley spent most of that year out attending the meetings and being very organized. The only way for me to remember the year, is to review my calendar and read my Christmas letter. I know I was busy but find it hard to fathom all the personal contact I had that year with other people.

I have never really personally been a people person, but many of my alters thrive on the contact. I let loose and let them take control. It was a great year.

I ran for Treasurer in Desk and Derrick and got elected the previous fall. I had monthly board meetings to attend and had to keep all the financial records straight. Shelley had taught herself accounting on the computer and was very comfortable with the responsibilities. All the quarterly audits balanced and the records were in better shape than they had been for a long time. Reports were regular and thorough.

I went to the Regional Desk and Derrick Meeting that was held in Salt Lake that year. Having been Bulletin Chairman the year before, my work was in contention for awards. I received the first place award for the region in Best Bulletin. From there, it was sent on to the national awards committee to compete with the six other regional winners. I did not make it to the National Convention that fall but did come away with the second place award in the Association for best bulletin.

I also had some experience that year with goal setting and long range planning. With the cutbacks the oil industry had experienced over the last few years, we needed a firm direction and objective for our existence. We had a marathon meeting on a weekend retreat in the mountains. It was a good opportunity to get to know some of the other women better and make some close friendships.

Friends were hard for me to make that were lasting. I can be friendly and have a good time when I am around people. Francie and a number of the others take care of that. My overall nature still resorts back to introversion and isolationism. I don't need people around me all the time to be happy and content. In fact, I'm more content when I'm alone and working on things that I enjoy. I'm friendly and enjoy the companionship when it is there, but I don't go out of my way to set up that environment. I almost never call anyone to go and do something together.

I continued to participate in the Chamber CEO Exchange program and NAWBO Round Table that I started in the previous year. These meetings and friendships were the encouragement I needed to keep my business on the right track. My business was not growing by leaps and bounds like everyone else's seemed to be doing. I just seemed to plug along. God saw to it that I had enough business to pay the bills and rent, but never enough to pay myself a salary. I still had to live off Social Security and live at home with my parents. I longed for the day that I could once again be self-supportive and move out on my own.

Speech tournaments kept me busy on the weekends during the spring and fall. I really enjoyed being around the different type of person that attended these events. It also gave me hope that not all of today's kids were growing up as lost souls in working families. I had really become discouraged with teenagers when I had my Girl Scout troop. These kids still had a wild edge to them but had more visible objectives with their lives and took an interest in the world around them.

Because of a slightly renewed interest in teenagers that these speech meets brought on, I decided to get a bit more involved in the community. Contract negotiations went on for the teachers in Denver public schools in the spring. They had drawn to a stalemate. The teachers were threatening to strike. The governor stepped in and acted as a mediator. He put together a plan that kept the teachers from striking but also set up governing committees in each of the schools. These were called CDM (Collaborative Decision Making) Committees. Each school would put together a committee of teachers, parents, administrative and business representatives. I contacted the state and Denver South High School to tell them that I would be interested in serving on the high school's committee.

I didn't hear anything back on the committee until May. I received a call to see if I was still interested in being the business representative to South. A meeting was set the end of May. We met just about every week through the summer and the rest of the year. A two day training was held in July that all committee members were required to attend. I tried to be optimistic about this process and feel there was help for the educational system. The school system had certainly changed since I was there eighteen years earlier.

My weekly calendar continued to be filled with meetings throughout the year. With what I have already mentioned, I continued to attend weekly support group meetings at a metro hospital for people dealing with bipolar illness. When I was at the office, I was alone and rarely had any contact with other people except when I met with a client or received a phone call. I could go all day and never talk to or be around another person. The meetings gave me the people contact to get through the days and weeks. I knew a lot of people, but never allowed myself to become close enough to really have someone to do extracurricular activities with. Everything was business. Nothing was ever for fun and just being with someone else. Even my regular therapy sessions were handled in a very business-like way. It was hard to address issues with feelings.

I never allowed myself to become close to anyone besides my family since breaking up with Gene. It took me three years to get over that relationship. I couldn't stand to go through the feelings of rejection again, so I did not allow myself to be put in that situation. Besides, when I do get real close to someone, they either die or move away and forget about me. It seemed so much easier and less painless not to allow a relationship to reach a point where that would ever matter to me.

I got called one day in November regarding a resume' I had sent out earlier in the fall. Carl was an employment contractor and owned a slide production service. He wanted me to fill in for his employees who were on vacation and because of work overload. It was to be working in the graphics department in one of the many U S WEST offices in downtown Denver. I jumped at the opportunity, because business was otherwise slow.

I worked in the office for about three or four weeks. I got some good experience doing practical graphics on a Macintosh. They all seemed to be very satisfied with the speed and creativity displayed in each of the assignments I was given. I told Carl that I would be happy to fill in for him any time he needed help. I really enjoyed what I was asked to do. The people were all great to work for.

At the beginning of the year, I was still self employed with my own little design studio. I still did enough oil and gas work to retain membership in Desk and Derrick. I don't know why, but I agreed to once again be editor of the monthly bulletin. This is always a major undertaking, because I took it seriously. I guess I am bound and determined to win the first place AIMEE that the Association awards annually through competition. It is the competitive nature inside of me. I always had to prove that I was the best. I wanted to prove to my mom that I was worth something. When I did win or accomplish something, her approval was sort of passé. I guess, deep down, I was really trying to gain my own self-satisfaction.

Once again the bulletin amounted to no less than 16 pages, and usually 24 to 28. I typeset and laid out the entire piece. I had a lot of help this year proofing it, because now I had a fax modem and could fax out the proofs to my committee. They would call me back in a day or two with corrections. The actual work on the bulletin took about two full days by the time it was copied and addressed and ready for the mail.

I was still looking for a regular job, because I was barely making it with my own business. I thought the work on the bulletin would give me practical experience that would allow me to apply for a job as an editor. Just one more category to submit my resumé to and broaden my chances at employment.

I was still the editor of my singles newsletter at church. I had typeset this newsletter every month without fail since February of 1990. I would edit it, lay it out and add art where and when it would fit. I then was sure to get it to the printer in time to be printed and back to the church for the man who prepared it for mailing was scheduled.

The employment contractor whom I had worked for the previous fall called me back late January to fill in while one of the guys was on vacation. I came in and worked on their equipment to get them started on a massive project the department had taken on.

At the end of the week, my boss, Carl, came in to see how things were going. They were bashing heads to see how they were going to get this job finished. They did not have another computer available in the office to devote full time to this project. I suggested that I could take it back to my office and work on it there. I had my own computer and laser printer. He talked it over with the US WEST manager and she agreed that that would be their best option. I had acquired their confidence in being able to work independently with little supervision and still do a great job.

The project was to take many of their training manuals and user guides and put them in a PC word processing program. They were on a word processor, but these had become outdated and difficult for updating. I would go down to the office once or twice a week as more material came in. When I couldn't make it to town, they had a courier service bring the work to me.

I typed eight to ten hours a day and five to six days a week on this project. I generated a lot of paper. It helped me to build my typing skills and speed. I also got to do some graphics to put into these manuals. They turned out far better than what they had originally been. It was a lot of hard work, but I really enjoyed this job. What was difficult was to find the time when one of my other clients would need my services. Fortunately, that didn't happen too often. I worked on this project from the first of February 1992 until mid-April on a regular basis.

The only disappointing part of this project was the pay. Even though I was using my own equipment and paper and office, I got the same pay I would have gotten if I had done it at US WEST. At least I didn't have to pay for parking every day. I could have retired for the rest of the year with this one job if I had gotten my full fee. However, when you are hungry, you will take just about whatever comes along without any argument.

It was a real let-down when the project was completed. I didn't have much other work come in. I made enough money off the job to become an exhibitor in the major business trade show held in the spring by the Chamber of Commerce. I had a number of people come by my booth, but no real prospects. I did get a couple jobs that summer that covered the expense of the booth and my time, but that was it. My business was not the best kind of business to exhibit at something like this. I was hurting for ways of exposing myself, though.

I spent much of the summer attending networking meetings and making cold calls to printing and oil and gas companies. I also got caught up on reading my magazines that I was six months behind on. I still sent out resumés just about every week, never giving up on the hope of getting a real paying job.

August came along and I had just returned from an interview. I felt good about how I had done, but I had felt that about many of the interviews I had gone on with nothing coming of them. That afternoon, I got a call from Carl. He asked if I would be available to come in and work until he found a new Art Director because he had just lost his. I told him I had just returned from an interview that looked promising. He said he wasn't aware that I was looking for a job and asked if I would be interested in his position. I told him I would like to try it for a week before giving him an answer. He agreed.

The week went well and I decided I would agree to take the job. I figured I would need at least $12-13 per hour to take it. When he said it would pay $11, I just said okay. No arguments or movement for negotiations to get what I wanted. I was just so happy that I would now have a regular paycheck and be eligible for benefits, that I didn't want to shake things up. I'm sure I could have gotten at least $12, but I was too scared to try.

One problem I have always had was to speak up for my rights. I have stumbled along taking what everyone dishes out to me, fallen and picked myself up and made the best of it. Again, it's the old programming that I can't be successful and that I should respect my superiors and not talk back to them. If I continue to let this programming run my life, I'll never get anywhere. This has and will be one of my biggest issues and obstacles to work through.

Not long after I took that job, I came home to find out my mom was going to take my father to the hospital. His condition was deteriorating and they needed to do some tests to try and find out where the pain was coming from. He had been on a very soft and light diet for quite some time. He just could not handle solid foods. One afternoon after work when I went by to visit, my mom told me that he tried to get out of bed and they thought he may have suffered a mild heart attack. They were going to watch him closely.

A couple days later he was having more difficulty with his heart rhythm and they took him down to intensive care. When I was there, he and my mom were talking about his will. She was telling him that she could not find his latest one that he had handwritten. He was wanting me to type it up and make it official. Because time seemed to be critical and he felt it was running out on him, he told me to take notes and put another one together. It was hard to understand him because he was wearing an oxygen mask at this time. He would take it off from time to time to clarify what he had told me. He had me read my notes back to him when he had finished.

That night, he called my mom about 10 p.m. He sounded better than he had for some time. He was perky and joking around with my mom. Her spirits lifted a bit after this call.

As it turned out, that perkiness was the calm before the storm. We got a call about 1 a.m. that next morning from the hospital saying that he developed great difficulty in breathing and asked to be placed on a respirator. That was Saturday morning of Labor Day weekend. I got up that next morning and told my mom that I would immediately go over to my office and get the will typed before going to the hospital. I had a contract project that I was working on and had to spend a little time with it.

I got to the hospital about two that afternoon. Roy did not look good at all. I told him I had typed his will and brought it with me. I read it to him and he motioned that he wanted to sign it. We called a nurse in to be a witness. The prognosis from the hospital staff was not very encouraging. They said he was deteriorating quickly.

My brother and sister-in-law were in town this weekend, but had to go back to Wyoming the next day. At least they had a chance to see Roy. They hadn't seen him for some time. Roger and Roy would spend hours out in the garage tinkering on the cars when he lived with my folks.

My mom called my sister in Albuquerque. She said she was going to fly in on Sunday. We all seemed to know that the end was near; that this time he would not recover. Roy had done so much for all of us in the past 20 years and was just like a real father to us. We were not ready to let go. Sue, his daughter came down from Cheyenne on Saturday.

Sunday, when I got to the hospital, he was struggling with trying to tell us something. He kept moving his hand and wrist in a circular motion. Finally, it dawned on me what he was trying to say. I had been in the hospital before on a respirator and I struggled with the doctors to get them to give me a pen and paper so I could write my questions and answers down. That's what Roy was asking for. We got a notepad and a pen. The very first thing he wrote was "Goodbye, I love you." Tears immediately began running from my eyes. He knew this was the end and he wanted to tell us that he loved us all.

He began writing up a storm. He told my brother what still needed to be done with the old car that he had been working on. He asked if Karla was coming. We told him she would be there sometime that day. He was relieved to know that everyone would be there in his final moments.

Karla was able to take the kids to Larry's store and leave them there so she could catch a flight to Denver. She showed up at the hospital about two or three on Sunday afternoon. A sense of peace came over Roy when he saw her.

I stayed at the hospital till after Karla got there, but I had work to get done and had to leave to go over to my office. Besides, the nurses didn't like too many people in the room at once in intensive care. Sue also came down that afternoon from Cheyenne. All of Roy's kids had come to see him at his bedside, except Tom, who was still in prison.

Monday was Labor Day. Mom and I took separate cars because I knew I couldn't spend all day at the hospital. I still had a lot of work to do because I had spent so much time at the hospital already. I knew I would have to leave sometime in the afternoon.

That morning when mom, Karla, Sue and I were all present, the doctor told us that he was barely breathing on his own. That the respirator was mainly keeping him alive. He told us what our options were and left us alone to decide what we would do. He said that whatever was decided would have to be agreed upon by everyone present. Roy came to long enough to motion us that he was ready to go and that he wanted us to cut off the life support.

Sue did not see this. She was out of the room when he did this. She could not accept that her father wanted to go in peace and that he was ready to give up. She would not agree to cutting off the life support. Karla and I tried to reason with her. After all, we had been so much closer to him over the last few years than she had ever been. She didn't even remember him on his birthday the last few years. How could she allow the doctors to prolong a life when he was ready to go?

Karla really got upset. She nearly made a scene in the hospital. Karla was closer to Roy than any of us kids; even his own daughter. She could not bear to sit by and see him suffer when he said he was ready to go. I went out of the room with Karla and tried to comfort her. She really blew up at Sue in the cafeteria at lunch time. We all tried to talk to Sue and explain to her that he would not suffer. The staff would see that he would go peaceably in his sleep and not in any pain. No matter what we said, this did not seem to sink in.

I had to go for a walk. Things were getting intense. Peggy was fighting her way out. She didn't want Roy to die, but did not want to see Roy suffer any longer. He had been her buddy like our real father. She knew she would miss him greatly.

Finally, about 4 p.m., we were able to bring Sue to her senses and see what she was doing to her father. The nurse talked to her and told her what it would be like for him. Finally, we were all in agreement. We gave the hospital permission to slowly shut off the respirator. They made sure Roy had plenty of morphine to keep him doped up and out of pain. It suddenly became a waiting game. The staff said it could take anywhere from a couple hours to several.

I asked if I could be alone with Roy for a little while. We all spent some time alone with him. They didn't know how long it was going to take, so my mom told me to go back to my office. She promised she would call when the time got close so I could get back to the hospital.

It was hard for me to concentrate, but I tried to get the work done. I got most of it finished when my mom called about 7:30 p.m. She said she wasn't going to call, but Karla reminded her that she promised she would. I told her that if she hadn't called, I would NEVER have forgiven her. I closed up my office and rushed to the hospital.

By the time I got there, his heart rate was all over the monitor and taking some big dips. I didn't get there any too soon. Peggy was there and I was there to hold and stroke his hand and tell him that we loved him and he would be missed. Within 15 minutes of my arrival, he was on his last breaths. My mom went out to get Sue to bring her in. She would not come. Karla and I were the only ones in the room when his heart finally stopped. I closed his eyes. We called the nurse and Mom. Mom and Sue came in. Roy was already getting cold and stiff. I reached over to give him one final kiss goodbye and I love you.

The nurse took the information necessary to call the mortuary. We left the hospital shortly after that. When we got home, we called Roger to tell him it was over. He was sorry that he didn't stay one more day. He said he and Linda would fly back to Denver in a couple days for the funeral.

Karla called Larry. He would take time off from work and drive up with the kids. They would be there on Wednesday.

I had never watched anyone die before. He was never in any pain. He looked so peaceful as the end came. I was happy I was there. I would have never forgiven my mother had she not called me to be there. I was not there when my real father died. It has been twenty-two years since then and some of my alters have still not completely processed it. They keep hanging on because they feel things are not yet finished.

With Roy's passing, I felt good about his finally ending the pain he must have been going through the last several months. I felt I could draw that part of my life to a close. I cried a lot in the hospital next to his bedside and in the waiting room. My grieving seemed to be short-lived. Roy meant a whole lot to me and I hated to see him go, but it was his time and I was ready to accept that and let go.

My real father's death was just thrown at me. I didn't know how to take it and work through it at the age I was. I never had the opportunity to tell him that I loved him and would miss him. I never had the chance to say I was sorry for all the bad things I had said to him and all the pushing and shoving. Peggy finds it extremely difficult to let go. She was very close to him.

Despite the arguing and fighting, my real father was a very loving and kind man with a big heart. He didn't know my alters but understood their needs and desires when they were presented to him. He was always giving to us kids and never really demanding anything in return except for us to be good at whatever we attempted in life. He tried to give us the world and then some, even though it was often beyond his means.

My father was manic-depressive. I see that clearly now. There were times when he would just go, go, go and spend all kinds of money that he didn't have. He would go on trips and drive for hours to bring back rental cars. He also had rapid mood swings. The only way he could deal with the torment of these mixed moods was to drink. It induced a numbing effect that would take away the torture of not knowing who or what he was. Even during the fights, there was a loving teddy bear underneath the shouting.

I can't help but think life would have been a whole lot different if doctors knew then what they now know about this illness. My life was chaos and torment until things became controlled and understood. The only way I could deal with my loneliness and depression and manic swings was to create alters who could take control of the situation. I have always had a reflective nature about me and rarely look to the outside for comfort and solice. I never needed alcohol or sex or allot of the vices many other people turn to.

I must admit that the cutting and other destructive acts I partook in could be considered as uncontrollable during that period in my life. I was confused and needed something to make me feel real. Seeing the blood brought me back into reality and told me I was alive and not dreaming. When I would overdose, Kim was feeling like I was not real and was indestructible. It was her way of testing the waters to see if I was really superhuman or just like any other human being. It was also a way to get people to show me how much they cared. If they cared about me and took measures to protect or treat me, I was a real person worth someone's attention.

I went to work the next day at my regular job. I explained what happened and asked if I could have time off for the funeral. They said I was entitled to three days of paid leave for a death in the family. I left Tuesday afternoon from work about 2:30 p.m. Other members of Mom and Roy's families were making arrangements to come to Denver.

The funeral would be Thursday. The body would be at the mortuary for viewing on Wednesday. Thursday we had a private ceremony of just family at the cemetery for burial. After internment, we went to Mom's church for a lunch and memorial service for friends and family. I did not go back to work until the following Monday.

It was hard to believe that Roy was gone. I thought that now Mom could have some freedom to go and do things. Roy didn't go anywhere and did very little his last year. He was plagued with a lot of ill health and his Parkinson's Disease got worse. He had very little energy to do anything but watch TV, but he did do that well.

Roy was a quiet presence in my life. This was even when I lived in the same house with him. We had some good discussions. I always respected his knowledge and authority. He was around when I needed him. He treated me like his own flesh and blood. He was the father I never had. My real father was an important figure in my life, but I had him for only 16 years of my life. Part of which I was too young to really know the man, the rest was a life filled with alcohol and arguing. Roy did not drink and despised arguments. Rarely did he ever raise his voice to anyone. Even when my mom argued with him, there would be only an inflection from time to time.

That year was not all work and suffering though some people would be willing to argue with that. Work is what you get paid for. When I donate my time and talents, I don't think of it as work, though it may drain me just as much.

During the spring, I took a class at the Community College of Denver that taught working with 3-D and animation on the Macintosh. It was a three hour credit class that met just seven Saturdays for eight hours. It was not an easy class but was fun. The time set up for the class was not near enough to really put a presentation of great worth together. I did not have the time to do anything real complicated. The answer was simplicity, but I did at least finish my final project and get an A in the class.

The previous December, I was selected to participate in the Greater Denver Chamber's Fast Track program for women and minorities. This was kind of a repeat of my entrepreneur course taken at Barnes. Only this time, the class had people who were in business or very close to getting into business. Seventy people started the class. I believe only about 39 finished. The final assignment was to write a business plan, as was with the other class. This program was well organized and had full community support. Anderson Consulting was going to review each of the business plans and make comments. I missed only one class and found it a great boost to the enthusiasm for my business.

I was hopeful of coming away with a business plan that would generate a loan to build my business. When I took the class, I had no idea that I would finally get a regular job that fall and decide to close my business. It was all I had to go with and I was going to make the best of it. With a bankruptcy in my past and being a service business, I had a couple strikes against me, but I just kept plugging away. I had to keep myself occupied or I would go absolutely stir crazy. If not that, I would risk falling into a very deep depression that would totally disable me again. That was one thing that I wanted to avoid at all costs. I was through with that kind of hell. I did not want to participate in that kind of life ever again.

I judged only a few speech meets in the spring. Saturdays were out in January and February when I was taking the class. When fall rolled around, I had my new job and it seemed that I had something else to do just about every weekend. I was still doing a little contract work and had mainly the weekends to work on it.

I continued with my responsibilities on the South High School CDM Committee. This program was really trying my patience. The committees were suppose to have the major roll in how the school was run, but the District administration and Superintendant always seemed to throw a wrench at us and was still dictating what we could and could not do. This was extremely frustrating. Everyone felt the frustration and many of the members began dropping off the committee. I refused to become a quitter but it got to be more than I wanted or felt I had to deal with. Besides, I had no kids in school and felt like my hands were tied. I resigned from the committee in January 1993.

There was a call for members to sing with the Early Singers at church. It was a choir that sang twice a month at the 8:15 a.m. service. It took a lot of prodding by the choir director, but I finally gave in. Susan was ecstatic. The only singing she had been able to do was in church and then she would bellow out the songs. I told her to be cautious, because Phyllis, the choir director, was serious about music. Members of the regular Chancel Choir had to try out for their spots. Susan is a natural as long as everyone else is singing on key. This choir turned out to be more of an ensemble. The choir usually had only seven to twelve members on a regular basis. Susan was one of three sopranos on many occasions.

With a new job and some money finally coming in, Mike got a wild idea. He decided to go out looking for a new car one night when I had full intentions of going over to the office to do some work. One thing led to another, and before I knew it, it was 9:30, and I came home with a new used 1989 Plymouth Grand Voyager van. I hate it when things like that happen. Alters go off on a tangent and making such big and expensive decisions without first talking it over with the others. Mike had this idea for some time and voiced it to the group, but we never expected it to happen just like that. I would have hoped he would have let a group go on a Saturday when we had all day to make a decision and negotiate a deal.

I kept the van. It was much nicer and roomier than my old truck. The truck was eight years old. That was the longest I had ever owned a vehicle. What got Mike thinking about a van was when Karla had helped me move some things from her house to storage. We could put more stuff in her van than I could in the back of my truck. It just made sense that a person that moved as much junk as I do have something that could do the job.

I had never bought a used car before, but a new one was way out of my price range. I learned one thing from this experience. You never buy a used car at night and without taking it to a service center for a thorough check out. I learned that the hard way. My brother was in town shortly after I bought the van. He checked it over then. He had to add a couple fuses to it and tighten the headlight. He also noticed that it was leaking oil and suggested I take it back to the dealership. Well, I did and it cost me just short of $300 in repairs in less than six weeks.

The other big change I had that fall came with my appearance. I was in need of visiting the eye doctor to get a change in my prescription. Before I made the appointment, I knew I wanted to try contact lenses again. It had been twelve years since I gave them up and figured technology had advanced enough that there should be some kind of lens that I could wear that would not be harmful to my eyes.

My alters seemed to think I was independently wealthy with this new job. They got me to make an eye appointment for being fitted with contacts. I wore contacts when I was in college and a few years after graduating. Technology was not there for soft lenses back then and I was forced to convert to hard lenses. After a couple years of wearing them and being in the drier Colorado climate, my eyes became irritated. My eye doctor back then strongly suggested that I go back to wearing glasses before the contacts damaged my eyes. I took his advice.

I went in the early part of November and had my eyes tested. I hadn't been to an eye doctor since 1988. I picked the doctor I did because he had seen me in the emergency room one Saturday in the spring when I had a bad eye infection. The prescription for the contacts was stronger than the supply house had in stock so they had to order them. I got my contacts the week of Thanksgiving.

I immediately started wearing them all day. It took awhile to get used to looking at the new me. The picture I got through my new eyes was not pleasant. The contacts allowed me to see just how fat I really was. Living with my mom and being on and off all the medication I had gone through the previous six years caused me to gain about 60 pounds. I was not pleased with my appearance, but I did not hate myself because of it. After my last hospitalization, I learned to love me for who I was. On the inside, my heart was solid gold. I just figure that someday, as done before, I will be able to lose the weight. In the meantime, I would do my best to remain attractive.

I had 90 days to decide about the contacts. I was having trouble with my eyes drying and vision blurring from time to time. I was having trouble reading close up. I went back to the doctor and he ordered me a new prescription for one of my eyes. This helped a little. I was bound and determined that nothing would keep me from wearing these contacts.

It wasn't until my check-up the following year that I realized why my vision would blur on me regularly. When I was sitting in the office after having had my eyes dilated, the blurring that I regularly experienced was comparable to the blurring I had when my eyes were dilated. I went to see Dr. Wilets right after that appointment and asked if any of the drugs I was on had the chemical that caused eyes to dilate. He looked it up, and as it turned out, everything I was taking had some of that chemical in it.

I knew that if I wanted to continue to wear contacts, that I was going to have to get used to this blurring. After three years, I still have this problem but have accepted it as the way things are and work with it rather than fight it. I have had to make some adjustments and find myself squinting or blinking a lot from time to time, but figure it is worth it. The freedom of not having to wear glasses is worth the adjustments I have had to make.

Christmas was just around the corner, and it looked like it would be just my mother and myself to celebrate the holiday and bring in the new year. A few days before Christmas, my mother got a call from my sister-in-law, Linda. My brother had become very ill and was rushed from work to the hospital. They thought he may have suffered a heart attack. They were going to transport him the next day by ambulance to Billings, Montana for further tests. My mom said she would try to get on a flight and meet them the next day in Billings.

Suddenly it was just me for Christmas. I didn't mind, though. It was going to be nice not having all the people around for a change. I had been alone only one other Christmas in my life. That was during the blizzard of 1982. I went to Christmas Eve services at church, came home and watched a little TV, and opened my presents. A nice relaxing evening.

I didn't know how long my mom would be gone. The day after Christmas, I decided to go out looking for a bed. I had decided it was about time for me to move out on my own again. After all, I knew my mom would want to sell the house once the estate was settled. I found a nice comfortable bed and placed it on layaway. I was tentatively looking to move out possibly in February.

Mom got back shortly after Christmas. She and Roger and Linda had sort of a falling out. Her domineering, take control personality, came on strong at the wrong time. Rog and Linda were not accustomed to her behavior and took offense to it.

After mom got back and cooled down a little, I broke the news to her that I was planning on moving out. She could accept it and help me look for a place or sit back and feel sorry for herself. Because of the blow-up in Wyoming, I felt kind of bad deserting her, too. But, I needed to get back out on my own again. I needed my own space to do what I wanted and come and go as I pleased. It was going to be tough finding a place that I could afford that would accept a dog.

In January of 1992, I joined a new support group for individuals with MPD. I had gotten the name of the group from my bipolar group facilitator. The name of the organization was Justus Unlimited. How fitting. This new group had an application process and waiting list. I received and filled out my application and sent it back. About three weeks later I got a call that there was a group I might fit into. The group met Thursday evenings in southeast Denver.

Having been in groups before, I was just a little nervous my first night. I wasn't sure just what to expect. I had not been around other multiples before and this was going to be a new experience for me. It was a relatively new group for everyone and so a lot of barriers were still being held by every one. I could see right off that this group could be good for me to explore and get to know my inner selves.

The facilitators openly encouraged alters to come to group if they had issues they needed to work through. I had never been in a situation like this before where my alters could show their full colors. I really felt this group could offer me what I was not able to get from Dr. Wilets or any of my previous therapy. I was looking forward to this.

Our key facilitator, Faith, and many of the other gals in the group were survivors of ritual abuse. I had a clear recollection of my childhood and knew this was not the case with me. Off and on, I questioned whether I fit into the group because of this. They kept insisting I was a survivor and had MPD and that was all that should matter.

Members of this group have come and gone. It still is a major part of my week and I get things there I don't get elsewhere. My alters feel comfortable enough to express what they are truly feeling. They have permission to speak out there when I might not listen to them during the rest of the week.

My mom never asked what went on at group, because she is still in denial that I have MPD. Besides, because of the confidentiality of the group, I would not have said much anyway; just general small talk.

In February, Mom and my trusty tape measure went with me on an apartment search expedition. I had a very small selection of places that would take Nikki. One was a little too pricey and two were not big enough to house me and my drafting studio. I had one place left on my list. It happened to be the first place I looked at. I didn't actually get in to see the type of apartment I was going to rent, because they had no vacancies.

I came home and took the two biggest units and laid out a floor plan. I measured all my furniture and proceeded to see how it would all fit. The place I didn't get in to measure seemed to have the best layout and most room. I filled out an application and placed a partial deposit to get on a waiting list.

I got a call the first of March telling me they would have a garden level unit available about the tenth of April. I told the manager that I would take it if I could get in to measure to be sure it would work. He lived in the same size of apartment and let me come over to measure his unit. It was going to work just fine.

I wasn't quite sure how Nikki would take to apartment living. She would not be able to go out during the day like at home, because nobody would be around to let her out. She would also need to learn how to work on a leash. She wouldn't be able to go outside and stay as long as she wanted on a nice day. Given time, I knew we would both adapt to the new environment.

I had lived in my parent's home this time for a little over six years. That was a long time. Longer than any time I had spent in any one place since being out of school. I only had my house for four years. I was ready for this change, though. My support group kept telling me that I needed to get out from the environment I was in if I was ever going to reclaim my identity and move forward with my healing. My mother was still reinforcing the programming of my earlier years while living with her.

By this time in my therapy, I had recognized my mother as the perpetrator, but also recognized that her behavior was not intentional and with ill-intent. It was the result of her upbringing and how she had been programmed. She was not willing to recognize this in herself, so felt there was nothing wrong. She was being the person she only knew how to be and thought what she was doing was for the good of all involved. She did not see just how overbearing and domineering she really was.

My mother is a very strong-willed person and feels that she can only do what is right and good. She does not have the ability to step back and look at what havoc she has created in the lives of the very ones she loves and mean the most to her.

I had reached a point where I could accept this in her. I knew that in this stage of her life, she was not going to change. I would have to learn how to deal with it in a healthy way. Just knowing what the situation is can make a lot of difference. I was willing to forgive my mother for her errors as a parent and person. Whenever I could, I would try to confront her with her behavior. I was not going to let the fear of hurting her intimidate me like it did. After all, she hurt me terribly.

The garden level apartment I got had nice big picture windows. It was kind of run down and needed work. Work that I quickly learned that the management could care less about. The move went fairly smoothly. I had two places to move. The furniture mom was giving me and my belongings at the house, and what I was keeping from the office. I had a couple yard sales prior to the move to try and weed out a lot of the stuff I no longer needed.

I moved on the Saturday before Easter. I hired an economy moving company. There were two guys and a big truck. They seemed pretty nice, but didn't move very fast. They didn't have the perception that professional movers had in how things fit together. When we got to my new apartment, they got the brilliant idea of moving the bulk of my stuff through the large bedroom window. It would save a lot of steps and having to go up and down stairs. I could see that it would cost me a lot more money if they had to go through the front door, so I told them do what would be most efficient.

We had a big project at work, and I was suppose to go in to the office after the movers left. Mom was out of town. She was down in Albuquerque spending Easter with Karla and her family. It was our birthday present to her in January. I was on my own to get everything done. Deep down that is just the way I wanted it.

The movers left at 4 p.m. I ran over to the house to get a quick bite to eat and let Nikki out, because she had been home alone since about ten that morning. I didn't know when I would get back to take her over to the apartment.

I got to the office about quarter to five. Laura, my supervisor, was winding down and getting ready to leave. It was a good thing she was still there, because I had left my ID badge at home. One other guy had left not long before I got there. Laura filled me in on what had gotten done and left, herself, about five thirty. I stayed and worked until around 7:30 p.m. I had a lot of work to do. I had just Easter Sunday to get my new place to a point that I could inhabit it.

I got over to my mom's around eight to pick up Nikki and her things. She didn't know quite what to make of the day. I got her over to our new home and gave her her first experience in some time on a leash. I had a retractable leash so she could go quite a ways without tugging. She didn't know what to make of this strange new place, but somehow she knew it was our new home.

The first thing I did was get my bed cleared off and made. It had been a long day, and I didn't know how long into the night I could go. I quickly found out that with a cable-ready TV, you need to have it connected to cable or an antenna. At this point, I had neither. I had totally spaced this little detail. Fortunately, I had a little portable black and white desktop set that had a radio. I at least had some noise and could watch the news. I finally peedered out around one in the morning.

I had too much to do the next day, so missed going to church. I got most of the kitchen in order and all the furniture set up. I still had a lot of boxes to go through, but that could be done during the week after work. Some of the boxes had been sealed since I moved out of my house and in with my folks. I had forgotten about some of the stuff that I had.

Knowing that I would have increased monthly expenses, I began looking for a second job about the same time I started looking for an apartment. I put in applications for part time work and continued to send out resumes for a better full time position. The search became complicated when Laura told me she would not switch schedules with me. She worked 7:30 to 4:30. This would have been perfect for having time to get home, let Nikki out and get a bite to eat and be at another job by 5:30.

I had not gotten another job by the time I moved in April. I knew I had enough money in reserve until mid-summer. After that, I would need that extra $150-200 a month that another job would bring in.

Finally, in June I got an awaited call. The Denver Post newspaper called and said they had an opening in my neighborhood to deliver papers on weekends to retailers and vending machines. I grabbed at the opportunity quickly. I started to work the next weekend. I was going to have to change my sleep routine on Saturday and Sunday. I would have to get up at 2 a.m. and be to the drop-off point by three. Saturday, I had a split shift. I delivered the Saturday edition early, but had to come back at eleven that morning to deliver the early "Bulldog" edition of the Sunday paper.

I had a supervisor go with me the first weekend to get me familiar with my route. We had to load our own bundles in our vehicle. Each bundle weighed about thirty pounds. We had to not only deliver the new papers, but pick up and count the returns. From time to time, we also had to place banner strips in the machines or signs in the front display plate. When we got back to the drop-off point, we had to bundle and stack all the returns. At the end of the weekend, we had to turn in our paperwork and time-sheets. I got good real quick with my mental addition. They expected the workers to be accurate with their figures on the returns and sell-outs.

The second week, I used my own van. I had to take out the middle seat. I left the one in the back where it was. My run was in the SE Denver and Cherry Creek neighborhood and shopping center. I had as few as thirty bundles for the Bulldog run and as many as fifty to seventy for the two early morning runs. It was not uncommon for me to move two tons of papers on a weekend. I was not sure whether or not my van would hold up to this torture.

I could tell right away that I was out of shape and overweight. I was huffing and puffing just by loading the papers in the van. I hadn't quite gotten over some bronchitis from January and would get real short of breath. I would sometimes cough until I could hardly breath, then feel like throwing up. I went to the doctor about this and he gave me an inhaler to use before going to work. That really helped.

I got to be quick at delivering my papers. I even did some driving that I normally wouldn't think of doing. I drove on the wrong side of the street and would go through red lights when there was no traffic to be seen. I had trouble at first with the hook that was used to open the machines but within a couple weeks got the touch just right. I only had trouble when I caught myself thinking about what I was doing. I finished my early morning runs by 7:30 on Saturday and 8:00 or 8:30 on Sundays. I was done on Saturday by one in the afternoon.

The only thing I didn't like was the bulldog run at noon on Saturday. By that time there was plenty of traffic on the streets. I had trouble finding places to park in the Cherry Creek shopping area to deliver some of my papers.

One September morning, I was going back to the drop-off point and passed a construction site off of Colorado Blvd. and Interstate 25. The sign had been put up just that previous week. There was a big computer store going into the shopping center. I thought to myself that this was something Denver needed badly and might be a fun place to work. A few weeks later, there was an ad in the paper for employees. I thought about it for a couple days, then made a call to schedule and interview.

By the first of October, I had a new part time job. It didn't come soon enough, though. The week after I noticed the sign, I was heading home but going to get some gas first. On the way to the gas station, a guy at the stop light said I was smoking underneath my car. I checked the heat gauge and the needle was way up to hot. Fortunately, I just had to go across the street. I pulled into the station and raised the hood. It was leaking coolant underneath. I thought to myself, great, I've cracked the radiator block. The Conoco station did not have any service attendants, so I went across the other street to an Amoco station to have one of the attendants take a look at it. We let it cool down. He flushed the radiator and put some no leak stuff in it and some more coolant. I told him I would try to get to the Amoco over on Colorado Blvd. because they had a larger full service department there. It took me an hour and a half to get over there. I could go about four to six blocks and have to stop and shut the engine off.

I was sure glad for one thing. This happened on Sunday after my paper route. I had a whole week to get it fixed. When I got to the other station, they, too, thought it was the radiator. I was there about 45 minutes. It had cooled down enough that I was able to drive home. I got home around eleven that morning. I just barely made it to my parking lot.

I got off work a little early on Monday so I could take my car to the dealer. The next day they called me with the prognosis. In addition to the radiator being cracked, the transmission was shot. It was going to cost me at least $1500 to get it fixed. I said I could buy a new car for less than that.

So I did. By Friday, I was driving a 1993 Plymouth Grand Voyager. It was an $18,000 vehicle and I was able to get 8% financing on it. My payments were more than on the other van by about $100 a month. There goes my paycheck from the second job. I wish I knew then that I was going to quit my paper route and take on a more lady-like job. I would have bought something less expensive.

My mom was not very proud of my second job with the Post. She did not let anyone know what I was doing. She was embarrassed that her daughter was a newspaper person. Just to show you how she felt about it, she didn't even tell her beautician who she tells everything.

In August, I celebrated my first anniversary with my full time employer. I was entitled to one week of vacation. I was hoping to take it over the Christmas holiday and go see Karla, who had moved to California. With my new job at the store, I knew Christmas was the biggest part of the retail year, and they would not let me off. The store had two weeks of sales training scheduled during the middle of October. I decided to take my week of vacation and use it for the first week of training.

Sales training began October 11. The first week involved basic selling skills and further orientation to the company. It was very informative. I was the only woman to be selected for the sales floor when the store opened. I fit in with all the guys. I was very active in the classes and, even though I was only part time, fit in the group like a full time employee. I missed the second week of training which consisted mainly of vendor training on the products we would be carrying. I was hired mainly to work in the software department, so wasn't overly concerned about what I was missing.

Soft opening for the store was October 30. That's when the store opened it doors for customers but did not advertise such. Grand Opening wasn't going to be until November 8. This gave all employees a week of working with customers and getting the feel for the job before the crowds descended upon us.

Grand Opening was a tremendous success. We were well accepted into the marketplace. Our sales were the highest for Grand Opening day for the entire company. We were beat out a few days later, though, when the store in Hawaii opened.

The crowds were overwhelming. I couldn't believe how many people were novices to computers, yet very eager to learn all they could. I bounced non-stop from customer to customer in the software aisles during each of my shifts for over a week. There was an awful lot of software to familiarize myself with; most being IBM compatible stuff that was foreign to me. I learned a lot about it, though, by reading the packaging with the customers and listening to what the customers were saying about products they were familiar with.

The most important part of selling is to listen to the customer. I learned that real fast. There was a lot of knowledge to be gained through listening. I became a very informed salesperson. My knowledge soon got around the store. I soon got the label of Queen of Software.

I had other valuable knowledge that was needed by the store. I had been working with Apple computers since 1986 and most of the other sales force were only IBM literate. They had knowledge I needed and I had something they needed so I gained tremendous respect from the other employees. We had a couple other employees that were practical users and knowledgeable about Macintoshes that usually handled hardware sales. I did get a lot of the phone calls from customers regarding Macs and software sent my way.

At times when none of the other Mac experts were scheduled, I would wander over to the Apple hardware counters. At first I was unsure of the knowledge I really had to share. It didn't take long, though, to know that I knew much more than the basic consumer who came in to browse or buy. It wasn't long before I had the confidence of being an informed salesman and could really help the customer. I began to split my time between Apple hardware and the software department. Besides, they had hired a couple other employees that felt more comfortable working the software aisles.

We were soon into the Christmas season. People were so eager to talk to someone who really knew something that they would line up and follow me around the store just waiting to have me help them. On Saturdays, I could easily have four to six people wanting to obtain my expertise. What an ego trip. I was flying on cloud nine. I got sucked into the whirlwind of this new demand for what I had to share. I began selling a lot of computers. I even sold my share of extended warranties which put extra money in my pocket.

For an overly introverted person, alters stepped forward that I didn't know ever existed. I was familiar with Francie, who was very outgoing and friendly, but I think her personality meshed with the unknown silent alter who engulfed herself in the world of the computer.

I've been so accustomed to alters evolving on demand to handle situations that become overwhelming to me. I have had a number of new alters just appear out of nowhere over the last five or six years. I had my old reliable group members from way back, but new ones were eager to come forth and take control. I welcomed them, but started to become confused as to who was who. Often, I didn't know who these new personalities were until I took the time to sit, meditate and ask them to identify themselves. This new alter that was wrapped up in the retail world is Connie. She loves computers and loves being able to help people. She loves to be around people. The other alters seemed to welcome her with open arms.

I was great when I was at the store, but I couldn't wait to get home to the peace and quiet of my own little world. Anyone seeing me in both worlds would clearly see that I had different personalities and more than one life.

I was totally addicted to the lift the store gave me. I asked for as many hours as I could muster into my schedule. I worked my 40 hours at US WEST and then another 27-30 hours at the store. It stimulated me into a semi-hypomanic rush. This high became very addicting. Dr. Wilets recommended that I cut back my hours, because it WOULD catch up with me sooner or later, and he didn't think I would enjoy another crash.

I had never been popular with peers before. Here, everyone was coming to me for help or answers to their questions. For the first time in my life I had an outlet for the wealth of knowledge I had accumulated all my life. I was on top of the world. For once, I was the focal point of attention. Connie ate it up. Myself, I would prefer not to have all that attention. I get embarrassed when the focus is on me. What a mix!

I still had some other activities in 1993 other than work. Again, most people would think the extracurricular activities were also work. Work is when you get paid. Relaxation is when you are doing what you enjoy and not expecting to be paid.

I was Membership Chairman for my Desk and Derrick Club. Because of all the time I was spending with my two jobs, I must admit I did a very poor job of it. My only accomplishment during the year was to get new members processed expeditiously and to design and print a new club brochure. I was really wanting to prepare a knock-out orientation program, but never got it finished. I worked on it during lunches during the day, but just couldn't quite pull it together. I wasn't as enthusiastic about the club as before, because I was no longer in the industry. I had gradually distanced myself from what was going on. I decided that I would not renew my membership the next year.

Working retail as a second job, my Sundays were tied up. I was not able to go to church on Sundays. I worked Wednesday nights so could not attend the dinner and program on those evenings. I still had my connection to the church. I would occasionally do special graphics projects. I was still the editor of the singles newsletter. This was something I had to fit in once a month. My schedule really got full and tight when that time of the month came along.

I think my mom didn't like me working at the store any more than she did the paper route. At least when I delivered papers, she saw me once in awhile. Now, she was lucky to see me one or two hours at the most a week. Mainly, it was to deliver and pick up my laundry. She was a lifesaver in that aspect. I would never have had time to do my own washing and ironing. Besides, I despised ironing. I always have. I freely welcomed the offer she made to do my laundry.

Nikki had to make some major adjustments, too, to all my hours away from home. First, she had to adjust to going out on a regular schedule and not whenever she got the urge. She did quite well with this. Better than I had ever anticipated. I guess I still thought of her as a young little dog; not one that was eleven years old.

When I took the job at the store, I realized I would not have time to dash home and let her out and feed her, let alone, myself. I had noticed in the apartment complex newsletter that a gal in the complex did pet sitting. I gave her a call before starting to work evenings. I made arrangements for her to come over and walk and feed Nikki on the nights that I worked. Nikki proved to be a one person dog. She did not take well to Sandy at all. She would hide from her when she came over. She had to carry Nikki outside to do her job. She often left her food untouched until I came home from work. This was quite a shock to her system at this time in her life. I needed the extra money at the time and had no other choice.

I noticed a big change in Nikki this year. She did not bark at the kids when they played outside my window. She didn't even bark during thunderstorms. She used to go absolutely crazy during a big storm. Now, she just laid there. I soon realized she must have lost a great deal of her hearing. Her eyesight was still pretty good, and she barked profusely when she saw people walking by. When I had her into the vet for her shots, the doctor said she had developed cataracts over her eyes. I said she seemed to see quite well and the doctor said, dogs adapt and learn to see through them. They have extra senses that are more powerful than we have that allows them to adapt. I made myself start to think about the day when she would no longer be around. I finally admitted that it could be sooner than I would want to think. From that point on I made myself do regular reality checks with Nikki.

It was clear that I was not going to California for Christmas, but there was a good airfare promotion that my mom couldn't pass up. She asked if I would be too terribly upset or lost if she went out to Karla's for Christmas. I told her not at all and that I thought she should go. Besides, she and Karla have always been closer and Stephanie and Daniel are her only grandchildren. She wants to share in their growing up whenever she can. I reassured her that I would be all right and could handle doing my laundry for the couple weeks that she would be gone.

I was really glad that she was going. As I mentioned earlier, I liked being by myself at Christmas. I'm not one much for celebrations and family gatherings. I felt like I was a rude freeloader whenever the family got together. I didn't help much with the meal preparation, did very little to help clean up. When the meal was over, I would usually wander off somewhere and go to sleep. This was not an occasional occurrence, but regular. It was almost like a habit. I would go along for the ride, so to speak. Actually, I would have rather been at home by myself, doing what I wanted to do; usually nothing. I was not good at socializing. Francie did not feel comfortable about showing herself to the family. Alters rarely showed themselves to my family. I don't know whether it was because they didn't feel safe or whether they didn't want family to know that I was anything but a quiet, introverted, depressed individual. Alters had been known to come out and play and present themselves when my parents were not visible. It usually happened when I was alone in the basement in my own dwelling.

My girlfriend, Joyce, had bought a townhouse in Denver, even though she worked in Louisiana. She wanted to have a place back in Denver that she could move to when she retired. She has another 15-18 years before that happens, but also wanted something to live for besides her job. She was a bankruptcy analyst for the Department of Justice. She despised New Orleans and couldn't wait to get out of there. She was going to be in town over Christmas. She was having the bulk of her furniture moved to her townhouse Christmas week. We tentatively made plans to do something on Christmas.

The store closed early Christmas Eve, so I did not have to work. I went to Candlelight Service at church that evening. I kind of revolted against my mom in a quiet way. I did not dress up. Dress codes nowadays are almost nonexistent. People came to this service wearing the whole gamut of attire. I put on a pair of my best dress jeans, a nice blouse and a blazer and went to church that way. No one really noticed. I was a little self-conscious, but tried to ignore the programming. I was doing what I really felt I wanted to do and didn't have anyone there ridiculing me for my choice and decision. This was nice, though awkward. I really felt strange and slightly uncomfortable. I know Alice, my mother alter, was scolding me in the background. No matter what I did, I could not get away from my mother's programming.

My support group was encouraged by my acts of defiance. They reassured me that these kinds of acts are really healthy as long as they are not carried to extremes. They told me that I had come a long way in regaining my identity(ies) since I first started the group. Despite this, they felt I had a long way to go with my healing. They didn't like the fact that I was trying to hide the pain and push the work aside by working myself to death. They kept telling me I needed more time to take care of my kids inside; let them have some fun once in awhile. I told them I didn't think anyone inside knew how to have fun. They responded by saying it's about time they learned.

I tried to heed the suggestions of the group. Peggy loved movies, so when I had a Saturday night off, I would rent three movies and have a movie marathon for her. Others enjoyed it, too, I know. That was about all that I would allow, other than getting a little rambunctious and playful with Nikki. Everything was so serious and focused around work. This has been our whole life. We don't know anything else.

I've known work since I was old enough to reach over the sink on a stool. I always had some chore that kept me from playing. When I did get to play, I did not have pleasant experiences. It seemed that friends were always wanting to take advantage of you in one way or another. It was no fun to play alone. It was better to be doing something productive. I learned to turn work into play. To most people, it would seem that I am not having fun, but a lot of the work I choose to do is what I enjoy and IS fun to me.

I guess that is why I don't have a whole lot of friends. It's the fear of being used. I have so much inside my head and in talents and skills, that I feel friends are only my friends because they know they can get something from me. I usually give it to them freely not thinking about my wants and needs. I have not learned to ask for something in return. I deserve things just as much as the next guy, but I can't humble myself to the point of saying I need help from someone else. I have been on my own since very young and had to get where I am by myself. It isn't pleasant when you know you are being used. I guess that's why I don't reciprocate the gesture. I know how it feels and don't want to wish it on my friends. It doesn't feel good much of the time.

Dr. Wilets says that I could always say "no." I told him that word was not an active part of my vocabulary. "No" means rejection to me. I have been rejected all my life for one reason or another. It's very hurtful to be rejected and an outcast. I feel so sympathetic to the other guy that I don't want them to feel the rejection I have felt. I am used to the pain it induces. I am used to being the punching bag. It is easier for me to go on feeling the rejection and hurt, because I have become numb to it and just accept it as a way of life. Others may not be so accepting of it.

I guess that's why I am so addicted to the atmosphere at the store. It is the only place I do not feel rejected. I do feel used excessively, but I am getting something back and it is not all one-sided.

We had inventory at the store shortly after the first of the year. I guess it did not go well. When it was audited, there was a big shake-up. The store manager and sales manager were let go. I had no clue as to what was going on. I came into work one day and the air was full of gossip and they were gone. The new store and sales managers were being promoted from the "baby store" in Colorado Springs.

More shake-ups would be coming down the pike within the first year of the store's opening. In February, the Merchandising Supervisor was let go. Because the company believes strongly in promoting from within, an announcement was made that interested employees could attend training sessions to vie for the position. Training would be from 7:30 to 9:00 on Friday mornings for five weeks.

I was definitely interested. I had accumulated some more vacation hours and requested to take that time and come in late on Friday mornings. I told them it was training for my new Lead position I had been awarded in January.

I thought retail management paid a lot because my brother-in-law, Larry, was able to afford a nice house for my sister and she did not have to work. Boy, was I wrong. Starting pay for the position was $17,000 with a profit bonus cut. I could potentially earn $25-28,000 in the Denver store with the bonuses it had paid out so far. I was making $23,000 at my other job. It would be a fairly even trade off with a lot of room for advancement. In my position as Art Director, I was pretty much stuck where I was. There was no growth opportunity. The only thing was, with the store I would be putting in 50-60 hours per week and would not have time to have another job. I could try to tutor on the Mac to bring in some extra cash.

I figured that salary would be temporary. Within a year I could promote up the ranks to a much higher paid position. Within two to three years, if I played my cards right, I could be a store manager. Somehow I would make do with that.

Towards the end of the training program the field was narrowed down to just one other guy and myself. The management would take a vote after we each had a group interview. They would announce the selection of the new supervisor at the last class.

I did not feel I did a good job in my interview. The other candidate said he thought he could have done better, too. I don't know whether he was just saying that to make me feel good or he really meant it. This is a cut-throat market and men will say anything to beat out a woman. I'm convinced of that through past experiences.

I really wanted this chance and was making plans for it, but had no clue as to whether or not I would be selected for the position. Before the last class, the store manager called me into the office. They said it was a tough decision, but he wanted to congratulate me on being selected as the new Merchandising Supervisor. I would assume my responsibilities the 1st of April. This was two weeks off.

I couldn't believe how things were working out for me. I had made the decision at the beginning of the year to increase my hours with the store so that I would be classified a full time employee with 35 hours. I basically allowed myself one night a week off, and that was really not a night off. That was Thursday night when I had my MPD support group meeting. Some kind of work was always involved in that meeting. By doing this management was made aware of how serious I was about my job with the store and my new career direction.

One thing concerned me, though. My lease on my apartment was going to expire the first of April. They did not have six month leases. By taking the management position, I would have to be open to relocation with the company. If on a lease, I would still be responsible for the time the apartment would be vacant. It could be one month or the duration of the lease. The latter was unlikely, but something I had to consider. The other concern I had was how I would move and be able to find a new place that would accept a dog.

I'm not an overly religious person but I do have firm beliefs. I believe that God is always looking out for our best interest and things will usually work out in the end. Nothing could be truer than that.

One Sunday around the first of March, I noticed a change in Nikki's disposition. She seemed a bit restless. She couldn't stay settled, but then would sleep for long hours. She didn't want to go outside. She had no appetite. I went to pick her up that evening and she let out a loud cry. This alarmed me, but I had no clue as to what was going on with her. It didn't seem too serious to rush her off to a vet. I thought I would just watch her for a couple days to see if it persisted.

The next morning I got up and she was panting regularly like she was out of breath. Again, she did not want to go outside. Now, I was concerned, but I couldn't stay home. I would call Sandy, my pet sitter, and tell her to call me that evening when she went over to feed her. If I had to, I would take her into the vet that night after work if she wasn't any better.

Sandy called me quite alarmed. Nikki was breathing very heavily. She was very listless. She did not want to go out. She had a glaze over her eyes. I wanted to come home so badly, but we had two people call in sick that night and there was no way they would let me take off. We were short-staffed to begin with on Monday nights.

I got home at 10:30. I immediately found the number for the vet that I had last taken her to. They did not have emergency hours, but referred me to a place over near one of the universities. I called and rushed Nikki over there. The doctor did not want to alarm me, but he let me know it was serious. He would put her in an oxygen tent while they ran tests on her. He promised to call as soon as he knew something. He said there was no reason for me to stay. She would be in good hands.

Somehow, on the drive away from the hospital, I realized that this might be it for Nikki. I knew what was wrong could be life threatening. I just kicked myself for not making myself stay home that morning and take her to the vet then. I guess my conscious was in denial to how old she really was and that this was when things start to happen to dogs that age.

I didn't go straight home. I went over to my mom's. I had to ask her if I could borrow some money to pay the vet bills. I did not have the money to cover the expenses and they expected to be paid up front. She agreed to loan me $300. After all, Nikki had been a big part of her life for the past twelve years. Mom had taken care of her each time I was in the hospital. In fact, my mom had the responsibility of her care within the first three months after I got her. She gave her one of her first toys, which she still had to that day.

The vet called back about 3 a.m. with the bad news. Nikki was experiencing major heart failure. They could put her on life support and try to correct the problem but it would not buy her much time. I said I did not want her to suffer any more than she already had. I thought the best decision was to put her down. I wanted to come back to the hospital and say goodbye to her before they did it, though. He said that would be fine. I immediately got out of bed and dressed and drove to the hospital. He brought Nikki out to me. She looked to be really suffering and asking for mercy. I said my good-byes. I knew people had been with their pets when they were given the shot, but somehow could not bring myself to ask for this.

On my way back home I kicked myself again for this. I remember how at peace I was with Roy's passing while being there for his last breathes of life. Here I left Nikki with total strangers in her last moments.

This gesture still haunts me today. I have not been able to draw my connection to Nikki to a close. I feel Peggy and Samantha are resenting me for this. I had Nikki cremated. Her ashes are still sitting on my dresser. I have a painting I did of her hanging at the foot of my bed. In my daily life, I don't miss her because of how my life has changed in the past year. I have moments, though, when her absence is clearly felt.

Nikki's death could not have come at a more ideal time. As I said, the Big Guy is watching over me. That very day of her death, I stayed home from work and went out looking for a new apartment. I now had no restrictions on where I could live. I was limited only by the space I needed and what I could afford. By the following Saturday, I had found a new place and made a deposit. It was closer to the store and a second floor apartment with a balcony. No longer was I going to allow myself to live in a basement or garden level apartment. I am uplifted and I need the brightness a day has to offer.

Now, there was nothing holding me back from advancing with the computer store. I could move anywhere without the concerns of a pet owner. Things were looking up.

I moved the first of April before assuming my new responsibilities. I had given notice to my other job and March 28 was my last day. I had given them only one week's notice. I felt bad about it but their interests were not with their employees, so I had to hold my best interests at bay.

I was pushed into my new position feet first. There was no formal training as to what was expected of me. The training I had gone through earlier was basic supervisor training. It was not specific to the responsibilities of the Merchandise Supervisor. They expected me to just know what I was suppose to be doing. I knew I was responsible for the appearance of the store and the monthly merchandising of aisle displays. I was also responsible for proofing the weekly ad. Other than that, I was expected to do whatever was dished out and assigned to me. No instructions as to the right or wrong way; just get it done. I learned the point of sale system in the systems room by trial and error. Anyone with a good head on their shoulders could have figured it out anyway.

I got along great with Klaus, the Sales Supervisor. Steve, who transferred up from the Springs, was my boss. We didn't quite see eye to eye. He was always pushing me and putting me down. He counseled me a number of times telling me how the employees said I was putting them down and being demanding of them.

I never put anyone down. I was demanding, but whenever I asked someone to do something, I would say please and then thank them for their performance. Isn't that what you are suppose to do? Steve would never give me names. It was always just hearsay. I told him if he could tell me who was feeling this way, I could talk to them and come to an understanding behind my intentions.

Yes, I demanded a lot from people. I grew up in the school that when you are at work, you are suppose to work; not stand around drinking coffee and shooting the bull. That comes when all the work is done that needs to be done. I can have fun with the best of them, but when there is a job to be done, I expect it to get done.

Retail is a male-dominated profession. Computer sales especially. There was only one other woman on the sales floor at this time. Guys get overly threatened when a woman is placed over them. Their ego gets bent out of shape. They are no longer macho if a woman is giving them orders. I have had to deal with this all my life. I was not going to let it get to me this time. Last time I gave in and stepped down. Not this time. I want this bad enough and nothing is going to shake me.

Corporate management had made the decision that Denver would have a second store within 18 months of the first one opening. The decision had not been made as to where it would be. Demographic records by our buyers would decide that. If the new store did come to be, it would be a chance for me to move up and stay in the Denver area. I eagerly awaited the decision.

By summer I had earned a week's vacation. I had not seen Karla and her family in over a year. I made the decision that I would take my vacation around the Fourth of July and go visit them out in Sacramento. My mom paid for the plane ticket so I could go. We got a real good fare from a local airline. I would spend five of my ten days out there.

Earlier in February, I came to the truth that I did not have enough hours in the day to do everything I needed. My lunch hours were going to waste. I had saved some money from my work and some of the last disability checks I had gotten. I also sold my old Mac IIsi computer to one of the guys at work. This gave me enough money to afford a notebook computer. With this money, I bought a PowerBook 180. I took this to work with me every day. I was able to keep current with my finances and do the singles newsletter when that time of the month rolled around. I also used it to write in my journal.

I had started these memoirs back in 1986, but got sidetracked and found I was not really ready for a project of this magnitude. However, now was the time. I made the decision that I would try it again when I started my vacation. I had acquired quite a lot of insight into who I was and what I was about since then through my therapy and group. I had also matured quite a bit. Finding the right combination of medications to treat my bipolar illness was really the changing point in my life.

I took my PowerBook to California with me to work on this book. I started it about four days before I left. I had a very peaceful visit. I got a lot written. I would write for about four or five hours a day. The rest of the time, I was out by the pool with Daniel reading over some of the papers I brought with me. I played some games with Daniel, my nephew, on my computer. I spent some time with Stephanie. She had really grown. She was now seven years old and making a lot of progress. She was still not walking, but had improved on her balance and could take three to six steps on her own. I couldn't understand her talking when I got there, but by the time I was ready to leave, I could figure out a lot of what she way saying.

The only thing that bothered me about the visit was the way Karla talked to the kids. She was my mom all over again. I was being triggered constantly. She would criticize Daniel and threaten him with punishment if he did not behave. She never thought twice about disciplining him. She was very stern with both kids. I knew it was necessary with Stephanie because she did have some very serious behavior problems. Daniel can try his parent's patience, but he was very polite and mature for his age.

I saw a lot of me in Daniel. I just kept hoping to myself that he doesn't experience the same difficulties I have had. He is too good a boy to have to go through something like that. He is very smart and very creative with his activities. He has a lot of talents. He is artistic and loves to write. He has had to take on a lot of responsibilities at an early age by having a handicapped sister. At eleven years old, he had a paper route and was doing well with it. Everyone on his route liked him and were generous with him at Christmas.

When I was hired at the computer store, I signed a paper saying I would not partake in activities that posed as a conflict of interest with the store. I had taken on a few tutoring jobs with customers, because we did not offer any Macintosh training at the store. This surely could not be a conflict. My problem was that I was not secretive about these extracurricular activities. I openly spoke about what I was doing. After all, I felt I was doing nothing wrong.

Nothing could have been further from the truth. At the end of my vacation, I had a job up in Aspen with a realtor who had spent $6000 on equipment. She wanted someone to show her how to use the software and computer she had just bought. She was going to pay me $30 an hour plus mileage. Not too bad for one day's work. It was certainly a lot better than what I was getting from the store.

This came back to hit me in the face in early August. On one of my days off, this realtor's friend called for me at the store. It got transferred to Steve. She said that I had helped her friend set up her computer and she told her to call me if she had any problems while her friend was away. A couple days later, I got called into Joel's office with Steve. They put before me a written disciplinary form. It said that I was not suppose to associate with customers after the sale and that such behavior was against store policy.

I was so intimidated by this ganging up that I couldn't stand my position. I did say that I was only tutoring her and that she had already set her system up before I met with her. I told them that I felt that since the store did not offer Mac classes, it was not a conflict to tutor customers. Their interpretation was that no employee would have any personal financial gain from activities outside the store with customers.

I felt like going to the Regional Manager with this issue, but decided to back down. The form stated that any further activity such as this would result in termination with the company. I did not believe their interpretation of the policy was correct, but I was not really in any position to argue. I had just been threatened with my job. Knowing how hard it was to find a good job, I decided to stand down on this one.

They told me to call the lady back and get the policy straight with her after I helped her with her problem. I did and the problem was nothing like what Joel and Steve made it out to be. Her question could have been the question of any customer. It amounted to a printer problem that a number of people had been experiencing. I told Joel about this, but he was not about to retract the action he had already taken.

Not wanting to jeopardize my future, I informed all my tutor customers that I could no longer help them out. I referred them to CompUSA or Random Access Training division. They were the only places I knew had regular classes in town.

This issue was raised a few more times by customers coming into the store. I tried to explain to them that I was informed it is not store policy for employees to participate in such activity. Then I would pass them on to Steve to let him explain to them why I could not provide the follow-up service they were needing.

I had another conference with Joel and Steve before this that was a little more productive. I told him that I had seen on one visit by our Regional Manager that the base pay for a supervisor in our size of store was $17,200. I told him I was earning only $17,000 and didn't think that was right. I told him I had full intentions of asking for $19,000 when I got the job, but was so happy that they selected me that I would wait for my 90 day review in the position. He informed me that reviews after your very first 90 days came only in January and that was when raises were given on performance. I told him I was making much less than I was at my other single job, let alone two jobs. With the hours the store was keeping and the fluctuating schedule, I couldn't work another job. I could not survive on the money they were paying me.

I explained that I had traded in my van for a smaller, cheaper car, but took a big hit on it because I had negative equity in it based on the trade-in value. As a result, I ended up paying $18,000 for a $12,000 car. My interest rate jumped way up and my payment only dropped $100 per month when it should have been two. I said I have made sacrifices and busted my butt to prove my capabilities at the store and they should recognize this and do something more for me. He said that he and Steve would talk it over and get back with me.

The mention of the new store came up in this conversation. I told him that I would be very interested in transferring to the new store. I felt I needed a clean break with all new employees to get away from these jealous rumors that were being spread about me. I told him that I could not transfer for any less than $19K. He thought I could have a lot to offer that store and would recommend me to Tom, the Regional Manager, with a raise to that amount.

The new store was going to be up by where Karla and Larry used to live on the way to Boulder. Negative vibes were flowing through the Denver store and I really needed to get away. It was going though major changes that didn't feel good to me. I knew starting up a new store would be hard work, but I could go in fresh as an authoritative figure and be respected by the employees.

It was first thought that the official transfer to the new store would be in September. As it turned out, it didn't come till the first of October. I was a little upset over how things transpired. Mike, who had since become my Sales Manager, was going to the new store as Sales Manager. We got along great and had a lot of the same beliefs. I would enjoy having him as my boss. He transferred his duties over the first part of September. The other manager that was going to the new store was David back in receiving. He was suppose to start the same time as me, but somehow pulled some strings and got moved over a week earlier than me. I was sure some "good 'ol boy" politics were behind it.

I struggled through my last weeks as Merchandise Supervisor at the Denver store. On my last day, I spent almost two hours with one customer. She was going to buy the extended warranty, but since I would not be in the payroll system when her computer came in, I was going to lose out on it.

The new store manager had come to the Denver store the end of August. He seemed like a nice guy. He came to the company from a warehouse retail establishment. He lost his job when a bigger chain bought them out.

A couple weeks before I was suppose to make the switch, Yvette, the Denver Administrative Assistant, gave me a copy of my personnel change record that showed my transfer and pay rate. I sat down and took a look at it, and found something terribly wrong with it. It showed me only getting a raise to $18,500 base and no position title.

The first opportunity I could get Joel alone, I explained to him that that was not what we had discussed. I told him that my rent increase and added car expenses to drive 40 miles instead of two would not be covered with this pay increase. I said something would have to be done. He said he would talk to Tom again and okay it with him. Three days later, Yvette came back to me and said she had completed the paperwork to change my pay rate and give me the title of Sales Supervisor.

I was informed that I would be teaching the Basic Sales Training course during the two weeks of sales training. I was disappointed that I would not get to participate in the hiring of the sales force, but because Mike interviewed and hired me, I felt confident that they would hire some good people for me to work with. I had basically one week to prepare for this. All sales associates were required to take a sales skill test and be certified within the first 30-60 days of employment.

I would spend the first week of training at the Denver store and participate in the training. Because our first receipt of merchandise would come the 7th of October, I would then be working out of the new store. I didn't miss that much, because not very many sales associates had been hired. There were eight associates that sat in on the first week of training. We were going to hurt real bad if we didn't get some more people hired, quick. This meant that sometime before the store opened, I would have to go through my presentation again to bring the new hires up to speed. This was just the first of it. Somehow, things would all fall into place. At least I hoped they would.

Just before I reported for my responsibilities at the new store, I attended the Trinity Singles Fall Retreat held at a local retreat facility in Evergreen. Everything seemed to work out just right so I could go. The direction of the retreat really interested me and I knew I could get a lot out of it if I went. I could have gone up Friday night when it started, but I was tired after a long day at the store and wanted to get a good night's sleep. I went up the next morning before dawn. I got there in time for breakfast.

Our presenter was a psychologist and a real personable guy. He was very open and willing to share his life's experiences as he would hope that we would. A great deal of the discussions focused around our relationships with family and friends. Not so much was on romantic relationships. I did quite a bit of sharing and became quite emotional at times. It felt good to share the things that were bottled up inside of me with a different group of people.

I had an immediate draw to the speaker and felt that this is a guy I could relate to and would like as a possible therapist. I approached him after the Saturday session and explained my situation. I told him I was looking for a new therapist and filled him in on my diagnosis and prognosis. He was very connected, but when I told him that I had MPD, he kind of backed off. He said, as a rule, he did not treat patients with this diagnosis. He referred them to other, more competent therapists. He said his office associate did work with this kind of patient. He did end it by saying that he would take what I told him and think about it.

I had talked to Dr. Wilets about finding another therapist. I came to realize that he was really uncomfortable working with me when my alters were involved. He never encouraged them to be present, though some of them showed up regularly. He could tell they were there but did not attempt to work through any of their issues with any sort of dedication. I guess the incident several years back with Ross Carlson kind of shook him up and scared him about what multiples were capable of doing.

After the Saturday retreat session, I asked Dale, the singles minister, if I could talk with him a for a bit. He agreed. I had told him about a year or two earlier that I had MPD, but he must not have absorbed that piece of information when I was explaining some of the trauma I had experienced. Anyway, I re-explained things to him and told him where I was with my mother. I guess I just wanted to spill my guts this weekend. I needed a good, strong emotional release.

I told him that I felt that people were using me and how I can never say no to anyone. I felt guilty when I would do something without expectations of reciprocation, then wonder when someone was going to do something for me. As a Christian, I felt that I should give of myself unconditionally, but deep down I really felt I should deserve to get some kind of compensation. This was something that haunted me regularly and bothered me deeply. He said that we are human and that only God and His son Jesus were expected to give totally and completely unconditionally. It was a human trait to have needs and wants. He said that I should not think any less of myself as a Christian for having needs and wants. He didn't think any less of me. He was totally understanding.

That weekend was just what I needed before having to dig in for the long haul of opening a new store. My Selling Skills presentation went very well. It took me five hours to present it. I just wish I had had a bigger group of associates to present it to.

That next week, the work really began. It turned from mind labor into hard, physical labor. We started to get freight in with a flurry. Our big shipment was due in on the 14th. It was our Ingram order and was said to consist of fourteen pallets of product.

I spent the first morning at the new store preparing the floor plan for where the product would go. I did a complete layout of the software and accessory departments. Before we could start putting out any product, we had to wipe down all the shelving. A lot of dirt and dust had accumulated from the interior construction. The construction crews were still at the store doing finishing projects and tying together loose ends with the fixture assemblies.

I had three or four temporary employees assigned to me to help prepare the floor to receive merchandise and to start putting things out. The regular store employees would not be there to help until the latter part of the second week. That week I was going in any half dozen directions. I would be working on one thing then get pulled onto something else. The temps would need more supervision and I was drawn over to help them. I was trying to put up signage on a ladder and stock the software that was coming in. The temps knew next to nothing about computers, let alone software. I was the only one who really knew what it was and where it belonged.

That week, we must have moved some of the accessory aisle products three or four times. The temps were getting frustrated. I knew what we had in the other store and tried to base the layout on that inventory. We had no clue as to how much we were getting of the different products. I suppose I could have studied the purchase orders, but I didn't really have time for that. We just kept adjusting as it came in and did the best we could to make room for everything. Mike, Charles and I walked the store every morning to go over our placement game plan for the day. Software stayed pretty intact from my original plan. About 80% of the accessory department changed that week.

It was a little more difficult to judge things in this store. It had an entirely different layout than the Denver store. We had more aisles for merchandise but they were different sizes. The aisles in the accessory department were at least eight feet shorter through the whole department than in the Denver store. We did have two more aisles, but somehow that didn't help matters.

Soft opening was suppose to be October 20. We had a lot of work to get done before that time and not a lot of time to do it. We needed manpower. The only problem was, with more people running around doing things, there was room for more errors to be made. I didn't have experience supervising 20 or more people all doing something different at the same time. I went from working five days a week 7 a.m. to 5 p.m. to working six and a half days from 7 a.m. to about 8 or 9 p.m. The day of pre-opening inventory, I worked from 7 a.m. to 12:30 a.m. Needless to say, I wasn't worth shit the next day. I got up late and didn't get into the store till 7:30.

Our sales force finally grew to an appropriate level by the week of soft opening. Now I had to find time to train all these new hires before opening. I had basically one day to teach them what the original group had two weeks of instruction on. My Basic Selling Skills presentation got cut down to two hours. There was no way I could really do justice to it, but that is all the time I could get. I still didn't get all the employees, especially the part timers trained. They were eager for it, too.

Few of the people that were hired had retail experience. Some had some sales experience. Most were computer enthusiasts and that was what brought them to apply for work. I can't say much about that, because that was what brought me to apply when I did. Oh, I had some retail background, but nothing in a high volume, high price product store like this.

I was exhausted by the time we were ready to open. Because of training issues and loose ends that needed to be tied up, we did not open on the scheduled soft opening day. I ended up getting only half the sales force trained and ready. The rest were going to have to "wing" it. We opened Saturday afternoon about 4:00 p.m. We had customers standing in line to get in. The ad in that day's paper made a mistake and had a map that said "Now Open." We were committed to opening on Saturday, ready or not.

The sales force and cashiers were not going to have a lot of practice time before our Grand Opening that was scheduled for October 26. Grand Opening would go off as scheduled. We did a lot of transfers between the Springs and Denver stores so everyone would have inventory that was in the big ad spread scheduled to run. I spent as much time out on the floor to make myself accessible to my guys if they had questions or difficulty meeting a customer's needs and questions. I was literally pulled in every direction from one end of the store to the other and going non-stop that first couple weeks that we were open.

All the corporate managers and executives that came to town for the Grand Opening were very pleased with the appearance of the store and commended the staff for a job well done. Our sales on that day were excellent for a computer store out in the suburbs in a field. They didn't come close to what Denver had the year before, but was an excellent showing, nonetheless.

This store in Westminster was in an emerging area that was across the highway from Westminster Shopping Mall. We were on the breaking edge of the development toward Boulder. West of us there was some industrial and a lot of farming acreage. It was growing and changing fast, though. The company compiles a database of shoppers from their stores capturing the zip code of customers. From this source they make their plans for future stores. We were in a new shopping center that had a Wal-Mart and Home Express that would open in November. A new PetsMart and Best Buy were going in between us and the other two stores. Rumors had it that another computer super store was going to put in a store across the road from us in a new shopping plaza that was being planned on that side.

My responsibilities at the Westminster store were double what I had at Denver. Here, I acted as both the Merchandise and Sales Supervisor. I was responsible for the ads and monthly merchandising program and the immediate supervisor to the sales force. I did all the scheduling and training and helped to keep the morale up on the sales floor. I was the first line link between those employees and management.

I felt lucky with the sales associates we had hired. They tended to be an older, more mature group of men than were at the Denver store. They showed a mutual respect for me and looked up to me for the knowledge and expertise I had demonstrated thus far. I knew what was going on in the store from my guys before senior management ever said anything to me; such as when my top sales performers were going to be transferred to business sales.

I made every effort to give the guys the schedules they requested and they showed their appreciation through performance. I demanded great things from them and they produced because, for the most part, we were a close knit unit. I had some complaints from time to time about the way some associates were dealing with customers, and I did my best to check things out and bring it to Mike's attention. He had the role of any disciplinary action that needed to be taken.

We lost a few employees on the floor the first few months, because they found better jobs, realized they weren't cut out for this kind of sales work, or just didn't want to be a team player. We didn't have to fire anyone. They all made their own decision to leave.

Our part time employees were one of our strengths. Many of them were top performers on selling extended warranties. Each employee selling a customer an extended warranty was entitled to a bonus. There was no fool proof way of tracking these and the way the cashiers were trained, some credits were not awarded. The POS software system the store used also had some glitches and some of the sales did not appear on the report I accumulated my data from. This tracking and award system was probably the biggest point of complaints by the employees. Some of them tracked their sales religiously. I tracked their sales to see who was performing well and to see who might need some additional training.

There was a terrible viral cold that made its rounds in the community and throughout the store. It took a while for me to accept and make the best of the situation when an employee called in sick. I sometimes had to get creative with my employee assignments. Everyone was good about pitching in though.

We were having trouble getting computers in the store. We had tons of monitors and printers but no computers to go with them. I couldn't figure out how corporate expected us to have the sales demanded without the main staple of our inventory. We complained loudly to corporate. Charles, was good about being persistent with the buyers in communicating to them our needs. By the end of November we had a decent inventory to go into the Christmas season. Not enough, though, to put our sales at the level we had the potential for. Fortunately, among us, Denver and the Springs, we were able to make it through Christmas. We missed quota in December by $26,000 and knew that we could have easily surpassed that amount if we only had the systems.

We opened the store without a Customer Service Supervisor. Around Thanksgiving, Charles and Kendall, the Ops Manager, asked me if I might be interested in the position. I thought it would make great cross training and give me an opportunity to learn that end of the store operations. I told them I would be interested, but my heart was still with the sales team. I felt a need for a presence to remain on the floor at that time. The employees were still coming to me frequently with problems and questions. Deep down, I knew it could get messy with me having split loyalties. I didn't want to think about the possibility of being tugged in too many directions. I had to have a job where I could stay focused.

Because the Christmas season was upon us and we really didn't need people learning new job responsibilities at this time, they gave the position to one of the customer service leads. I had no hard feelings whatsoever. Kendall told me that after the first of the year, we might get into a cross-training situation with management.

Before the Christmas season swung into gear, I had two weeks where I had two days off. From the 11th of November until after inventory the first of the year, management would have only one day off a week. We worked eleven hour days. I spent most of my days on the closing shift. I worked from 1 p.m. to whenever we got done after closing. When the store stayed open till ten o'clock, this could be as late as 1 a.m. This was rough on the back to back days that I closed and then had to be in the next morning at 7 a.m. I managed without much difficulty, though.

My mom thought that the winter driving up to the store would be difficult. I tried to explain to her that we don't normally have many days where travel is really difficult with our semi-mild winters. Even though it was twenty miles each way to the store, it was a quick, easy drive. I had only about ten blocks of street travel. The rest was all highway. It only took me about twenty minutes to make the drive. I rarely drove it in rush hour, and I usually was going against the flow of traffic. In fact, I found it to be a very relaxing drive.

Christmas was upon us before I knew it. Time just whizzed by. My mom was going back out to California for Christmas again to be with Karla and her family. She still had this feeling that I needed her and would be lost without her to do my laundry. I reassured her that it was only for three weeks, and I could manage. I tried to impress upon her that I was not helpless and could take care of myself. I sometimes feel she still thinks it is ten years earlier when I was somewhat incapable of managing on my own because of my illness.

I used to have great difficulty around separations. Something would get worked up inside of me and I would act out by doing something stupid. Things like cut on myself, take an overdose or get very depressed. I was in an entirely different state of being now and I actually needed that freedom to fend for myself once again, instead of have a mother hen look over me. I needed as many opportunities as possible to prove to her that I was a healthy, productive adult capable of taking care of herself.

I was scheduled to work Christmas Eve. I was hoping we would get out of the store early enough so I could go to the Candlelight Service at church. I was not getting many opportunities to attend church on Sundays and didn't want to miss this service. Business was slow, so we could do early closing preparation. We closed at seven and I was able to get out of there at eight. I took a nice blouse with me that afternoon to change into for church. I got to the church by just a little before 8:30. I had plenty of time to sit, relax, and meditate.

During my time of meditation, an idea came from nowhere and hit me straight on. I was getting the message that maybe I should open a computer store of my own. An Apple computer store to be more specific. I don't know what initiated this thought. It came out of the blue. There was no premeditation that led to this at all. I took it as a sign from God. After all, it came while I was in His house. I spent much of the rest of the evening thinking about this idea. I even came up with a name for this store, Apple World.

When I got home from church my mind was whirling. I couldn't think of much else. I was so excited that opening presents was not a thought. I decided to leave them for Christmas morning. I had a very restless night. I got up at 6:30 the next morning.

I didn't know where to begin. I started by checking out a U.S. phone directory I had to see if anyone else had the same name. Apple Computers was the closest thing that I could find that really dealt with computers. I got the names of some of the distributors that I knew we dealt with and numbers for Apple. I was off on Monday and hoped that I could reach some of these companies, especially Apple.

On Monday, I drove around southeast Denver looking for possible retail storefronts. I found about five possible locations. I would try to connect with these people that week for rates and square footage.

My original plan was to sell mainly software and peripherals. I really wasn't wanting to go so far as to carry the computers themselves. However, the more I thought about it, the more I realized that this would not be as strong a venture if I did not carry at least some computers. When I got a hold of Apple, they steered me toward some of the major distributors and the application process to become a Value Added Reseller (VAR). That was my original direction.

I told my mom and my sister-in-law about this plan I had on Christmas day. I told my mom that I did not expect a penny from her or any time commitment other than moral support and a non-negative encouragement. She kept saying that she had no money and couldn't bail me out if it didn't fly. She would not hear what I was telling her. NO INVESTMENT, mom.

This first few weeks I was a bit overwhelmed by the contemplation of such an endeavor. I was on again, off again with the idea. I had to find someone that would work with me. This was not a project I could accomplish by myself. I needed someone with knowledge and encouragement that was just as excited about the idea as myself. I thought real hard about who would be a possible candidate. Then it struck me. There was one guy at the Denver store that had become their Apple expert when I left. I racked my brain for a week to try to remember his name. It finally came to me. Russel would be the candidate. Now, I needed to figure out how to approach him. This took another ten days. I had called Ingram, one of the industry distributors. They said they could not send out a recent catalog until I had opened an account and furnished them with a tax ID number.

I was still uncertain as to how far I wanted to pursue this idea. I had mentioned it to a few of the older guys at the store, who I knew had businesses of their own and were some of our top salesmen. They encouraged me to go for it. They thought it was a fantastic idea and something that was certainly needed in the Denver market. These comments gave me the added push that I would need to really start moving with this project.

I knew the first thing I was going to have to do was incorporate. To do that, I would need at least a second name on the incorporation documents. I couldn't wait any longer. I first tried calling Ike Garst from a few years back that had served on my board when I had my design studio. He was really into something else that was keeping him busy, and suggested I try my other choice, Russel.

It took a couple days to actually make contact with Russel. I didn't realize his wife had recently had a baby. Because I didn't want to talk to him when he or I was at work, I had to schedule sometime when we were both at home. I actually had to get him one morning after he had a long night with the baby. He seemed genuinely interested on first approach and said he would talk it over with his wife. He got back with me the next day and said he was genuinely interested in pursuing this project with me.

The business, Apple World, was incorporated on January 31, 1995. The next thing I had to do was get a federal identification number and then a sales tax license. I had to wait for the first before I could apply for the second. I could not get through to get my ID by phone so had to wait for it through the mail. The very first business day after getting our FIN, I went and applied for the state tax license. I had to make a $50 deposit to get this set up in addition to the license fee.

Having done these three things, I was now able to classify myself as legit and could make application with the national distributors. One other item of business needed to be dealt with before submitting these applications. I had to open a business bank account. This took a little longer, because I didn't have any extra money to spare. Since going into management, I was making way less than I had at U S WEST. Bonuses were not up to what I was told they would be. Fortunately, I got a contract drafting job with one of my long time clients. Just as soon as I got my check from Max, I went straight to the bank.

The money from the drafting job was not enough to put much in the account. In fact, I had to take some of the money that was suppose to be used for my car payment and add to what I had. Between this and the sales tax license, I put myself a month behind in my car payment. I sure hoped that I would get enough back on my taxes that I could get things back on track.

Finally, I had all the information necessary to submit my applications to the distributors. Finally things were beginning to roll. The first account I opened was with Ingram Micro. The second was Tech Data. The third one took a little longer. It was with Merisel.

Merisel required each of its prospective customers to place an order with them before sending out a catalog. There was a mix-up and the order didn't come for two weeks. I finally called them back to find out the problem. They said they needed my application before they could ship the order. They couldn't get through on the fax. I gave them the number at the store and got things moving again with them. One thing good about the delay; I had given them my VISA card number and I knew my payment had not been received when I first placed the order. I was afraid the transaction would not be approved.

My VISA was maxed out. Each month, something came up that I had to use it for. I needed it for groceries on a number of occasions. For a few months, I had to pay a penalty for going over my limit. This account had been set up with my inheritance from Roy. It was the one way I could think of to not spend it and have it go for something of value. I opened this secured credit card account. I needed to rebuild credit and was getting interest on the money at the same time.

I wanted to do some market research to see just where the market was. I had made a number of calls to find an acceptable mailing list. I was able to get through to the people who maintain and sell the MacWorld magazine list. It was going to cost $600 for a minimum list of 5000 names. OUCH! I was going to have to find some other way. I had very limited resources. Russel was not going to be of help because he had the new baby he was paying for.

I had gotten a business phone directory on CD-ROM the previous summer. I figured I would go through it and get names for design studios in the Denver area. I wound up with a list of just over 200 when I selected certain zip codes. Now I had to design a survey and print and mail it. This required more money. I had a little left from my car payment fund and used it to buy the stamps. I used the rest of the funds remaining on my VISA to buy the paper. It would not have been my first choice, but was readily available, plus I got a discount on it, and the price was right.

The surveys went out and I anxiously awaited the response cards to come back. I got the first one back within three days. I also got what ended up being the kind of response I was not wanting to see. A "Return to Sender" response from the post office. Many of these businesses had moved and their forwarding order had expired. That told me right off, that the data for this list on the software was just a bit outdated. I was getting a 3:1 return on undeliverable pieces over actual responses. I decided to spend another stamp and look in the phone book for a good address. I should have referenced this in the first place. Getting the name was the hardest part. But that thought had not occurred to me when I was in the process.

My goal was to have my business plan completed by the first of March. I missed it by a week. I was wanting to send it out to a venture fund in Boulder. They required the plan to be no more than ten pages in length. For Katherine, that was very difficult. She tends to be a very wordy writer as you can see from this book.

As always, the financial figures took the most time to put together. This was much easier, though, having had the experience of writing plans for my other businesses. Each one gets shorter. I mailed the completed plan March 8.

I played phone tag with the President of that fund for the whole month of March. I finally got an appointment to meet with her April 3. She told me she would give me an answer within the week. I talked with her the following Monday. She said my venture was more than they were investing in at the time. She suggested going to the Rockies Venture Club and said that she would call if she heard of any good leads.

That night I mailed out my business plan to the Rockies Venture Club for review. I was hoping to get the opportunity of presenting my venture at one of their meetings. The following week I was on vacation to do a lot of running around on this project. I got a call Monday night from Jim from the Venture Club asking if I could be a presenter that next evening. I said of course; no problem. Now I had to write a five minute speech. Piece of cake. I'm great at spontaneous presentations. Or at least Karen is. This was going to be my big chance to tell the business community of my plans and the enthusiasm behind it.

The presentation went quite well, no thanks to Karen. She was nowhere to be found. I had to stand on the podium with my quivering voice and rubber legs. I got through it and had some accolades from members of the audience. One problem, though, I had only one person come up to me after the meeting asking to see my business plan. I thought, okay, they got my phone number, they'll call later like the last time. I ended up getting only one call from the presentation.

I'm still very upbeat about the whole thing. I know this business is going to fly. It's just a matter of when. I have all the confidence in the world about it. I really believe. I spent about five hours at the library researching other venture capital firms. I called some of the companies in the Denver area and got an uninterested response from them. They did suggest I go to the Pratt Guide at the library. I did, and got a lengthy list of companies around the U.S. I spent the last day of my vacation faxing out letters and Executive Summaries. I changed my summary to my speech which was converted into a document.

I feel my life is just beginning. So many opportunities are opening up to me. The bleak, black past is behind me and there is a whole new life out there for my taking. It will require a lot of hard work, but is in reach and for me to explore.

I will be in therapy for some time to come and I will be on medication the rest of my life. That is a given I have come to accept and will live with. The message I want to spread to all survivors is to not give up. You need to wake every day with the attitude that these struggles that we have to deal with are only temporary. We are God's chosen warriors. You can't be a warrior without having battles to face. We must look at the battle from every perspective and devise our tactics to come out the winner. We would not have been chosen if we weren't found to have the strength to carry the burden that we were thrown into early in life. Survivors have a true gift if we just open it at the right time. My time is here. It was a long time coming, but the struggles and battles I faced made me that much more valuable a person to society.

The storm will subside. Our one true virtue for survival is patience. Gene told me the first night we met that "Patience is a virtue." It has never been so true as now. Fight for your rights, and whatever you do, don't give up. You have made it through the worst of the worst. Lift yourself up, dust off the dirt and show your true colors. Life is wonderful. Make the best of what time you have left. Seek your purpose and fulfill your dreams.

THE SORORITY

MICHELE – The depressed core and host personality

WHISPERING OWL – The Indian Wiseman who is responsible for the Group's evolution

CHRISSY – A protector; the holder of the checks and balances for the Group; spokesperson

THE BIG GUY – A protector; the father figure for the Group; holds some anger and rage

MIKE – The tomboy, muscleman and outdoorsperson of the Group

SAMANTHA – The smallest of the Group members; she is 5 years old

PEGGY – Another child in the Group; attaches herself to male figures

KIM – This is the alter with the self-destructive behavior; she is the one that holds most of the anger and rage

ALICE – The mother identity of the Group; takes after my real mother and grandmother

KATHERINE – The Group writer; one who likes to dig for answers

BONNIE – The precision artist and drafter

BOBBIE – Bonnie's twin; she too is an artist but really works in crafts and fine art

DIANE – The geographer/geologist of the Group; loves the outdoors

CAROL – The teacher in the Group; she holds the greatest amount of patience

ELIZABETH – The photographer; sees inner beauty in everything she captures on film

SUSAN – The Group vocalist and musician

KAREN – The thespian and public speaker

CORY – Least known member of the Group; fearful of the touch of anyone

SHELLEY – The brain of the Group; also the businessperson; very proper

NICOLE – The computer whiz; loves to tinker; would spend every minute of the day on the computer

CONNIE – She is the personable salesperson; enjoys being around people and helping others

FRANCIE – Group historian; also the socialite of the Group; loves to be the hit of the party

SALLY – The conservative alter with sexual tendencies

MONIQUE – The nymphomaniac; has issues of control in her sexual behavior

There are other fragments of personalities within the system who share bits and pieces from the alters listed above. Many act as transitional alters. When the appropriate alter is unable to surface at the appropriate time, for whatever reason, these fragments hold things together until that alter appears. Sometimes they get stuck with the dirty work. For the most part they are nameless.

MICHELE

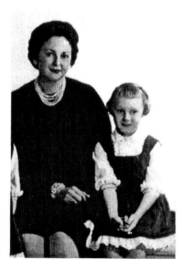

Help! I'm a little girl trapped in a big fat woman's body! I still see myself as a five year old who is quiet, lonely and depressed. My world is cold and dark. My mom is always there but not really there for me. I am her little girl to all her friends. I want to be liked by kids my age. Not by all the adults my parents associate with. I'm just a cute, sweet little girl to them.

I haven't done anything wrong. I'm always a good little girl on the best of my behavior. I'm scared to be punished. As long as I am not in trouble, I am loved by my parents. I just know I am.

I want my parents to pay more attention to me. I don't want them to argue. I hope I don't make them argue. I do everything I am told. The only thing I don't like to do is eat. That, I do get in trouble for. They would make me late for school because I wouldn't eat my lunch.

I want to be liked and accepted by people, but I am terribly afraid of them. People are so unpredictable. You never know when they are going to be nice to you, or when they are going to treat you badly.

The only real friends I can trust and depend on are my special secret friends that nobody knows about. They keep me company when I am lonely. They cheer me up when I am sad. They do things for me when I can't or won't do them because of how I have been taught. My secret friends have done a good job at growing up and making something of this person I am trapped inside of.

I say I like to be liked by people, but I am happiest when I am all by myself. When I get sad, I go to my bed and wrap myself in a blanket as tight as I can. That blanket protects me from the bad feelings I have.

I hope my friends will get me to a safe place that I will feel good about. I think it is time I grow up, but it isn't quite safe yet. Life is too complicated and confusing right now. I am afraid of being a failure. If I am a failure, my mom won't love me any more. I need to have love from somebody.

When this system becomes successful in all aspects of our life, it will be safe to grow up and resume my core responsibilities. In the meantime, my Group is doing just fine getting me by. I am confident about their abilities. I have all the time in the world to grow up.

Thanks for letting me come out of my bedroom and share this information with you

Michele

WHISPERING OWL

I am Whispering Owl. You might call me the Genesis and Creator of the Group. I don't really consider myself as a separate entity, but rather as a floating spirit of the whole. I am a spiritual being and was when I found Michele almost forty years ago. I'm very old now and don't recall things as well as I did long ago. I was in my early 60's when I first encountered her. I am over 100 now.

In real life, I was an Indian tribal wise man. It's hard to really pinpoint the tribe, but I was of the Cherokee Nation. I was a teacher of sorts and an advisor to numerous tribal chiefs. I had a lot of depth and insight into life and the way things should be.

I was in Sheridan, Wyoming during the late summer, early fall of 1955. I was there to gather with other spirits and tribes participating in a large Indian gathering. It was at this time I felt the whispers of a small cry, of sorts, for help. It was a lonely little cry which I could not rid myself of. It came from the small child, Michele.

You ask, how could I detect this sort of need from someone so small? Well, there was something about Michele's inner sights, soul and needs which reached out and grabbed me. I saw something special in her which sparked my curiosity. This child was unique; so good, so bright, and very promising as a person. I knew from the beginning that this was someone who could use some wise guidance and support.

Somehow, Michele knew there would soon be a new addition to her family and that things would change for her. My gift of wisdom was such that she was given the will and determination to be a survivor. This new little being would not jeopardize her existence but build her into a stronger, independent being. I gave her guidance and nurturing until she was big enough to understand and need like companionship. Until she was old enough to learn the importance of how other Group members created from her being could grow with her, enrich her life and help her to be a survivor of her world.

You might say that I was Michele's "Guardian Angel" until she was three. That's when I created and introduced her to a playmate who was much like herself. This was Samantha. Then came Mike, Bobbie and Bonnie. They were the first members which enlisted some of her many talents. Peggy was another young friend I introduced her to. Bonnie didn't really show her full attributes until junior and senior high school.

I remember things beginning so simply and innocently. I never imagined how the Group would grow or how it could ever get out of hand. My workings were sincere and in Michele's best interest, not for near destruction. Chrissy was created as a stabilizing member. One to keep tabs on things like in a checks and balance system. I guess I didn't spend enough time teaching her the proper way to take control if things were to ever get out of hand.

I didn't create all the Group members. I just got things started and showed Michele how easy it was to take her talents and give them to another part of her which, in turn, could grow and develop and make her that much stronger a person.

I left her when she was five and came back every year for several years in the late summer to see how things were progressing. She was slow and shy about creating new Group members. She did develop the ones I started her with to varying degrees. Samantha; however, never did grow up after I left the first time. Maybe that's good, or maybe that's bad. I don't know in this day and age.

I pretty much lost track of Michele when her father died and she moved away from Sheridan. It's just been the past few years that I've refound her. I'm so old that I don't know how much more wisdom I can bestow on her. I get tired easily and don't think as clearly as I did when I first met her. The Group can sometimes blow like a whirlwind and really send me hurling away. I wish I could have been around to help maintain and guide Chrissy's part in the Group. She has come up against some very difficult times and could have used a wise shoulder to lean on.

I feel, at times, when Francie fills me in on what has happened to Michele, that I failed her somewhere along the way; that I forgot to tell her some important things. My senility now gets in the way and I sometimes lose track of my wisdom and responsibilities. Yes, spirits do lose their strength and power in time. We grow old, too, just a little slower than others.

I am going to try and regain a closeness to the Group. I may be old and forgetful but still have things to share. The Group has matured so much over the past few years that I think what little I can contribute will be welcomed and put to good use.

Well, I'm growing tired now, and my mind is starting to wander. I hope I have given you the information you need to understand who I am and the role I play in Michele's life.

Whispering Owl

CHRISSY

There is no picture of me because I am ever-changing and have never really evolved into a true image that has been captured on film. I have a little bit of everyone in the Group in me. You could look at all their pictures and see some of me.

I have probably led the most exciting and difficult life of any of the Group members. Before I go any further, I want to make one thing perfectly clear — I despise hospitals or confinement of any sort. I have a real issue with control, and find that these situations make me vulnerable and take away my control.

My life began when Michele was around five years old. I evolved as the control element that would guide and grow with the system. Things were pretty easy for me to cope with until other Group members gained more personal strength.

I helped Michele deal with the frustrations she encountered being left alone because of her level of intelligence. That's where I and the Group shine. We were her companions and she soon grew to accept her isolation from being different than a lot of the other kids. She knew we were close and there when she needed someone to talk to.

I guess my abilities gave Michele enough confidence in her support system that she just pulled inside herself and let us take off once I came along. She gave me the encouragement to take over for her and step into her shoes. She wanted to stay behind until we built her a world where she would be loved and accepted by those around her outside of the Group.

We all tried real hard to make a go of things and make a new life for ourselves. We learned how to create new alters to assume responsibility for new talents we discovered we had. As Michele stayed behind, we became more independent of her. I tried to incorporate Whispering Owl's wisdom to keep the Group focused for the betterment of the system.

I'm the type of individual that tries to make the best from the status quo. I don't like to "rock the boat" so to speak. Not some of the others. They have a mind and will of their own. Take Kim, for example. She was too ashamed of her inability to control her behavior that she disguised herself as me. Because I was the stabilizer of the group, she had everyone believing I had gone off the deep end. That I had lost control. In a sense, I had, because I did not know how to control Kim. She had so much rage built up inside her, she was a walking time bomb. I was scared that I might really drive her over the edge by standing up for my rights and taking control. That's why I allowed her little game of imitating me to continue. I was freaked that I was not in control of the Group, but very fearful for our lives.

Finally, after her second nearly fatal attempt at coping with her anger, I said enough was enough. No longer was I going to just sit by and take this behavior. I told her that if she did not come to grips with her anger and learn how to deal with it in an appropriate way, we would abolish her from the Group. We would no longer recognize her as a member of the system. I was firm and truly committed to this ultimatum. She knew I was serious and would do as I promised. She finally came out and showed her true identity, and asked for help.

For nearly all our life, I have taken on the responsibility of the core person for this Group. The real Michele insists on staying in the background until we have succeeded as a team effort;

until we have fulfilled her dreams for her. She shows herself every now and then to remind us who we are working (living) for and what our goal is. I have convinced her that as a reward when this happens, she will not integrate us. We will continue to live an existence side by side in perfect harmony and cooperation. We have been through way too much to just melt into the background.

One critical step in accomplishing this goal, is in having finally found the proper medication that has taken away the depressive tendencies of most of the Group members. Michele even comes out of her bedroom from time to time because she is not as burdened with that heavy cloud of depression.

I have tried my best at keeping the Group together through a cooperative nature. Some shine through more than others and I give them a long rope to work from. I am managing the Group from day to day and stand in when others go off into their own little world. It is tough having to explain the actions of the others, especially if they are inappropriate.

I act as a bit of a traffic cop for this Group. Also as the glue that holds things together. I won't admit that I am great at what I do, but the job somehow seems to get done. More so lately. My biggest problem is that I am not a very good listener. If I would just ask the others to talk to me on a regular basis, I think things would all fall into place. I need a vacation. I hope I can guide this system to the place Michele is looking for soon so I can sit back and be an observer for a change. I am really getting burned out and don't know how much longer I can remain pleasant and smiling. That's why I am not talking to the others. They have more demands than solutions and I'm clean out of answers.

I know I haven't said a whole lot about who I am. I've more or less filled you in on my role in this system. I am being worn to a frazzle, but I am committed to this Group for the long haul. Somehow, I will find the strength to fulfill my responsibilities until Michele is ready to get back on top.

Chrissy

THE BIG GUY

I am Michele's father replacement. When her father became more and more distant from the family through his drinking, I stepped in to give her firm guidance and someone to talk to. I appeared around the time that she was in junior high. At that time I was about 45 years old. I have aged some but not in physical years. I am now about 60.

In general, I think Michele kind of fears me. I am a strict disciplinarian and firm with her. I don't let her get her way all the time. Don't get me wrong. I'm not cold towards her. I can be very loving and considerate.

I have not been a major player in Michele's life until most recently. When she was younger, I gave her the courage to continue working toward her dreams. I wouldn't allow her to throw the towel in when things got rough.

I guess I got a bad reputation during her roughest years when Kim would act out destructively. I kind of led Kim to perform some of her actions. Not the overdoses mind you. I played a major role in her cutting on herself. I felt Michele and Kim needed a lot of reality checks back then. By doing the cutting, it allowed them to release some of the built up anger, but more importantly, the sight of the blood made them feel this nightmare was not a dream. They had a habit of getting caught up in the feelings and losing touch with reality. No telling what they would have done had I not made them aware that what was happening was real and they had to be responsible for themselves.

I played an active role in Michele's life when the Group was away at college. Along with Mike, I helped get the Group through the AFROTC program she participated in. Alone, she would never have made it through the Silver Wing pledge program. I gave her the discipline to be an outstanding cadet for which she received awards for. I guess my middle name is discipline.

I am the real authoritarian for the Group and I guess I have gotten in Michele's way this past year. When she is placed in a leadership role, I kind of step in and try to run the show. My ways are the old-fashioned ways and my people skills are not what is needed in today's society. I am making her progress in her present position very difficult. I have good intentions in what I do, but today's young adults have to be babied. They want the soft life. They don't want to do an honest day's work for an honest dollar. I think people should enjoy their work, but I can't bring myself to accept the possibility of having fun at work. Fun doesn't really register as a part of my vocabulary.

Michele is having problems in her management positions with the store. I am at fault for these problems. It is hard for me to accept this. I have always meant well. I guess I need to get with the program and do some changing. I surely don't want to keep Michele and the Group from their dreams and goals. If I weren't so dominant in her background and looking out for her, I guess I would just slither away and hide until there was a more appropriate time for me to be around.

Michele allows people to use her and walk all over her. This hurts me deeply. I know she wants approval and acceptance from her peers. By sitting back and taking all the shit they will gladly dish out to her is not what she needs. She needs to be in control. The whole Group, aside from Michele and a few others, have strong issues with control. We need a sense of having control over our life or we will revert back to a life of rejection and loneliness. We have these even when in control, but it is perceived in an entirely different light and more acceptable.

I am participating in Michele's therapy and trying to listen to some of the tapes she has to help me change my ways. I want us to succeed in life and I don't want to carry around the guilt that I was the reason for Michele's failure. I don't like the idea of failure any more than the others. You can teach an old dog new tricks; it just takes a little longer.

MIKE

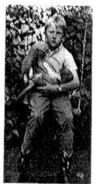

The picture to the left was when I was fairly young. I have grown up since then and am in my early thirties.

My idol was and still is John Wayne. Mainly because he was strong and looked a whole lot like my dad. Or my dad looked a whole lot like him. My newest idols are Sylvester Stallone, Chuck Norris and Arnold Schwartzenagger.

I guess I'm suppose to tell you just who I am and what makes me tick. I was born when Michele was three or four. There weren't many girls in the neighborhood, so Michele needed someone who could understand guys and get along with them. She also needed physical strength to endure. I used to think of myself as a hard-core tomboy. I do not want to be called a dike. I am a man in a woman's body and that is all there is to it.

I enjoy fishing – when I catch something. When young, I loved to go fishing and to the mountains with my dad. We would often go to Teepee Ranch in the Big Horn Mountains. My dad knew the Fordyces and they allowed us to fish their streams and lake any time we wanted. We always caught fish there. My sister, Karla, hated to fish. One time she had a fish on her pole and dropped the pole on the bank. I ran over to save the pole and wound up with a good-sized fish. My dad would also want to take off fishing sometimes after he had been drinking a lot. I was concerned, so insisted on going with him. His driving up that dirt mountain road sometimes got scary.

I used to play just about every sport made available to me, even when this body got fat. I love the out-of-doors and to build things, too. When young, I'd climb anything around. I love the labors of gardening and yard work, but don't care that much about eating what I grow.

When I was real young, I loved to play with Legos and Tinker Toys. I spent a lot of time in the backyard and sandbox. In kindergarten, I would play in the coat room with the building blocks and other boys. It was either cowboys and Indians or army. You wouldn't catch me dead playing house, dolls or grocery store with the girls. I liked things that dealt with exterior and interior force and strength.

When I was old enough to go out of the yard by myself, I'd be off playing with Rusty or Johnny. We would spend a lot of time over at Taylor School climbing on the fire escape. I'd collect pigeon feathers. When I got big enough, we would climb on top of the boiler room roof. I thought I was big stuff to meet the challenge of making it to the roof. It was just one story, but tricky to get up onto. Sometimes I'd go over to Rusty's house and we'd climb and play on the storage shed at the back of his house.

I couldn't wait till I was big enough to climb the small tree on the corner of our front yard. I'd climb on top of the fire hydrant and reach that first branch. I wanted to climb the big cottonwoods, but wasn't big enough while we lived on Fifth Street. I also liked to climb the swing set in the backyard of our first house. I called them monkey bars. We also had a tree swing tied to one of the big trees that I loved to swing on.

I started working in the yard when I was very young. I had my own rake and shovel. I got to help mom plant bulbs and keep the garden weeded. Even when we moved up on Thurmond, I got to take charge of the gardens. I got to have my first vegetable garden. When big enough, I did my share of the lawn mowing, watering and snow shoveling. I also did some hedge trimming.

I liked to visit my neighbors across the alley on Fifth Street. They had tons of flowers, a big goldfish pond and frogs in their yard. They would let me help pick flowers and clean the fish pond.

I guess my mom and dad knew how much of a tomboy I was, because when they came back from a trip to New York, my sister got a Barbie doll. I got a Ken. I spent more time, though, playing with my brother's race car set and his electric train than with my dolls.

I liked Whispering Owl. I could really relate to him. I have this fascination with the old West; the cowboys, Indians and settlers. They were all hard workers and survivors in their own right. I love to go to rodeos. I love horses and animals. I used to get up at the crack of dawn and hang out of my bedroom window watching the sheep and horses be herded from their different pastures in the spring and fall. They would go right past the front of our house. We've always had pets of some sort; usually dogs.

I had a little Yorkshire Terrier for twelve years. She died last year of old age and heart failure. When in junior high and until we left Sheridan, our family had a black poodle named Sheri. She was basically my dog, because she slept with me and would wait for me in the front chairs when I'd go away to camp.

When we moved up on Thurmond, I got real active. I put most of my weight on then, but didn't really let it stop me. I played tetherball, kickball and, when in the fifth grade, started to play dodgeball with the older kids and the hard soccer ball. They had no mercy, either. When you got hit, it usually hurt.

There was a big hill next to the playground at Linden Elementary. During the winter, we'd slide down the hill on our feet without a sled or tubes.

I got a lot of teasing because of my weight. I was called things like "Cyclops" and "Sherman Tank," in addition to the usual. Some days I'd get mad and chase the guys who would be teasing me. One day, I chased a guy all the way around the school and would have caught him if he hadn't chickened out and ducked into the boy's restroom. I was going to beat him up because I was so mad at him.

I had a friend, Wendy, who was also a bit of a tomboy. She was my competition. I was always trying to beat her in everything, but she was just a little bit better than me. In everything but Girl Scouts, that is. That program was one of the highlights of my life. I earned more badges and went to more camps than she did. During intramurals, we usually wound up in the finals against one another. It's a good thing we were on the same basketball team in high school.

Wendy and I had a brief falling out incident in the sixth grade. She and some of the guys were teasing me. I got mad and chased them up the hill and around my old kindergarten teacher's house. They were throwing snowballs at me with rocks in them. One hit me. I was furious. I finally caught up with Wendy and knocked her to the ground in the backyard. She slipped in some mud and the rest is history. The fortunate thing was that she and I didn't hold this against one another for long. We remained friends and competitors until I left Sheridan.

During junior high, I wasn't getting teased as much as in grade school. There were more kids and they came in all sizes and shapes. I didn't stand out as much. One guy used to follow me down the halls singing the Beatle's song "Michelle" when it came out. I hated it. To top it off, he kept punching me in the arm. He had a crush on me or something. Anyway, one day I got so fed up with this little ritual of his, that I turned around and gave him one swift punch that threw him across the hall into a locker. Of course a teacher saw it and I got in trouble.

In grade school during P.E., there always used to be more girls than boys. Guess who got to play the guy when we had dance lessons? I got so used to leading that when Sally would go dancing with guys, I found it hard to refrain from taking the lead. Sally does okay, anyway. She has some pretty good moves.

When still in grade school, my sister and I got to go up to Montana to spend some time during the summer on my aunt and uncle's farm. It was great! We got up in the mornings and got to gather eggs and help milk the cows. We didn't get to ride any horses, though, because my uncle had all but a couple of them at the ranch somewhere else. We spent the Fourth of July there and it was my first experience with firecrackers. I really enjoyed that summer. It was like being a settler in the old West with some modern conveniences.

I spent two weeks at Girl Scout camp near Casper, Wyoming, when I was thirteen. I had a great time. We got to ride horses and sleep outside in platform tents. Wendy went to camp with me and we got in the same tent. We took some day hikes and found some pieces of arrowheads. I liked that, the horses and campfires best.

The next year, I applied for two Girl Scout summer camps that took only a select number of girls from all over the state. I was first alternate to the Wyoming Game and Fish Conservation Camp and second alternate to a Covered Wagon Trek. As luck had it, I wound up going to both camps. I found out about the Covered Wagon Trek the night I was suppose to be on the mountain with the other girls. I had one night to pack and get my gear together for this primitive camping experience. They were great. I met a lot of neat people and made new friends.

At Conservation Camp, we slept in two-man pup tents on cots. We got to build a dam to create a fish pond and swimming hole. It took a lot of work finding and placing rocks two feet thick and about ten to twelve feet across the stream. We also got to electrocute fish in a stream to see how big the fish were and what species they were. I got to help round up geese in an air boat and band them for the Game and Fish Department. They even took us to a game preserve where there were a lot of wild baby animals and some which had been hurt or deformed. This camp lasted a week.

The Covered Wagon Trek was the ultimate in a camping experience. We stowed all our gear in an old covered wagon that had been rigged with rubber tires for easier pulling. It was pulled by two big team horses. We walked alongside and behind the wagon. We'd cover 10 or 15 miles in a day's hike trekking across the hills and mountainsides of Wyoming. We covered about 65 miles all total. We'd stop for a couple days at each campsite. We got to see an old deserted mine and mill, and some pretty countryside. We roughed it in that we slept on the ground without tents, cooked all our meals over a campfire and used homemade latrines. We got good and inventive with some of the unique latrines we built.

I got a chance to ride one of the team horses at one of our campsites. I rode that big hunk of horseflesh bareback. I'd never ridden without a saddle before. I did great while the horse was walking. On the way back to the camp from my ride, there was a little hill to go up. The horse decided to canter, then broke into a gallop because he wanted to get back to camp. I couldn't keep my legs wrapped around him tight enough and fell off. I got quite a jolt and my pants full of sand. I dizzily walked back to camp. I definitely saw stars after this experience.

On one of our final day hikes, I came across a little garter snake crossing the road. I caught him and carried him for awhile. The trek counselors happened to drive by in our outfitter's truck on their way to our last campsite on the edge of the Girl Scout National Center West. I stood in the middle of the road waving the snake at them. They rolled up the windows and sped past me. Shortly afterwards, I put the snake down because he was beginning to smell. Soon, I caught up with the counselors. They were still in the truck with the windows up and doors locked. I couldn't convince them that I had let the snake go. Just about that time, I heard a loud rattle, screamed and jumped in the back of the truck. They were certain I had the snake for sure, then. Actually, what I had was a four foot rattlesnake about five feet away from me.

The highlight of the trip happened the very next day. It was in July of 1969. I was viewing a beautiful canyon and could see for miles, while at the same time, the astronauts had just landed and were walking on the Moon. What a beautiful place to share one of the greatest events to happen to mankind. Chills ran through my body.

The next summer, my Cadette Girl Scout troop took a trip to Canada. We went in a car caravan. We went to Vancouver Island, B.C. When we went through Idaho, we got our pictures taken and made the newspaper. We camped out at various campgrounds along the way and ate off Coleman stoves. We took a ferry across Puget Sound and saw the Butchart Gardens. The night before, we stayed in a campground on the island of Island County, Washington. Most of us slept in the cars because when the dark hit us, we were invaded by giant slugs. We were chopping off their heads with our hatchets and pouring salt on them until the ranger came around and told us to stop. That's when we decided we'd be safer in the cars. Our plans were to take us across southern Canada to Banf National Park. The trip got cut short and we never made it there, because our leader and one of the drivers had illnesses in their families back at home. It was fun while it lasted and was the first real long trip I'd ever taken.

Next to all the intramural activities in high school, I got the most enjoyment playing basketball and watching my brother, Roger, play. He made the varsity team his sophomore year. I was so proud of him. I still am. I respect and admire him a lot. He's a hard worker and a great brother.

I had some real excitement on one of Karen's speech team trips. On the way back to Sheridan from Billings, Montana, our bus hit a car that drove out from nowhere and across the highway. It was on the Indian reservation. I watched the car drive cross country to a farmhouse. I watched that house so intensely that I either saw or imagined I saw the Indians trying to find a place to hide from the highway patrol and reservation police. Ever since then, I've had fantasies of being an investigator of sorts. That's why I got into Air Force ROTC in college. I was hoping to go into intelligence.

When I was a junior in high school in Billings, I got to take part in a police "Ride Along" program. Any interested student could sign up to ride along with a patrolman for four hours on a Saturday. I found it quite interesting. Another boy from the other high school was in the same patrol car that I was in. We didn't have any exciting chases or stuff like that, but we got to hear about some on the radio. If the policeman got a dangerous call, he was suppose to let us out of the car anyway.

The best and hardest times I ever had was in AFROTC at ASU. As a freshman, I pledged an organization called Silver Wing. It was very military, but once through the pledge program, there was the true closeness of a real fraternity. The pledge program lasted a whole semester and was real tough. They used hazing like at the academy; anything to get you upset and to break. My class was the first to have women in it. Two out of three of us made it, but it was hell. My pledge brothers accepted us and treated us just like one of the guys. I liked that. In addition to all the memorizing and drilling, we had a weekend FTX (field training exercise), Butte Watch, a Hell Night and Final Test Boards.

The FTX was an experience in the desert. Our first night was relatively easy; just a little hazing. Saturday and that night was a real test of endurance. We were broken down into three groups. Each group was given two quarts of water for the whole weekend. We had to wear full backpacks and follow a map course through the desert. We'd hiked about eight miles through cholla and prickly pear in 80 degree temperatures. When we got to our third map coordinate, we were given one more coordinate that would lead us to our pledge symbol that the actives stole from us the night before. It led us to a large granite mountain. The actives dropped it off the top and we had to find it. Our pledge symbol used to be an old hollow bombshell until the FTX. When we recovered it, it had been filled with sand. The night before when they got it away from us, it wound up in the fire.

It was dusk when we got our pledge symbol back. Our next assignment was E & E (escape and evasion). We had to split up into smaller groups to make our way through three miles of desert, at night, to get back to the base camp without being caught by an active. Our only light came from the moon. We were able to come into the base camp the five minutes before and after the hour between 11 p.m. and 1 a.m. If we got caught, we were interrogated like a POW. Fortunately, I made it into camp during the free period. They tried to convince me that I had been caught, but I gave them a good, strong argument over the matter and they gave up. They didn't want to admit that a girl could get through their defenses, and they had all sorts of plans for interrogation. I laid in a gulley for an hour by myself before making my way in. I hadn't had any food all day nor water for about 6 hours. It was a tough day, but I actually enjoyed it and learned a lot about the desert; especially during the E&E.

I would describe the rest of the program, but as a dedicated alumnus, it is an obligation of mine not to give any secrets away. Some of the program has changed, but not all of it. I don't want any prospective pledges to know everything that lies ahead of them.

Silver Wing was just a freshman and sophomore organization, but once a Silver Winger, always a Silver Winger. As a sophomore active, I was permitted to join Arnold Air Society. It's not nearly as military and its pledge program is quite sedate compared to Silver Wing.

I didn't make it into the Air Force because I failed the eye qualifications during my physical exam. I was too near-sighted to qualify as an officer. The Colonel who was the Professor of Aerospace Studies tried to obtain a waiver for me but failed as they had too many officer candidates who qualified for the program.

I did learn a lot about the Air Force and received several awards and two medals of merit for the two years I was in the program. I was "Cadet of the Month" one month and got a free jet ride in a T-31. I got the experience of negative G's in a barrel role. I even got to man the controls and fly the jet for a few moments.

I have a fascination with airplanes and enjoy flying. I got to fly Bryan's dad's Cessna on a couple occasions. I've even had some fighter simulator time. I get a thrill seeing jets flying in formation from Buckley Field east of Denver. I used to go to all the air shows.

I tried to develop the nasty habit of smoking cigarettes on a few occasions but never came to recognize the thrill or necessity of it. Maybe that's why I'm so fat. My grandpa let me try his unfiltered Camel when I was super young but didn't care for the tobacco in my mouth. When in junior high, I belonged to a small secret club that met in one neighbor girl's home. At certain times, we were suppose to steal cigarettes from our parents and bring them to the clubhouse to smoke. The girl's brother said you don't just puff on a cigarette. To really smoke it, you have to inhale and swallow the smoke. Well, I tried it and got real sick. I didn't try smoking again until college, cuz my roommate was a smoker. She was trying to quit so bought a pipe to smoke and chew on. She said I could try it if I wanted to. I did and got a few thrills, then just quit. I hate the taste that smoking leaves in your mouth and on your breath, and the way it smells up the air. It's funny, because everyone in my real family smoked. I'm the only one that never took up the habit.

I do have a very good tolerance to alcohol, though. When in ROTC, I found that I could drink some of the guys under the table. I can easily have a whole bottle of wine or about five drinks before I start to feel intoxicated. I must have gotten my tolerance from my father. At least, I used to. Because of the medication I am on now, my tolerance level has dropped quite a bit and I try not to drink very much any way.

Getting my new house in 1982 was the best thing to happen to me since college. I couldn't wait to put in the fence and yard and start decorating inside. I enjoyed decorating my condo, but the house had it beat by a mile. I was painting the guest bedroom the day the movers came. I slept in there for about a month until I painted and wallpapered the master bedroom. The gardens were next, along with preparing the yard for sod. I laid the sod in May. I always had something to do. I even enjoyed mowing the nearly 4000 square feet of lawn that I had. If that wasn't enough, the summer before I lost the house, I mowed my lawn, two other people's and my parent's yards. I also trimmed some people's evergreens and shrubs in addition to my own.

With Bonnie's help, I designed a deck and had it built for a hot tub that I had gotten. I felt kind of lost after the bankruptcy and when I moved back in with my parents.

I'll admit that I'm not all that perfect. I do have my own faults. I've done a few things, spontaneously, that have put a financial burden on Michele and the Group. My love of the out-of-doors is to blame.

After driving the better part of 4500 miles in less than ten days, I put a lot of strain and wear and tear on my Chevy Malibu which, for six years, was my pride and joy. I had to do something before "Betsy" died on me. I traded her in on what the other Group members kept telling me was foolish and insensible – a truck. Something I had been dreaming I wanted since I had to give up my 1962 VW Beetle I had in college. Just one day out of the blue, I stopped at the local Datsun dealer and bought myself a shinny, new yellow, 1984 Nissan 4x4 King Cab truck. I called her "Buttercup" and dearly loved driving her. She saw the heart of Texas and the flatlands of Saskatchewan, Canada. I had her for eight years until she was worn to a frazzle. I never did much four-wheeling with her, just drove her hard.

The Group recognized that the truck was not all that foolish. We have a habit of hauling a lot of stuff around. It came in real handy for that. It hauled the wood and dirt for work on the yard of our house. Most of the four-wheelin' that I did was in town during the winter snow storms. Too bad I didn't have that truck during the Christmas Blizzard of 1982.

One night in 1992, when Bonnie was going over to the office to do some drafting, I persuaded the others to make a stop at a local Ford dealer. I wanted to look at vans. Karla had one and could fit more in her van than I could in my truck. This is what I decided would be my next vehicle. Because of the bankruptcy, it was not going to be easy getting financed. They would not approve a loan for an $18,000 van with my credit history and since I had just started another job. Instead, the salesman sold me on a 1989 used Plymouth Voyager van. It seemed clean and well kept. I learned quickly, though, that you don't buy a used vehicle at night. You need the light of day to thoroughly check it over; especially to look underneath for oil leaks. I ended up spending $250 on repairs the month after I got it.

God, I love to drive. If I had anything to say about it, I would be an over-the-road truck driver seeing America. I had so much fun driving my bug in the desert. The Group now only lets me drive them around town and to and from work. I had a great time when I had my paper route. I did some illegal driving, but I think newspaper people are given a little leeway on the rules because of the nature of the job.

I blew the transmission on the van I had when I did the paper route. I had traded it off on a new 1993 van before finding out that I would quit my paper route and we would go to work for the computer store. Because of the financial hardship we were faced with going into management with the store, I had to trade that new van off on a car that would give me smaller payments. Right now, I have a little five-speed Dodge Shadow. It's okay for getting us from place to place but not the kind of car I want to have for a long period of time.

The other dumb thing that I did was when the Group took a retreat to Silver Creek near Grandby. It was a free weekend for the cost of a promotional tour of the development. Despite the rain and snow and cold, I fell outwardly in love with the area. I even did some of my first real four-wheelin' in the area. It was gorgeous. So much solitude and beauty. So many places to explore. I was hooked on the place and made a contract on a $25,000 parcel of land. I had no control over myself. I knew we didn't have the money, but somehow felt that I would find a way to get it. No such luck. Because of the bankruptcy and the scam that the developer was trying to pull, we ended up only losing $500 of our own money on the deal.

I had done something like this before and should have known better. But I don't get that much time to spend camping in the wilderness. I had bought a Cutty's membership. Even before I had my truck and camper shell. That piece of poor judgment cost us $800. I saw it as an opportunity to go camping on my own, alone, and feel safe. I never got the chance to use that membership, and because I was a bit manic at the time I signed the contract, I was not thinking rationally.

I spent a lot of money on doing things around the house. The fence, the biggest lot in the cul-de-sac, the lawn, my ever-changing gardens, the flowers and seeds and trees, etc. And then there was the inside of the house. I'd decorated everything but the smallest bedroom and finish off the basement. I did turn the basement into a very workable art studio for Bobbie and Bonnie, though.

I didn't agree with Kim's methods and actions, but gave her the physical strength she had. Without my strength, she would not have been able to put up the struggles with the hospital staffs that she had. I must admit, I got some pleasure out of those struggles.

I had a gun once. I bought it to have when I went camping for protection. Kim found out about it and began making threats to Dr. Wilets and my mom about it. They finally convinced me to turn it over to Dr. Wilets for my own safe keeping.

I bet you wonder where my strengths and loves come from. They come from the five men who have taken time to teach them to me. They are Whispering Owl, my real father, my stepfather, the Big Guy and my brother, Roger.

It was my dad and brother that got me interested in cars and driving. With the gas station and car rental, I got to wash and be around a lot of cars. I had fun with this and asked to help out whenever there was a chance. Funny, though, I never learned how to pump gas until I went to college. When first learning to drive, it was they who had the faith in my ability and the guts to let me behind the wheel. My dad having had a bit much to drink sometimes created an opportunity for me to drive on the highway. My mom didn't seem to think I was capable of driving. She still questions my ability because of the medical problems we have had. She worries when I have to drive great distances. I think I have enough good sense to know when I can and cannot handle a car.

Only on one occasion did I really find myself in a situation where I could barely drive. It was in 1984 when I drove Elizabeth down to New Mexico to take some pictures about 25 miles from Las Vegas. On the way down I felt spacey a couple times and as if my truck could fly if driven off the highway. It was like I was in a tunnel of sorts. After Elizabeth took most of her pictures and we were driving back to Las Vegas, I began to feel a bit nauseous and dizzy. It was almost like someone had dusted me with some sleeping powder, cuz I was not very alert to what I was doing. I was almost numb. I ended up driving back about 25 mph and along the side of the road. The first thing I did was find a hotel and lay down. Things kind of spun around for awhile, then I passed out for a couple hours. When I woke up, I was a bit groggy but felt a lot better and went to get something to eat, but brought it back to my room. The next day I was fine on the trip back to Denver.

Whispering Owl gave me the love for animals and the out-of-doors. I'd never become a hunter unless it were a matter of survival. I couldn't even bring myself to kill a bird. I got upset hitting a prairie squirrel on the highway one time. I might have second thoughts if placed in a dangerous situation, but I'd try anything to avoid a confrontation. I do eat the fish I catch, but that is the extent of my hunting instincts. I eat meat and fowl, but at least I didn't know the animal or see the slaughter, so I don't think of it as an animal. In general, I'm not afraid of any animals. I do detest most insects, though. The wilderness is so free and peaceful. Sometimes I fantasize about going off into the mountains and becoming a recluse with the Group.

The Big Guy gave me strength and the lack of fear I have. He also gave me the natural know-how to do things with my hands. I would be more skillful if I didn't have so many inhibitions by having my mother so close. It took me two months to get up the guts to knock a hole in the wall of my own house for a doorway to the studio. I was afraid of what she would say. It wasn't the neatest or best thought-out project, but I did feel good about it when I finally did it. I just took a hammer one day and knocked a big hole in the wall, then took my saw to cut out the doorway.

Well, it's not every little tidbit that I've ever done, but it is pretty much my story. As you can see, I have played a very major role in Michele's existence. I have had more time around than many of the others. I am probably the oldest and most active member of the Group today. I appreciate getting the chance to tell my story.

Mike

SAMANTHA

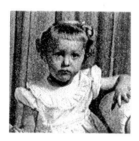 Michele and Whispering Owl gave me the name Samantha. It stuck, but I like Sammy Jo better. I am five years old. Katherine is writing this for me from what I tell her cuz I can't write or spell much yet. I know the alphabet and some numbers, and really only spell my name very well.

Whispering Owl introduced me to Michele when she was about two and a half. I was her first real playmate and close friend. We would play dolls and just talk to one another. I kept her company when she wanted to be alone or away from other people.

I like simple things, and nature and animals. I really liked to go over to Avis and Bob's across the alley and sit and watch the big goldfish. Sometimes I'd get to feed them. I liked to go across the street and sit for hours listening to Mr. Peck tell stories of when he was a kid and young man growing up in the West when things were hard but kinda simple.

It was more fun when Peggy came along. We made a great threesome. We would play house with our dolls and tea set on one of the two porches we had with our toys. We are all very much alike, but Peggy likes being around people more than Michele or me.

Most of my toys are gone now. Michele gave away or had to sell a lot of my stuffed animals before our move. I didn't play with all of them, anyway. Michele let me keep my five favorite: Mr. Popples, Mickey Mouse, Honey Bear, my unicorn and Pegasus. I just recently got a new puppy dog that sits on my bed. He is nice and cuddly and reminds me of Nikki, who I miss very much.

I like horses. I used to try and ride Mr. Hobby's pony, but mostly would just pet and feed him grass. I could never pass up the pony rides at the carnivals that we'd go to. I always dreamed of having a horse of my own until mom and one of Michele's friends explained how much work is involved in keeping a horse – and the expense. I'm not around enough to devote the time to a horse, and we don't have enough money.

I've gotten plenty of enjoyment from the animals that the family or Michele has had. We've had lots of dogs, some cats, fish, turtles, birds, hamster, mice and rats. I think animals are neat to watch. My grandfather had some neighborhood squirrels trained so that they would crawl right up his leg and take nuts from his hand.

I especially got close to the two dogs Michele had of her own – Toshi, from college and Nikki, the Yorkie who died last year. I really loved Nikki, cuz she was the best behaved and trained pet we have known. Nikki was the playfullest thing and longest lasting pet Michele ever had. I sometimes thought Nikki was human because of how loving she was. I miss her very much. I made Michele have her cremated so I could hang onto her ashes. I won't let her spread them anywhere just yet. I even make her hang the painting Bobbie did of Nikki at the foot of our bed.

I like Mike a lot. He is very caring towards me and Peggy. We're his little sisters. He lets us help him do things and he takes us places. I like to go on trips with him cuz he's fun. I even used to like to help out in the garden. I think it's neat to watch flowers and vegetables grow.

I'm pretty much a homebody. Except for going on trips with Mike, I like to stay close to home. I especially don't like hospitals. I don't like being around a whole lot of people and strangers. That's why I'm just five still. I didn't want to grow up and go to school with all those other kids and people. I went to Arizona with Michele and the Group, but stayed mostly away from the campus and people. I would go with Mike and Francie and Katherine to the top of the Butte at times, though. It was so pretty and peaceful up there. But, most of the time, I would usually just stay in the dorm or around the apartment buildings.

I don't know what else to say about me, cuz I'm so simple and there isn't a whole lot to me. I don't spend that much time out and about anymore since Nikki died. Michele and my other sisters have more important things to do with our time. I like to play with Michele's nephew, Daniel, but he is growing up so fast and I don't see him that much now that they don't live around here any more. I sleep a lot, too.

Sammy Jo
(as told to and written by Katherine)

PEGGY

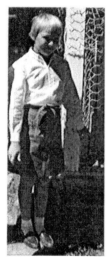

I'm probably the Group's most visible young alter. I like to be around people, but most of all, I like to be around the other Group members. I learn a lot from them. I'm very smart for my age. Some people think I'm a genius. I'm modest about it, but I do know a lot. I like imitating what I see and I can make good deductions about how things should be.

I came around when Michele was very young. I was one of Michele's best playmates, but tended to like being around Mike more. It took me a long time to grow up to eight years old. I have grown some more lately. I'm now about twelve.

I have a tendency to attach myself to people that mean a lot to this system. One was our real father. He seemed to understand us and wanted to see us experience some of our dreams. I hated to see him drink like he did, but I know it was his only way to deal with the demands my mother placed on him. She can be a very critical person and be hurtful to the ones she loves. I don't think she does it on purpose. I think it was because of the way her parents were with her.

I was deeply hurt and lost when my dad died. I was just really getting to know him. I had a warm spot in my heart for him. I cried an awful lot when that happened. I kind of resented my mom for awhile, because I felt it was a lot of her fault that he drank himself to death. I was glad when the priest asked me to find some passages in the Bible that reminded me of the way I felt for him. I feel there is a reason for why things happen, and I now feel that there was a reason for my dad's death.

My life has been really screwed up when he was alive and since he has died, but his death offered me so many more opportunities I would never have been able to experience if he were still alive. I would never have been able to meet and get to know Roy, my stepfather, had he not died. We probably would not have been able to go to college in Arizona and have the best years of our life. I could go on and on, but I think you get the picture.

Since Roy's death, I have become closer than ever to my mom. I have grown to love her more for the person she is today (though not much different) than the way I saw her years ago. She has opened up some of her vulnerability to me. I have been able to see inside her and the good intentions she really has. If it weren't for the other Group members and our support group, I would probably move back in with her. They keep telling me that time will come sooner than I think and to just be patient. As it is now, I only get to see her once or twice a week.

I enjoy the outdoors and nature a lot. I really like the seasons. My favorite is the spring and summer with the thunderstorms. They excite me and dazzle me with their power. The wind has been blowing all day today. I have made Michele keep the balcony door to our apartment open all day so I can listen and meditate to the sound of the rustling cottonwoods around the complex.

Next to being in nature, my favorite pastime is watching movies. I love exciting action-filled movies. I like new movies mainly, but like some of the good old ones from ten to twenty years ago. I don't get to go to the mountains very often, so when Michele has a little extra money, I harp on her until she gives in and gets five movies from the video store to do a weekend movie marathon. It doesn't happen very often but I have patience to get me by until the opportunity is there.

I like to ride with Mike to and from work during the week. Now that Michele has turned the radio off while she is in the car for meditation, I can talk good ol' times with Mike. We relive the memories of going to the mountains and some of the long trips we have taken. We talk a lot about the good things both our fathers had in them.

I have really become intrigued with the computer business the others are in. I like to talk with Nicole and help Connie out when she is on the sales floor at the store. I like to spend as much time as I can learning about new things and being around other people in need. Customers sure are in need of a lot of help.

Like many of the others, I am very introverted. I do like to be in the presence of other people but I like to sit back and observe them. I don't like strong interactions. I find people to be very interesting and often quite humorous in the positions they get themselves into.

I could probably dazzle you with all the philosophies I have developed on life, but don't want to bore you or show off. The doctors at NIH couldn't believe that someone my age could be as smart as Michele or Shelley. I learned a lot from them. I paid attention in class. I went to school, even college, but just decided to remain young and innocent. Like Samantha, I like simple pleasures of life. I don't like to get caught up in the adult whirlwinds.

I guess that is my story. I guess if I could have anything to do all over again, it would be to relearn how to play. Play for a kid was simple. Adult play is too complicated. This system is extremely wrapped up in adult play; or should I say work. Work for this system is play. The only play they are good at.

Peggy

KIM

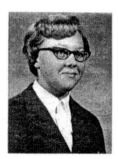

My life began when Michele was around five years old. I evolved as a control element for pain, anger and frustration. The only problem was that Whispering Owl failed to give me all the necessary wisdom and judgment needed to strictly control these feelings. I had to feel my way through the situations I encountered. Michele had to be a brave little girl to make it through some of the early events of her life.

Things were pretty easy for me to cope with until other Group members gained more personal strength. During Michele's early years, about all I had to deal with was the pain incurred from bumps and bruises and the frustration of blackout spells we used to have. Michele had a tendency to be somewhat clumsy and uncoordinated. Then, there were those shots she used to get for something or other. I got to enjoy those shots and needles, but had a dreadful time convincing her to like them. I loved to give blood when I got old enough and wasn't ineligible because of medications. I have great veins and give blood just about as fast as anyone can.

I also had to help Michele with the frustrations she encountered being left alone because of her level of intelligence. That's one thing I was good at. Me and the Group, that is. We were her companions and she soon grew to accept her isolation from being different than a lot of the other kids. She knew we were close and there when she needed someone to talk to.

Sixth grade was when the conflicts really began to get out of control. That's when our father's drinking problem started to get bad. He was considered to be an alcoholic at that point. The next four and a half years became a living hell that we all tried to ignore. We began to develop and go in separate directions, each concentrating on what we did best.

I had to look to the Big Guy for guidance in this situation, because Whispering Owl was not around enough, especially when I needed his support. The Big Guy became the father we had essentially lost. He gave me the sense that I was indestructible and that I could handle anything Michele would have to face in her life. But I wasn't really prepared for what was ahead.

The anger and hatred that flowed through the family was so intense that I found myself in a position that I was unable to appropriately deal with in a rational manner. The strength which was exhibited by Bobbie, Shelley and Katherine made things even worse. They strengthened their talents and began to over-involve themselves with school projects and Girl Scouting. Not only did I have unbearable conflicts on the homefront, but conflicts arose at school. Since Michele didn't have much of a social life other than scouting, that was one area that gave me little trouble on top of surmounting turmoil.

Things got so out of hand that I began to experience a sense of nonexistence; I was not real and felt as though I was dreaming everything that was happening. I had my first real void feelings during junior high. Somehow, slamming doors, yelling back or just going off to be by myself no longer worked. They didn't make me feel real again. I had to do something; something to identify myself and Michele. After an especially despairing day at school, when Michele got into trouble for things other students were doing, I was compelled to do something that would give Michele back a sense of identity. I took a comb and, during the afternoon at school, proceeded to carve an "M" and an "N" onto the back of each hand. My first act of self-mutilation. Michele was appalled and couldn't understand what had happened. Explaining it to her parents was even more difficult. Needless to say, with all this turmoil, communication within the Group was beginning to fade.

The arguing and fighting at home got worse than worse. The words got louder and uglier and things got physical; pushing one another around the house into furniture and against doors, and food being thrown across the table at mealtime. I was frustrated. Michele, the Group and I became torn and confused. We loved our father so much, but couldn't stand to see what it was doing to our mother, even though she didn't help matters with her defensive antagonism. I needed help. I didn't know which direction to go. I had no one to really advise me. I could take pain and self-punishment, but couldn't cope with the frustrations and anger that was present. Aside from the engraving and bedroom door slamming, all I could do was withdraw with Michele. We withdrew more and more with a feeling of hopelessness. I am suppose to be the strong one in the Group, but certainly couldn't demonstrate it back then.

When our father died in 1970, I wanted to die, too. That was the first time I ever felt vulnerable and as if I *could* die. The whole Group mourned the death and withdrew for quite some time afterward. Michele's depressive behavior became more intense. I began to feed on it. Not to hurt the Group, intentionally, but to try and re-establish my strength. The Group was becoming more separate and independent of Michele. I didn't know how to pull things back together. I was in a personal crisis.

I thought things would be different when we moved to Billings that next summer. When fall came, Whispering Owl was no where to be found. I had to rely on the Big Guy more than ever at this point. I had to regain my strength. He offered me a source. A man's strength. Unknowing to me, however, he began to steer me in an unrealistic direction of power. He really had me believing that I was free of pain and that nothing could ever hurt me again.

We all tried real hard to make a go of things and make new lives for ourselves after the move. It was an opportunity to be reborn. We were, yet became more independent of Michele. Michele was still depressed. Not as much, but it was still there. Next to Francie, I was the only Group link Michele had, and neither of us was all that successful. Michele started to become somewhat footloose, like Francie, and not care what was going on around her. She became lost in another world. Her grip on reality was fading. I held her together until our mom developed her relationship with Roy. We all felt it was much too soon after our father's death for her to become involved with another man.

Michele started to lose a grip over this. The Group tried to ignore it by getting involved again with school. They wanted to escape reality, too. My frustrations grew. Michele became suicidal in her thoughts. I tried to intervene. She wanted to slash her wrists. I stepped in. I cut our wrist, but just deep enough to draw a little blood. That's when my fascination with blood began. It gave me a feeling of rejuvenation. Seeing that blood made me feel that we were still very much alive. Licking the wound and the taste of the blood made it just that much more real. I saved Michele and had a renewed sense of purpose and existence.

Michele failed with her attempt, but I succeeded in demonstrating the strength I was created to have. I may have succeeded with crude-like behavior, but the important thing was that I saved Michele's life with little incidence. When asked what happened, we just said a cat scratched us.

I got Michele and the rest of the Group, with the help of Shelley and Alice, to rationalize and realize what a blessing in disguise it was for mom and Roy to be getting married. It meant a brighter future for all of us. A chance to pursue our dreams and develop our talents. It also made the thoughts of going to college a more realistic plan and idea.

Things settled down and my job was easy when we moved to Denver in 1972. Group members developed further and pursued their talents, but this time, not as an escape. Michele made a new vow to start over and get herself straightened out.

Michele was able to attend the college of her choice, but I was back on the job for a brief period. Eight hundred miles away from home caused some anxiety and separation issues for Michele to cope with. Alone, in strange surroundings and a new lifestyle called for survival tactics. Again, Michele was plagued with depression and Group members taking off in separate directions. Withdrawal and suicidal thoughts once more came into the picture. I convinced her to go for professional counseling. She saw a psychologist, but the depression and suicidal thoughts grew more intense. The psychologist recommended that she seek help from the university psychiatrist, who could prescribe an antidepressant. Dr. Bohn prescribed Elavil for the depression and set up regular psychotherapy sessions. Mike was going through an intense pledge program which put a lot of extra stress on the Group. This undertaking, the others' pursuits, in addition to depression got to be overwhelming. One night I got the idea to take some extra Elavil. It caused us to be drowsy and I felt that if Michele could just go to sleep, the turmoil would subside and she could get some peace. The next day I went to Dr. Bohn to explain what had happened. She prescribed a few days in the school medical center with some sedation and a bit of TLC. This was my first experience in a hospital setting. I hated it. I was absolutely bored and felt too restricted. We were so doped up that I didn't really remember much about it, though. Michele did get a number of visitors of concerned school friends. I think that helped her to feel her wanted and in a more friendly surrounding.

The overdose was not serious, but left me feeling strange the next day. It was a new experience for me and made me feel strong that I came through it okay. I felt that nothing could hurt me.

Things settled down after that first semester. Michele was still slightly depressed but no longer felt it necessary to see the school psychiatrist. The rest of the Group took over and lived very prominently for the remaining time we were in college. Each one did their own thing, with little conflict, and really became separate identities in the sense of multiple personalities.

Things started getting rough again during the fall of 1980. A new supervisor had been assigned to Bonnie's department at work in April. She was having difficulty adjusting to the man and felt that she could be doing a better job than he. She was also experiencing a number of manic-depressive episodes. Michele went to the company psychologist for some help in adjusting. He overlooked the seriousness of the work problem and placed emphasis on the quivering relationship she was beginning to have with Gene. He sent her back to Employee Relations for the difficulties at work, who, in turn, sent her straight back to the problem. For her social difficulties, the company doctor recommended a local psychologist in private practice.

Michele began to see that psychologist. Shortly afterwards, she attended a cousin's wedding in Billings, Montana. With Bonnie's serious difficulties at work and Sally's falling relationship with Gene, a wedding was the last thing Michele needed. She was becoming more depressed over everything that was happening. I was frustrated with this rut we were in and needed to get us some relief quickly. Michele had some Tylenol 3 w/Codeine she had gotten for a strained thumb. One day in September, things got overwhelming for me to control. I got that void and senseless feeling. Michele was getting little help if any to relieve her problems. She was becoming desperate and having suicidal ideations. I thought about the incident back at school with the Elavil. It worked then, why couldn't something like that work again. The next thing I knew, I was taking eleven of the Tylenol 3's. Of course, I thought the power I had would prove that nothing was going to happen. Remember, I'm invincible. The Tylenol 3 didn't help much with the pain in her thumb and extra strength Tylenol did nothing for headaches. I figured we'd take the bus home from work and sleep the feelings away.

About thirty minutes passed and I was beginning to feel a bit shaky. I wasn't expecting to feel something this quickly. As I was at the bus stop waiting for my bus and feeling this way, I thought it would be a good idea to get to the doctor's office and somehow explain to them what I had done. I caught the next bus that went past his office. The girls in the office rushed me over to the Denver Presbyterian Hospital emergency room. They induced vomiting, but the Tylenol had been in my system for so long that I don't think they really accomplished a whole lot. While in the ER and when they were taking me to my room, I was having uncontrollable shaking and body jerking. I spent the night in the hospital under observation. I was so sedated from the Tylenol that I wasn't aware of things enough to hate it.

A psychiatrist was called in the next day for a consultation before they would release me. Michele showed her severe depression and spoke of her suicidal thoughts. The doctor recommended an evaluative hospitalization at Mt. Airy Psychiatric Hospital. He released her to our sister, Karla, with whom we spent the night before entering the hospital the next day.

The next thing I knew, I was having my things searched and I was being left in a locked ward at Mt. Airy. Michele was assigned a Dr. Whittington to treat her. His diagnosis was that of depressive neurosis with schizophrenia and suicidal behavior. I tried to persuade him that there might be something physiologically wrong in addition to the depression. At times, our limbs would twitch and go numb and we had this feeling of lost time. They did some tests, including a neurological exam and EEG's which came back borderline. Michele's continued depression and suicidal thoughts were not convincing them that there was a physiological reason for her dilemma.

Anger and frustration with Michele's behavior continued to grow inside me. I didn't know what to do. This anger and frustration got the better of me and I began to have impulsive and compulsive feelings. My behavior started to get irrational. I felt I had to do things which ended up making matters worse. After a period of confinement in the hospital, I was compelled to do things like put my fist through a non-breakable glass window and beat my fists bloody against a brick wall. At one point when I was trusted to leave the ward, I hid from the staff and tried to escape. I was having real difficulties with the control issues. I was not in control.

Dr. Whittington didn't see me one day and I had some important things I wanted to discuss with him. I left word with his office to have him call me. When he didn't return my calls, I got very angry. I then started to threaten and play games with the staff. I had to show myself I could be in control of the situation. They put me on fifteen minute watches. Between the times the staff checked on me, I removed the light bulb from the lamp in my room and broke it with a towel. I hid some of the glass in my bra to be sure I'd have some if they should somehow catch me with the rest and take it away from me.

I had the strong desire to cut on myself to make sure that all that was happening was real. The staff came in a found me trying to cut on myself. They tried to take the glass away from me but I wouldn't let go. I kept clenching my fists and cut the palms of my hands. The staff joined forces (3 or 4 of them) and drug me to the isolation room and put me in four-point restraints. The cuffs were loose enough that I was able to pull the glass from my bra and proceed to cut on my arms. It looked bad when they found me, but things were actually superficial. This caused Dr. Whittington to put a 72-hour mental health hold on me. I was demanding to be released with the argument that Michele came in voluntarily.

My need for control started getting in the way. The hospital staff was not going to give me the satisfaction. My behavior worsened as my confinement frustration grew. I wanted out. Michele was still talking suicide. All this wound up getting Michele placed on a 90-day court hold.

Michele's insurance ran out shortly afterward and we were transferred to Bethesda Community Mental Health Center. Michele was assigned a new doctor who really knew little about what was going on and had transpired at Mt. Airy. I tried a new tactic to get out. I took complete control of myself and the situation and gave Michele very little time to express her feelings and desires. Within a couple of weeks, I had the doctor and staff convinced that the medication was finally doing Michele some good and that she no longer had suicidal thoughts. We were released the end of October. Bonnie returned to work on a half-day schedule for a couple weeks.

Michele was actually still depressed, so returned to Dr. Whittington on an outpatient basis. Bonnie lost her position as Lead Drafter. Despite the reduced pressures she was suppose to have, things had not really become any different. Even after trying to work things out with Nenad through the aid of the Employee Relations department, things seemed to get even worse. I had to share some mighty hard words with Nenad on a number of occasions. During one such session a geologist, in passing, made the comment that they thought they were going to have to send an ambulance for one of us before the session was over. After we came to some satisfactory conclusions, he had the gall to reach over his desk and pull me towards him and shake my hand. I felt he was just about ready to lay a kiss on my cheek when he actually kissed my hand. Michele couldn't handle the ensuing confusion and contradictory signals she was getting from the work situation and her private life. This set her up for another hospitalization of about five weeks in the psych ward at St. Luke's Hospital.

I was cool this time, because Michele was just confused and depressed. She didn't outwardly express any inclination toward suicide. Depressed enough, however, that she couldn't function. Katherine and Bobbie kept her thoughts under control and tried to depict them in words and through art.

Things were definitely very unfriendly when Bonnie returned to work. In fact, they acted fearful of her and took a number of her responsibilities away. To top it off, Michele and Gene had ended their relationship after three and a half years.

Dr. Whittington put Michele on Parnate, an MAO inhibitor for her depression. The rougher life's situations got, the more frustrated I became. Dr. Whittington must have thought Michele hopeless, because he turned her over to his associate, a psychologist, and put her into a group therapy program with no more private sessions. I don't think that was a wise move. We were losing contact with reality. I was getting desperate again. Things were going in circles and nothing was seeming to get resolved.

While on Parnate, you have to be careful with the amount of caffeine and alcohol you consume. In August 1981, I reached a point to which I could no longer handle the daily frustrations. One morning I got desperate enough to begin a game of Russian Roulette. I took my Parnate times two for the day plus drank a lot of coffee and took a Dexatrim diet capsule which was loaded with caffeine. I left work early to attend group therapy at Dr. Whittington's. Before going into therapy, I took three or four good shots of straight bourbon. By the time the group started, I was very quiet. I said very little during the session. I was in a bit of a daze. When the group was over, I was like a zombie; real tired and dizzy. I didn't think anything could affect me like that. I asked to stay for awhile in the doctor's office and fell asleep for at least a half hour or so when the secretary came in to wake me and say that I would have to leave. All I can remember is that I couldn't move. I felt paralyzed. I was so groggy and what speech I could get out was slurred. I didn't know what was happening to me.

Dr. Whittington came in and thought I was faking my symptoms for some attention. He threatened to put me in the hospital if I didn't get up and leave. Well, my frustrations grew to an overwhelming proportion filled with anger. I was not going to the hospital. I staggered to my feet and crawled along the walls to leave his office. I could barely open my eyes to see where I was going. I thought that if I could just make it to my car, I'd sleep it off there.

The next thing I knew I was outside in the parking lot hanging onto a pole. The psychologist from the group came out with the building guard. Suddenly, I found myself in a wheelchair being pushed to the emergency room at Mercy Medical Center across the street. The last thing I wanted. I was enraged. I grabbed the Parnate bottle from my purse when no one was watching and dumped 10 or 15 more into my hand and then into my mouth.

I soon lost consciousness but was somewhat aware of what was going on. I felt nothing and couldn't respond to anything that was being said to me. I was a limp noodle. They put a tube in my throat but I didn't feel it. The next thing I remember was being moved from the ER to a room.

It seemed like such a long trip. I later found out that I was in intensive care. I still felt nothing. I then reached a point when I felt my body was no longer breathing on its own. I remember my parents talking but couldn't respond. I finally had a feeling of inner peace. The anger was all gone. There was a calm about me that I never experienced before. I almost felt like a spirit out of my body.

It wasn't long after this incident that I was referred to Dr. Greg Wilets by the physician who was attending me at Mercy. I decided to go see him, because I was not really comfortable with the arrangement with Dr. Whittington and his office. I felt comfortable with Dr. Wilets from the start and was glad Michele decided to start seeing him regularly.

The peace I experienced from the Parnate overdose didn't last long. Things were almost back to where they were before then; the aggravation, frustration and despair. Work was becoming a war zone for Bonnie. I was losing touch with reality – no more control. I felt as if life was a dream. I began cutting on myself again. The sight and taste of blood made me regain some sense of realness. If the cut was not deep enough nor produced enough blood, I would suck it like a vampire. I needed that taste. Our arms and wrists have cross-hatched scars from all the cutting I have done. I didn't, and still don't fully agree that this act is self-mutilation. I might consider it more as a form of self-punishment for losing control of life.

Soon the cutting got to be old and didn't satisfy me. My next act was to try and repeat the same sense of peace and calm obtained from the Parnate overdose. I was no longer taking the MAO inhibitor, but Trilafon. I survived one severe overdose so felt I would have no problem with another. I just wanted to find peace and control. I was confused after taking the pills, so put in a call to Dr. Wilets. I know I was not very rational when he called back. In fact, I think I hung up on him when he recommended the hospital. I was angered by his threats of intervention, but felt that I didn't have enough of the drug to get the results I was looking for. Dr. Wilets put in a call to 911 and had an ambulance and paramedics sent to my condo.

I had forgotten to lock my door, so the paramedics had easy access to my place. I was a bit out of it when they arrived, but remember arguing that I didn't want to go to the hospital. I was too weak to fight them. They drug me down to the ambulance and took me to University Hospital for the normal overdose treatment. When stabilized, Dr. Wilets had me transferred and admitted to the psych ward at St. Joseph's Hospital and placed on suicide precautions.

This hospitalization lasted from October to December 1981. I was resistant, yet cooperative at first. As time passed, so did my patience and control. That's the way it was with most of my hospitalizations. The confinement and restrictions placed on me were against my nature. I demanded freedom to do as I pleased. I couldn't handle the thought of someone else doing my job and taking control.

I've had six additional psychiatric hospitalizations since the one above, which was my first under Dr. Wilet's care. Turmoil erupted with each confinement. My control issues would always get in the way and keep me from having a productive encounter. I would act out and the hospitalizations would drag on. One lasted over two months.

The way I would maintain a sense of control is by being defiant and seeing what I could get away with. Usually my acts of defiance were destructive. You see, I had a lot of anger trapped inside me and I had this thing about hurting other people – I couldn't do it no matter how badly they may have hurt me. Instead, I would direct this anger inward against my own well-being. I still had this feeling that nothing I could do to myself could hurt me as much as other people have hurt me in the past. My system was armor-plated.

My two main acts of destructiveness were that of taking more than the prescribed quantities of pills and cutting on myself. I had that thing about blood for the longest time.

The worst act of self-mutilation was when I was in the hospital in 1982. I was so bad that Dr. Wilets talked me into undergoing shock treatments. I'm not quite sure whether I had anything to say in the matter or not. I draw a pretty strong blank to nearly that entire experience. Shock treatments have this horrible affect on the mind. It makes you lose your memory. I think it affected me more than the normal person. For years afterwards, I had problems trying to find the right words to communicate with other people. I know the words were there once. Even today I often have instances where I can't put the right words to what I want to say. The flow is rigid.

Anyway, on with what I did. Upon review of my records I guess I ended up taking overdoses of prescribed and over-the-counter drugs three or four times. Worse than that, though, was my cutting gestures. I always seemed to find a sharp that would give me the gratification I was seeking for a release. One day out on the rooftop patio, I noticed that the edge of the metal furniture was relatively sharp. My thoughts were with thinking I could climb the fence and jump off the fifth floor roof. A couple of failed attempts got me interested in the furniture. Over the course of a day, I continued to rub my right wrist along the sharp edges. I remembered seeing it get redder and redder, but have no recollection of it ever bleeding much. I'm not certain whether it ever did, or whether I just can't remember the incident that clearly. Whatever was done put a big enough gash in my wrist that it created quite a scar. When I came to after my treatments, I remembered having a butterfly bandage on it. It may not have been deep enough for stitches, but sure made a nasty scar. I'm very self-conscious about it today.

During one of my later hospitalizations, one of the technicians commented about it and asked if I had carpal tunnel surgery. With so much of that going around and someone in the medical profession thinks I had it, I just hope that other people who see it think of something similar. For people who ask about it, I just tell them something to the effect that I gashed it on some glass or barbed wire when I was young and don't quite remember which it was. I play it as a childhood accident.

Another of my common activities when in the hospital was not eating. I would go on a hunger strike as a control action. When that wouldn't work, I would eat so the staff saw me, but when I would go back to my room, I would make myself throw up. This worked on a couple occasions but was short-lived. I didn't get as much satisfaction from it as the other activities I partook of.

I'm not really all that bad, mind you. I just have not been properly taught how to vent my anger and frustration in a constructive manner. Something changed that, though. During my last hospitalization, I realized just how vulnerable I was to my actions. I had control issues, but this time I got out of control by being totally naive to what I was doing. This was in the fall of 1989.

You see, I have this problem with my sleeping when in the hospital. Different noises, smells, bed and perceptions would not allow me to get restful sleep. I would go days on just two to four hours of sleep. I was always getting up and going to the nurses station in the middle of the night for a repeat on my sleeping medication. Even with that, I would not get the sleep I needed. There had to be a better way.

One day, I got out on pass to pick up or deliver some work that Bonnie was doing for a client. I went home and thought that I would pick up my sleeping medication that was home and bring it back to the hospital and have a stash. Not to overdose on, but just for helping me get some needed sleep. Before I could go on pass I had to make a contract with the staff that I would not do anything out on pass that would jeopardize my well-being. That wasn't my style. I never did anything out on pass. It always had to be in the hospital. When I was out on pass, *I was in control.* Anyway, when I got home I was surprised to find all my medication gone from my room and bathroom. My mother had confiscated it. I thought I would go up to her bedroom to check to see if she had hidden it there. My father had just come home from the hospital and was in their TV room next to their bedroom. He was awake and spoke to me. I was hoping he would have been asleep, but because he wasn't, I couldn't check their bedroom. This made me furious with my mother. How could she not trust me? I became a desperate person, looking for anything. I went back to my bedroom and came across some Fiorcet and a few antidepressant tablets she had missed. I had gotten the Fiorcet for some migraine headaches I was having a year earlier. I really had no clue what kind of drug it was. I decided to put the pills in one of my rolls of socks and take them back to the hospital. I was still furious with my mom when I returned to the hospital.

The staff searched me and my belongings when I came back to the hospital. They did not find the pills. The rage inside of me became obsessive and I couldn't think of anything but taking the pills. There weren't very many; only about a dozen. The next thing I remember was standing in the bathroom with a cup of water and pills in my hand. I looked at them then myself in the mirror. I couldn't see myself, just the rage. I was numb. Before I knew it, I had taken all the pills. The next thing I remember was going to my occupational therapy session. About halfway through the session, I was beginning to feel very strange. I felt like I was in a bubble and had cotton stuffed in my head. I certainly was no longer enraged with my mother. I had problems with my speech – it began to slur. I couldn't focus my eyes or concentrate on what I was working on. The sounds around me became indistinguishable. Things started to spin slightly. I couldn't wait for OT to be over with. When it was, I went to my room. I thought I just needed to lie down and sleep this off. It was kind of what I felt like when I took the Tylenol with Codeine. I put my headphones on to listen to music and laid down on my bed.

The next thing I remember was someone shaking me to get me up for dinner. I told her I was too tired and not hungry. My speech was still pretty slurred. She sensed something was wrong and rightly so. I could not keep my eyes open. I couldn't even sit up on the side of my bed. She asked me if I had taken anything. I was evasive, but more than anything don't think I could have told her if I weren't. She called another nurse in to go through my things. They found the prescription bottle. They began to monitor my vitals and made several phone calls. At this point I just remember sensing several people in and out of my room. The decision was made to move me to ICU for medical intervention. Because I couldn't sit up, they put me in hospital gowns and moved me to ICU on my bed. I was fading in and out of consciousness.

Dr. Anneberg came in at one point and helped try to get me intubated. My throat was already beginning to swell shut that it took them three or four tries before they were successful. A half hour longer and they would have had to do a tracheotomy or I would have suffocated. I was in and out of it throughout the night. I heard bits and pieces to what was being said or done around me but I was pretty limp and unresponsive. They spent much of the night pouring charcoal down a tube in my nose. It seems that every time they got some down me, I would spit it right up. I was a black mess. I was alert enough early in the morning when a male nurse was trying to clean me up. I remember opening my eyes for awhile and feeling embarrassed by the whole ordeal.

The hospital staff saved my life that night. Who would have thought so few pills could have done me in? I don't know what it was, but that fit of rage did something to change me. Maybe it made me realize I was not as invincible as I had once thought. The nurses kept telling me that 30 minutes later and I would not be alive today. That thought scares the shit out of me. Even though Michele and I often say we wish we were dead doesn't mean we really mean it. It is just a cry that we are hurting deeply inside and desperate. If I have my way, I will live beyond 100.

When I was moved back up to the psych ward I was immediately placed in isolation. I would later find out that a patient had succeeded in killing herself the few weeks before I came in. I scared them shitless. They would never live down two suicides in one month. This ordeal was somewhat of an awakening for me. I no longer posed as Chrissy. I wanted me known for who I was and face up to the torment I had put this body through. I was not proud of previous actions. It was the only way I knew how to cope with the ball of fire in my gut that I had carried all my life. I was ready to ask for help. There had to be a better way.

Over the next week or so, the nursing staff helped me to get in touch with that anger that was eating away at me. I was angry at Dr. Wilets for refusing to talk with me and the staff for shutting me away by myself for two days when I was hurting. They showed me how to work through the anger and analyze it. They showed me how to constructively confront the people who made me angry. I confronted Dr. Wilets. He said he was angry with me because I was being gamey and splitting hairs over the contract I had made before that pass. The nursing staff came down on him pretty hard for not knowing what I would do on pass. I had a lot of trust from him and by doing what I did, I erased that trust. I was scared I had ruined the patient/doctor relationship we had. I had too much invested in our relationship to send it down the tubes. Once I faced him with my issues and we both laid everything out on the table, I found my anger diminishing and I ended up apologizing to him.

He and the staff talked it over and they felt that trying some biofeedback may teach me to redirect some of my anger. We were kind of skeptical that it could work, because I tried it once before with little success. Regardless, I was ready to try anything if it might help me. It was time to grow up and change my ways. The biofeedback did seem to work this time. Since that orientation, when I begin to feel the least bit of tension, I try to sideline it just long enough to get into my relaxation space to chew it up and spit it out. Since learning this technique, I rarely find myself getting into fits of rage or worked up such that I have to do something destructive to relieve the pressure. Rarely does anything anger me for more than a few moments. More than anything, it turns to frustration and then shrivels up and disappears. I kinda think some of the medication I am and have been on since then has had something to do with this also, because I find myself not getting angry when I have every right to do so. My attitude is in a state of so what. It happened, I lived through it and it isn't important enough to get angry about. I will handle myself differently next time.

Our system has been in a good way since this near-tragic experience. Medicine has developed some drugs that have finally been able to control my depression and not given me a reason to hold the weight of the world on my shoulders. I have become more of a protector than a destructor; however, this now seems to be getting me in a different kind of trouble at work.

Even though the medication I am on keeps me from bottling too much up, I still live a pretty rigid life. I am not a people person and it is having an affect on Michele's ability to move up the ranks at work. I see a job needs to be done and it needs to be done quickly and efficiently. My boss says that's okay for me but that isn't the way I should come across to my people. I need more latitude and need to throw my rulebook away. This is so hard to do because of the lifelong programming that has evolved into my perception. This is going to be another tough one to get through. I know it needs to be done and I need to change, but I have some mental resistance to it. I guess if Shelley can learn to not be such a perfectionist, I guess I can also learn to be not such a hard-core driver boss. All I ask is that everyone be patient with me. I have forty years worth of living this way to chisel away at. I hope it doesn't take too long that it will ruin things for the others.

Well, that's my story. I hope you can see what a different person I have grown and matured into. I no longer want the reputation of the Demolition Man of the Group. I can be warm and cuddly if just given half a chance.

Kim

ALICE

As Katherine said, I am the mother hen. I probably have more traits that take after our real mother than anyone else. The only person that I know acts more like my mother than herself is my sister, Karla. I have the homemaking skills. I can cook when I have to and do a darn good job of it. Both my mother and grandmother are (were) good cooks. I also have some perfectionistic traits in me. When I do things, they have to be done just so. No one can do them as well as I do things. I am also a fairly rigid disciplinarian. I feel people should know what to do and if they don't do it themselves, not complain when it doesn't get done. People should also do what they are told by their elders or superiors.

Since the microwave became such a dominant aspect of our lives, I do very little cooking. When I do, it doesn't amount to a whole lot, because I am cooking for just one person. When we go over to our mom's or someone else's place, they are in charge. If they ask me to help, I gladly do so, but I don't volunteer to help. I do a job when it has to be done, otherwise I'm pretty lazy. Besides, a number of the Group members don't care for me because I am so stern. They keep telling me to give them some slack.

I don't know what makes me so rough around the edges. I guess the Group needed someone like me to stand up to our real mom. She was always telling us what to do and never praising us to our face. It seemed that no one could ever do right by her. No one is good enough for her. She is always putting people down. I know I am bad and a lot like her but not that extreme. As they seem to say – "Like mother, like daughter." I guess it is true.

Kim is not the only one who is making life difficult for Michele at work. I have a bad case of ogeritis. I can't seem to find anything good in the people at work. I started the job with good intentions, but I get so wrapped up in seeing that a good job is done, that I lose track of people's feelings and needs. It's hard to give praise if you don't know what it sounds like. Like Kim, I would like to soften around the edges but this affect is so drilled into me, I don't know if I can be any different.

I am very judgmental and I need to stop it. I am so quick to find everyone's faults and not the good in them. In the past, I used to do everything at any cost. Now I would like to be liked by other people. I would like to rid myself of the reputation I have acquired. I would like to be more like Michele's grandmother was. At least, how we saw her. She could be stern when she had to but for the most part was a very kind and loving person. I don't know if that is how she got in her older years or if that was how she always was.

One thing I am not like our mother is that of a bigot. She judges people by their affiliation and not by who they are as an individual. I judge one person at a time and don't lump them together by race religion or whatever.

Despite my rigidness, I can be very caring at times. I can feel the hurt others may be feeling. I just have difficulty in showing it. It is so hard for me to find the words, "I'm sorry," that I almost think they don't exist in my vocabulary.

I can see my faults, because I can see them in my real mother and sister. I don't want to believe that is how I am, but the truth has a way of hurting. I'm trying to work on my behavior, but again like Kim, it won't come quickly or easily. I just hope I can sideline some of the damage.

I don't know what else to tell you. I was necessary for the system to survive, but now that Michele has learned to forgive and take away the blame, we are all feeling a need to mellow out and change our responsibilities to the Group.

Alice

KATHERINE

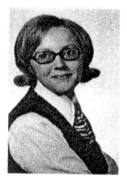

I wish this were all my story but it's not. This book has been for the total benefit of the whole system. I was here just to put it into words for everyone so we could reflect on it and see where we were and how far we have come in the past forty years.

I have such a way with words and feelings that I tend to amaze myself often. I certainly amaze the Group. I will write something and when they read it, they can't believe it came from the same person. Of course it didn't. It came from my heart, soul and perspective.

Let's see. I guess I am here to tell you *my* story. I arrived early on, but didn't get to the point of putting my thoughts down on paper until junior high age. I was gathering research, you might say. I would go to the adults in the neighborhood and listen to their stories with some of the others. I would take their stories and create visions in my mind. I would build a library of the mind.

When I got into junior high, specifically the eighth grade, I developed the burning desire to put down some of what I had heard on paper. I became the school newspaper editor. I did 90% of the writing for this paper, but loved every minute of it. I was a bit of a procrastinator, though. I would wait until right up to the deadline to finalize my work. I seem to work best under pressure. With Bonnie's help and the help of one of the school secretaries, the paper was a pretty decent piece of literary achievement for the audience it had. I did a series on smoking, drugs and alcohol that won recognition for scholastic achievement. I got my picture in the community paper for it.

In high school I didn't do as much writing as later on or in junior high. I spent more of my time reading. The others hate reading and I didn't get a lot of opportunity. I focused more on poetry than anything else. Because of the brief times I would have out, I couldn't risk reading a whole book. The others should have given me more time, because I would have helped with English and literature classes. They were all so gung ho and eager beavers, I didn't want to ripple the flow.

College was when I got my big chance. It was full of new experiences and responsibilities. It was serious business, because it was costing us money. I had plenty of opportunity to read, but didn't do all the reading. Some of the others did it by default. They wanted to be out and reading had to be done. Needless to say, they didn't comprehend things or take as much interest in it as I would have. I also got plenty of opportunity to write. Most of it was done in my composition class, but I had other opportunities.

I wrote one piece of prose that I was really proud of and got an "A" on. The only thing is I no longer have a copy of it. I don't recall what was done with the typed copy that was turned in, but I knew it may get lost and copied it in my journal. Little did I know that Michele was going to let someone read my journal. She wanted someone to understand her and where she was coming from. Anyway, she gave it to her psychologist of only a few visits and he supposedly lost it. I personally don't think he lost it. I think he realized what a treasure it was of a confused, sick mind and kept it for a thesis he was planning to do. These guys have a tendency to do that. I know how it is when you get the itch to write. You collect anything you can put your hands on that you may be able to reference.

That piece of prose was a reflection of all my senses one day up atop the butte behind the football stadium. This was the first real time that I experienced every sight, sound and smell that was around me. I really got in touch with the world around me. I woke up and began viewing the world in a different light that day.

I never have been greedy with my time out until I started this book. I made the others commit to giving me so many hours a week...and that was the second time around. I had attempted to write this back in 1986, but we still had some growing, healing and resurrecting to do. This past year, I felt we had reached that point where we were all ready to contribute to the story of our lives.

Authors nowadays are able to crank out biographies in a matter of weeks. This has taken me just a little over a year to write. It has not been easy reliving the past, but I think I have a level of maturity and respect for what we have been through to be able to tell the story. I know other people who have had more difficult and darker lives than we have lived. What I am hoping to convey in this book is the sense of hope that people who have led troubled lives can look toward uplifting themselves and healing.

The important thing is to be able to give forgiveness to your perpetrators. Until you can stop blaming others for your troubles and accept what has happened as something that just happened, you won't be able to get on with your life. We still don't agree with everything our mother says or does, but we are accepting of her for herself and who she chooses to be. We all have choices. We are the only ones who choose to be miserable. People need to learn to make the best of every situation.

One thing this system has learned to do is forgive others for their actions. We don't condone their actions. We are better in God's eyes if we are able to turn the cheek. I purely believe that we all have a purpose in life. Those with the difficult lives to be lived are God's chosen ones. They are not weak if they recognize the suffering they are in as a strengthening process. By coming to this understanding, I have more depth in what this life is about. We are still searching for our purpose and it is a difficult job, but no one has ever told me life would be easy. The survival mode we have been in exemplifies this.

My goal is to help others to see this light through my writings. Everyone seems to have such a doom and gloom outlook on life that their lives are miserable. I want to write poetry that reflects the true beauty of this earth that we are on. I want to write stories and books about how we can enrich our lives to live them to the fullest. I have reached one milestone by getting this book written. Another will be when it is published. It will all be worth it if I can touch just one person's life and give them hope for recovery.

I guess I will get off my high horse now and let the others get on with their stories, so this book can really get published. God Bless.

Katherine

BONNIE

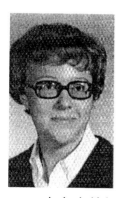

I am one of the perfectionists in the Group. Not hard-core mind you, but just a little sharp around the edges. I am the artist with precision. I do the technical drawings that Michele is asked to do. While in the oil and gas business, I was around most of the time. I am also very much a realist.

I don't know just exactly when I was born. Bobbie, my twin has been around since Michele was six or so. I would have had to been around about that time, too. I was just present in the background for a long time. I would come out every now and then and build houses with the Legos and log cabin blocks.

I really like to design things. If I had any say in the matter, I probably would have been an architect. My first real treasure was an old sailing schooner that I made out of twisted wire. I did it when I was a junior in high school. I had over 100 hours of love and labor in that piece. I still have it today. I've thought about selling it before but always put such a high price on it that no one will buy it.

College was most interesting. Bobbie and I were at odds with one another. She was present most of our freshman year. The bulk of our art classes were studio art classes. I would sneak in when she did her sketchbook classes and push the realism into the items that were sketched. I would insist on a high degree of accuracy in the work. I wouldn't let her go very far with creativity. I would always nudge in some of my details even when she did get to exhibit her creativity.

Things really took off for me when Michele changed her major to Physical Geography. I really got intensely interested in the cartography classes. If I couldn't be an architect, this was the next best thing. There was a touch of creativity in how a map was actually portrayed, but it had such an exactness to it. Being accurate with your rendering was the most important factor in drawing a map. The scale differentiation was tremendous. Bringing a global perspective down to something a human could comprehend was a real challenge.

I did very well in my cartography classes. Things got real difficult when the class changed from utilizing pen and ink on paper with my hands to generating a plotted map through the use of a computer. Needless to say, I had big problems conceptualizing how to tell a computer to draw a map for me. This technology was more complicated than I could comprehend. I ended up getting a "C" in my computer mapping class.

My cartography professor thought I did such a good job that he recommended me to one of the other professors who was writing a book on Mormon migration. I ended up drafting the map for him then printed the final map for his book on one of the presses in my graphics class. I never did see how the finished book turned out. I kept plenty copies of the map though for my portfolio.

I did most of the work in the graphics and printing classes because the work that was required was more precise than what Bobbie really cared for. We almost decided to change our major again, but put that idea to rest because we all wanted to get on with our career. At least I did.

Before leaving Phoenix I was planning on taking the government civil service exam to see what grade level I could qualify for with the USGS. I was really hoping to get a job out at the Denver Federal Center with the Geological Survey. The news that our parents were not going to let us take our dog, Toshi, back to Denver was such a heartfelt blow that we couldn't concentrate on the idea of taking a test.

Since I was the one with a bonafide trade in hand after graduation, it was up to me to find a job we could list as a career. The first place I checked was out at the Federal Center. They had nothing I was eligible for available. I took a week off before going out looking for something else. I played navigator while my mom drove me all over town to fill out applications and answer ads. It was rough not having a car, but Roy had put the bug off limits since it was pretty much a lost cause and in such disrepair. It never was the same after that last Christmas when the engine was stolen out of it.

A couple oil companies had ads in the paper. Roy suggested I give serious consideration to them. I questioned him, because I didn't think they had much to do with maps. That was before I learned about the business. I called on an ad and went in to talk to a man in the drafting department with one oil company. We hit it off right away. His daughter and I had both been selected to Who's Who in college. I had to take a drafting test. Boy was I nervous. My palms sweat so much I could hardly hold onto the pen. Regardless, he thought I did a pretty decent job. I went out of the interview fairly upbeat.

Later that afternoon I got a call from Jim. He asked me if I wanted the job. Butterflies were leaping around in my stomach. I was in a daze. I said, "Are you kidding? I'd love to have the job." He asked when I could start. I said, whenever. I went in the very next day, which was Friday to fill out the paperwork. He said it was an entry level job and paid only $900 a month. That was $100 more than I ever expected. This really shows our age by saying $900 was a lot of money.

Monday was my first full day. Since I didn't have a car, mom drove me to and from work each day. I fit right in like a natural. Diane picked up on the terminology and science behind the work right away, too. This made my work easier, because I knew what it was that I was drafting. I was quick to find out just how much oil companies relied on maps. The whole basis of the business revolved around the graphics I created. They couldn't sell their prospects to the company or partners without a good, clear picture of the prospect's viability.

It wasn't long that I became Jim's pride and joy of the department. I was a hard worker and very fast at what I did. He had me sitting at the front of the room behind his desk. He just piled the projects on my table and I worked on them several at a time. I had a natural tendency when it came to juggling multiple projects.

I was happy as a lark until the atmosphere in the department changed. They got employees in the department with attitudes and personalities that clashed with me and Jim. Morale started to take a nose dive. I was there to do the work, but worked at a distance. I had control of the hands that did the work but let others step in to hear and witness the disruption in the department. I could not stand to be around people who would not work and were not disciplined. I enjoyed going to work just as long as I didn't have to hear the grumbling.

One day I guess we got into a disagreement with one of the other employees. All I remember is hearing him tell me to "fuck off!" That was more than my precious ears could stand. I had to do something. I did not have to stand for that kind of treatment. I started looking for another job. I was even more set on finding something else when Jim told me he wanted to keep me in the building with him rather than send me over to a satellite office. I was one of his few allies.

About a month later I had a lead on a job with another oil company. I left my job to go to that company for only $50 a month more. I thought anything was better than what I came from. That didn't turn out to be quite so. Once I really settled in and got to know my new supervisor, I discovered very quickly that he had peculiar habits of whistling and telling stupid jokes. This got on my nerves. Once again, I distanced myself into the background to make work bearable.

I kept in close touch with Irene, one of the drafters back at my old job. She called me one day a few months after I left and told me that the guy that was sent to the satellite office was making a mess of things and Jim was going to replace him. She said not to be too surprised if Jim didn't call me and try to get me back. She also suggested I make it worth my while to come back. Sure enough, later that week, I got a call from Jim. He asked me what it would take to get me back. I quoted a figure that was $300 a month more than what I was making when I left the first time. He didn't pause or flinch. He just asked how soon I could start. I told him I needed two weeks. Actually, I would have liked to have said the next day, but that wouldn't have been fair to my new employer. Three months after leaving, I was back to work at my old job.

I loved working in the new Anaconda Tower with new equipment. I did all the drafting for the engineers and one geologic team. I was in heaven. I was my own boss. I got along great with the guys I worked for. When I got my work done, I offered to help Jim with some of his backlog. That didn't last too long because some big projects popped up. I was putting in overtime.

Over the course of my career with them, we made two more moves building-wise. After the first move we were storing our maps in the big wardrobe boxes that they were moved in. No one made any plans for setting up a filing system in the new filing cabinets. This seemed like a job for me, Diane and Shelley. It required close attention to detail.

The first task was to figure out how we were going to file hundreds of maps in the nine slot filing cabinets. We in no way had enough cabinets for all the different sets of maps that we had. We swore that we would not file the maps in voluminous roles when we got to the new building. I did some tinkering and thinking and came up with a design for an insert that would turn the nine slots into 36. Jim thought it was a great idea and sent me out to get bids on the cost to have all the inserts made. I don't remember how many cabinets we had, but I know we had at least sixty. Each cabinet would require eighteen slotted dividers that would have to be assembled and secured in the cabinet.

This project turned into an eighteen month pursuit. I devised the filing system, Diane logged the titles and descriptions and categories of maps and Shelley typed all the cards for the index file. It was true teamwork in its purest form.

I worked on my regular drafting projects during the day, then worked about four hours a day of overtime and weekends on the files. We were living with Gene in his Victorian at this time and this didn't say much for our relationship. Francie and Sally were having fits that they couldn't spend more time with him. He had lots of friends from work that he was able to do things with.

Morale continued to drop to an all time low. Some of the employees caused Jim to be ousted as the primary supervisor. A new guy was brought in from the California office to be our supervisor. He and I did not see eye to eye to say the least. He came from a different school of cartography and didn't have the art background that I had. We were opposites on a number of theories and techniques.

The situation did not improve any with him as supervisor. I was lead drafter at this time in charge of geology. He followed me around the department. I thought that the people working under me had a good relationship with me. Nenad had a bad habit of giving my drafters directions that were just the opposite of what I had instructed them. This really confused them. Who do they listen to? A lead or the supervisor? The situation was becoming futile. Other drafters were ridiculing Nenad, yet stabbing me in the back. This created constant turmoil.

I became extremely confused and frustrated. Anger was building up inside me without a way to release it. I passed it on to Kim, and you know what she did with it. This did not make the situation comfortable. Me being out sick regularly. Out for mental health check-ups. When we wound up in the hospital, I demanded that I be trusted enough to go to work. I needed to stay busy. I was losing face as it was. Soon my responsibilities were gradually taken away from me. My performance deteriorated to an embarrassing low. The environment became counter-productive. It was bad enough that I was fighting depression. To top it off, I had to develop a seizure disorder. My life was sheer chaos. I didn't know which way to turn. Things were falling apart all around me.

Soon, Nenad was relieved of his responsibilities. He was still a supervisor, but one of three under the direction of a new department head that was hired away from Coors, I think. I was going to be in charge of the new computer drafting department, but it came at the time of a hospitalization. I said I did not think I could handle the stress that job would produce. Besides, I did not agree with the computer system the company decided to buy. Even after the work I put into getting it, I was relieved that I would have no part of it. With my problem of depression, I did not need to spend eight hours a day in a cold, dark room.

Work no longer had meaning for me. I mustered the best I could to do a good job with what tasks I was assigned. The seizure activity began to become as big a hindrance to my performance as the depression. I was wasting away. My career was going down the tubes.

One day in April of 1985, I was called into the department head's office. I was then given a written warning. They were bound and determined to make an example out of me. They said my absenteeism was excessive. If I missed any work again in the next 6 weeks for any reason, I would be suspended. After that, I would be terminated. Two weeks later I got a serious eye infection. Puss was oozing from my lids. I had to go to the eye doctor. As par for the course it had to be during working hours. My supervisor was on vacation that week, but the time off was documented on my time sheets.

Once again, I was called into Jim's office. This time they were suspending me for two weeks without pay. It couldn't have come at any more an opportune time. I was scheduled to go to Canada for a Desk and Derrick Regional Meeting during my suspension time. Now I wouldn't have to take vacation time. Regardless, though, I wasn't going to get paid for it.

Before my departure, the company had announced that it was going to do some drastic downsizing. The oil and gas market had taken a nose dive and the bottom was dropping out. If the company was to survive, it would have to have major cutbacks in expenses. My department was union represented even though we were not required to join. The union and company had not decided if the same severance incentive would be available for represented employees were they to voluntarily leave. Just in case, I took all the information about the program when I left.

My first day back to work was May 30, 1985. That morning, I was informed that I was eligible for the retirement severance. I decided right then and there to take the money and run. I immediately began processing the severance paperwork. My first day back was also my last day at that job.

I didn't really wonder what I was going to do right then. I had started my own drafting company back in 1983. Incorporated it and everything. Due to a possible conflict of interest, I could only do freelance graphics. Nothing pertaining to the oil and gas market. I did some work for some landmen at the company. They had developed a marketing scheme around Texans and the Colorado ski industry. I designed t-shirts, a poster, bumper sticker and an embroidery design for them with Bobbie's help. It wasn't much but generated a little extra income.

After leaving that job, I immediately felt a sense of renewal. A big weight was lifted off my shoulders. Yeh, I worried about how I was going to make a living and be able to make my mortgage and car payments. I took a couple weeks to regroup and put together a plan. Shelley had taken a small business management class at the community college and we had devised a marketing plan. I got a copy of the *Rocky Mountain Petroleum Directory* and began doing some mailings. I was still in Rocky Mountain Energy Drafters and made some contacts through that organization with other drafters. I also hoofed the pavement and passed out marketing packets on a walk-in basis.

My first real client was an accident. I was in a building to meet with another drafter. On my way out of the building, I noticed an oil company name on the door. It was Sheffield Exploration. I didn't have my materials with me, but made a mental note of the place. The next time I was downtown, I stopped in with a packet. Not long after dropping the info off, I had a meeting with the geologist, geotech and Vice President. They were impressed with my samples. They said they could see a definite opportunity for a working relationship.

The Vice President of the company was a Dr. Max Sommer. He was originally from Switzerland and had a strong accent. We eventually developed a very strong working relationship. Sheffield has since gone by the wayside, but Max is still around and I am still doing odd jobs for him today. We have become good friends. He appreciates my work so much that when I have had health interruptions, he has delayed his deadlines so I will work on it for him. I tried to pass him off to other drafters, but he would have nothing of it. That is true loyalty. There is a bond there that is lasting.

I began getting other jobs. Long term temporary projects to work on. I even went to work for another drafter who had his own company. I was getting $8 an hour. A far cry from the almost fifteen I was getting earlier. Every bit helped, though. Some jobs that I got on my own paid me twenty. I had one that lasted for a couple months at that rate.

Most of the work came from answering ads in the paper. The small independents were getting away from their own drafting department and hiring contract labor on a prospect by prospect basis.

I don't quite remember how I got it, but I landed a big drafting job with a mining company that was wanting to market itself for a possible buy-out. This was my first venture at placing a bid on an entire project. Based on their original explanation of the project I gave them what I felt was a solid bid. Once the project got started, they began making all kinds of changes on me and adding several exhibits. Before it got too far out of hand, I made an amendment to my original bid. They had also bumped up the completion date for the project. When that happened, I knew I would have to bring in additional labor to get the job done.

The stress got to be too much for me. I wound up in the hospital in December that year. It was only for a few weeks, and I was allowed to leave during the day to work, or bring my work into the hospital. The February deadline was getting close. I couldn't afford to screw this one up. $9000 was riding on this job. I told Dr. Wilets he had to work with me on this one. My seizure activity began to intensify because of the stress. The first of February came and I got the job done. Don't ask me how, I just did.

One week later, I ended up in the hospital. Kim had to have a release and took a large dose of sleeping pills. This time it was Halcion. I was shook up by it and called my mom. She got me to call my neurologist because the overdose was triggered by the frustration of increased seizure activity. He convinced me to come into the hospital. My mom drove me to Porter Hospital and had me admitted. I was taken to ICU, because I had enough Halcion in me that it was causing irregularities in my heart rate. This time I did not resist the charcoal. I tried to take it but couldn't get it down. They ended up putting a tube down my nose and pumping it into me that way.

The rest of the hospitalization was a big blur. I remember doing terribly on some IQ tests. I couldn't concentrate or pull any thoughts together. I had trouble just getting up to go to the bathroom. I was so weak that the nurses insisted I call them whenever I got out of bed. I was bedridden with the rails up. I felt like a vegetable.

What was so bad was that my niece, Stephanie, was born when I was in the hospital. I needed to be with my sister and I was no better off than her. I cried and prayed a lot that day for little Stephanie and my sister.

That year I was no good to anyone. I struggled with whatever came along. I did not look for any additional work. I was in and out of the hospital five times in 1986.

The real turning point in my life was after my hospitalization at the National Institute of Health. Was I ever relieved to find out that the seizures I was having was due primarily to stress and my inability to cope with it. I'm not going to discount the fact that I never had a real seizure. I'm sure I did. My body must have realized what a release of pressure it was to go through that twisting and turning and jerking. So much so that it began mimicking the process when I had to get a release.

I gradually worked to rebuild my strength after that. The bankruptcy paperwork was filed and I knew I was going to lose the house. Fortunately, I had my parents to turn to. They were always there for me when things got rough. We tried to sell the house but there were no takers. The market was depressed at that time. All I could do was try to sell what I really didn't need and prepare to move back in with my folks. That happened January 1987.

We were still having some bad depressive episodes and got on disability after returning from NIH. The problem was that I could no longer afford my health insurance. It had climbed to over $350 a month and was very limited at best. I had to stay out of the hospital. We all made a pact to help each other get through the down times. We cut back on our sessions with Dr. Wilets and just rode out the doom and gloom episodes.

We would go for weeks without getting out of bed but to eat and go to the bathroom. I must have slept twenty out of twenty-four hours a day. It was never a very restful sleep. I was having fantasy dreams that were anything but pleasant. Group members would think of something or hear something and the dreams would take off on whatever it was.

In the summer of 1987, I got another wind. I began to climb out of the deep depression. I got excited about looking for work again and started making calls. I put together a revised marketing packet and started sending it out. Slowly the jobs started trickling in. It didn't amount to much. Certainly not enough to make a living. It was just enough to occupy my time and to keep me from feeling worthless.

I felt good enough to start looking for regular employment. I worked on my resume and started answering ads in the paper. I answered one with the Battelle Institute that had an office out by the airport. Unfortunately, I didn't get the job. I did make enough of an impression though, that I started getting some contract work with them that fall. I was brought in to work on a major government contract.

The amount of work began to grow to overwhelming proportions. I knew I would have to bring in help on this one. I began looking for a place that I could move my office. I found a place downtown across the street from the ARCO Tower. It was an old converted parking garage. It had a beautiful atrium that led to the roof. Shelley put pen to paper and informed us that with this project, we could afford to set up a real drafting studio. She signed the contract. It would be February of the next year before the suite was ready to move in. I anxiously counted the days and weeks.

I went out and searched for some additional used furniture and another drafting table. I got a desk, flat file table and large format light table. I even went out and bought a copier. Before I knew it, it was moving day. I hired a local moving company to take the things from the house and to make a stop at the used furniture store. Everything was going smoothly until they tried to get the flat file table up the elevator. It was too long. It was eight feet high and the elevator could only handle seven. They had to come back the next day and take the desk apart. That was four more hours of time I had not counted on.

Once I got settled, I began looking for additional help. I called all the drafters I knew but they were all busy with their own business. I did not want to run an ad in the paper so I started calling the drafting schools. They sent out students to interview and test. I was not overly impressed with what I had to work with but I was desperate. My deadline was coming up and I had a number of additional maps to create. I ended up having about four students help for a couple weeks, then kept two others on for a month. I would run out to Battelle every couple days to give them maps to look at.

Finally, it was the weekend before the project was due. I began looking over the last set of maps. I was not happy with what I saw. The lines were all shaky and weak on many of the drawings. There was no compromise, I had to redo them. I ended up spending two days that lasted fourteen hours at least and an all-nighter to get the drawings done to an acceptable appearance.

I sure learned my lesson on this one. Don't wait till the last minute to get help. They are not likely to be the caliper of person to do the job to my standards. I had let one of the students do a map for Sheffield. Max said if I hadn't told him someone else did it, he would have thought I had been drunk when I did it. I ran an ad in the paper for contract help in hopes of having back-up help should another project like this come down the pike.

I was not prepared for the response that I got from the ad. In the two weeks after the ad, I received responses from almost 120 individuals. I ran the ad only one day. I was very specific in what I advertised for, but got a wide variety of responses. Very few of the applicants had mapping experience. I took the best respondents and sent them an application I had prepared. When they came back, I began scheduling interviews and testing. Another job did not come along that required additional help, but I did have a couple names I could call on should the need arise.

That summer, I got a call from a headhunter out of North Carolina. He was looking for a cartographic supervisor to run a U.S. mapping operation for the Michelin Corp. At first I told him I was not interested, but after thinking it over, called him back. Business was slowing up considerably and I was uncertain of where my business would go. This would be a sure thing with a regular paycheck and a way to get back into the workforce. I sent him my resume and samples of my work. He called back for a telephone interview. A week later, he called back and said they would like me to come out to Springville, NC to interview with his client. I prepared for the journey.

I was not prepared for the weather. It was hot and humid and that was at 10 p.m. I got off the plane soaking wet. I picked up a rental car and found my way to the motel where I was going to stay. When I got to my room, I called the headhunter. He came to the motel and met me. We went out for a drink to get acquainted and for him to tell me what the next day's schedule would be.

I got up early and drove around to check out the town. I went to a couple apartment complexes to see what the community had to offer should I get the job. That afternoon I went over to the Michelin office for my interview. My first interview was a real disappointment. I met with the manager from their French operation. His English was very broken and difficult to understand. I was uncertain of some of the questions he was asking. In other words, I made a lousy impression. The other interview was not so bad, but blowing it with the big guy was not cool. I had a migraine when I left. It sounded like a marvelous opportunity but I was not very hopeful. I checked out and went to the airport for my flight home.

I came home relatively depressed. I tried to think of ways that I could rectify the mess I may have caused. I waited for a week and got no news. About ten days later, I got a letter saying someone else was chosen for the job. I began getting depressed. Partly due to not getting the job and partly because it was turning into fall and that is what happened on a regular basis.

By September, the days were becoming unbearable. I forced myself to go to the office, but found myself locking the door and going into one of the interior rooms to lay down. Work was almost at a standstill. It was difficult to do what little I did have. Fortunately in August I became eligible for Medicare. I wasn't overly concerned should I wind up in the hospital.

The first of October, I got a memo from the management company saying that the Post Office had bought the building and tenants on the upper floors would have to move. God must have been looking out for me because it was becoming more and more difficult to come up with the rent money. I didn't want to give up though. I kept thinking that things had to get better. The company said they would pay for me to move. I began to look at other office space downtown.

During one of my visits with Dr. Wilets, he suggested that maybe I not move into another office. He said it didn't make sense with my depression and lack of work. He suggested I move my office back home again at least until the next spring. Reluctantly I knew he was right and took his advice. I prepared for another move. I contacted some companies to sell some of my furniture to. I sold just about everything. Even my good oak drafting table. The other members of the Group convinced me that I should give up trying to have a business. I was too depressed to argue.

The winter was long and dark and blue. I kept my drapes drawn and on some days never got out of bed. I was not going to go into the hospital though. I was going to ride this one out on my own. I decided to close my business the end of the year.

In January, I was feeling stronger and was getting some energy back. One day I got a call from a company I had sent some information to the year before. They needed a drafter for a special project. I told them I didn't have my business any more but would be interested in some contract work. I went in to talk about the project and show him samples of my work. He liked what he saw and agreed to pay me $18 per hour. I would work in their office but would have to bring in some of my own tools. I started a couple days later.

As I had my energy back and got into the flow of things, I slowly began to become hypomanic. The Group and I began feeling real good about things. Voices were swimming in my head as I tried to work on the project. I was fantasizing about a new business I wanted to start. Soon, I kept a notepad next to me on the table to jot things down as they popped into my head. One day I saw an ad in the paper about an Entrepreneurship Program at one of the business colleges in town. I went to check into it. I knew that if I was going to start a new company, I was going to do it up right and know what I was doing. No more flying by the seat of my pants.

We all went to check out the program at Barnes. It sounded just like what we needed. The others pushed me to apply. I was accepted and was approved for a school loan. Classes would begin in March. Fortunately the project I was working on had to be done by the end of February for a hearing. I told the others this was not my forté and they would have to take the responsibility of school. They agreed.

Shortly after school started, we took another leap. We started our new business. This time Shelley did the paperwork to file the incorporation documents and draw up the bylaws. She typed them all out on the computer. We were back in business!

In June of 1989 after school was out, I answered an ad for a temporary drafter. It was to replace the company's drafter when he went on vacation for two weeks. I got the job. It was to work in their downtown office. It was a company that did geologic microbiology studies to predict good prospect areas for oil companies. This was new to me. I used the skills I had but did an entirely different kind of work than I had done for so long. They were very pleased with my performance.

I was called back to the company a month later to give a bid on a massive project they had decided to take on. It was to involve the drafting of extensive, detailed cross sections. After doing some research and thought the project through, I said I thought I could handle it and told him the approximate cost of each cross section for the project. They told me they were still collecting the data and would call me when there was enough to get started.

In the meantime something tragic happened. We ended up in the hospital that fall in 1989. Things got to be too much or overwhelming or something and some of the others felt they wanted to die. This time there was no overdose, but a lot of desperation. It could have happened. My mom and Dr. Wilets talked me into going into the hospital. Dr. Wilets was finally going to start me on this miracle anti-depressant he had been talking about for months. Kim nearly screwed things up by taking a near fatal overdose on some barbiturates. We survived, fortunately due to the quick response of the hospital staff at Presbyterian Hospital.

This hospitalization after that incident turned out to be the best experience we had ever had. We learned a lot and grew up from this experience. Due in large part to the scare Kim created. We got out of the hospital toward the end of October.

In November, I got a call from Micro Strat that they were ready for me to start work on the project. The initial phases of the project were to put together the graphics that would be repeated throughout each of the cross sections. I decided to experiment and see if I could do them on my computer. I could and they turned out pretty neat. I found I could improve and increase my skill through utilizing the computer. I used to be a real skeptic about the possibilities with this technology but quickly became a believer.

As this project got further under way, I realized it was going to be much too big to work on my little drafting table I had gotten. I was going to need a bigger six or seven foot table. I was also going to need more room to spread out. Work did not really pick up to require those needs until the next spring.

July of 1990, I once again decided I needed an office. I began looking around for space close to where my folks lived. I did not want to pay the high price of having an office downtown and have to pay for parking on top of it. I was going to be a little more conservative. I found a place about two miles from my folk's. It was about as big as my other office was but layed out differently. It was a garden level suite so I didn't have a view. That was no big deal, though.

About a month before I was to move in, I went to an office furniture auction not far from the office. I ended up getting some chairs and a desk. Now all I had to do was find a good used drafting table. These were hard to come by if you didn't check the ads early and jump on it. I found one for what seemed a decent price and called the guy at 8 a.m. He was way out west toward Golden, but I got it. Good thing I had my truck.

Moving day was the first of September. I had scheduled the movers in plenty of time, but by 9 a.m. they hadn't shown up. I called the moving company. Somehow I didn't get put on the schedule. I said I had to be up and running by Monday and had to be moved that day. They said they would check with their sister company and see if they couldn't get someone out there after lunch. The movers finally showed up at 2:00 p.m. I told them I was not going to pay them overtime if the move went past five. They said not to worry, I wouldn't have to. The movers pulled out from the office complex around 8:30 that night. I had stuff from the house to move and stuff that was in storage. I had collected a lot of stuff in the five years I had been freelancing.

When I wasn't working on the Micro Strat project, we were going to meetings, networking and putting together brochures for marketing purposes. Shelley did the bookkeeping and we had a darn good set of books. They even did some cold calling for me. I tried calling some past clients to see if they had any upcoming projects. I tried to contact Battelle. I found out they had moved and changed their name. They were now SAIC. The Battelle Denver operation had been sold to another environmental firm. Many of the same people went to the new company so I had contacts. I was able to renew my relationship with them and got some small jobs to work on.

Even though I was bound and determined to make a good go of things this time, I constantly had a nagging in the back of my head telling me to get a real job. I continued to read the paper and send out resumés. Drafting was drying up and I started enlisting the services of Bobbie to do some graphic and desktop publishing work. She was really into the computer thing and I encouraged her to expand upon her skills.

Bobbie ended up taking a contract job doing desktop publishing and computer graphics that eventually led to a full time job with a client in the fall of 1992. Because we were into something regular that looked permanent, I gave in and closed the business the end of 1992.
Clients have come and gone and I have lost touch with most of them. Max keeps coming around now and again for me to do some drafting with his own business. I have also done a few small jobs for another independent geologist. I guess I get about six or seven small jobs a year. I try to do as much of it as I can on the computer if it is small enough. My activity level has really diminished considerably as of late. There isn't a whole lot for me to do. I draw floor-plans whenever we move and when my mom moved into her new apartment after our father's death. I also worked on the floor-plan for our retail store idea. These piddly things pop up now and then that I get to shine on. My business now is pretty much a hobby. But, I guess that is the sign of the times. I don't mind the relaxation. I think I am due for some time off.

I think I have probably written my own little book here, but there is so much that has happened in the last ten years that Katherine forgot to mention, that I felt just needed being said. Bobbie and many new alters have come into the light and dominate the scene now. I wish them the best and ask that they not forget me. I know they won't. And, that is my story.

Bonnie

BOBBIE

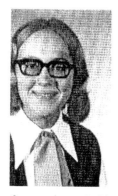

I have been around for a long time. Just as long as Bonnie, but my activity level hasn't been as great. My time out comes in spurts. A little here, a little there. More or less when everyone wants a change of pace and scenery.

When I was little I loved to color. I first got a small box of the big crayons but outgrew them quickly. For one, they were used up quickly. The other thing is that they were too big for me to color all the nooks and crannies in the coloring books I got. I went in a little for precision and detail like Bonnie, but that was only because the lines were already drawn for me.

I really got rolling with my talent when I was in kindergarten. Here, I was given a blank sheet of paper and told to create a picture from stories we had heard in class and at home. I didn't get too many stories at home.

My first pride and joy came from the story of Little Red Riding Hood. I drew a picture with Little Red Riding Hood and the wolf. My teacher was really impressed and submitted it to the annual spring art show at the junior college. I won a first place ribbon with that painting. It was one of my first experiences with paint.

After kindergarten I kind of disappeared for awhile. I next remember a strong showing when I was in the third grade. There was lots of art time there. I really liked my teacher. She encouraged me to test my talent. We used a lot of new media that I wasn't accustomed to. I did a horse's head out of rice. That's the only picture that I clearly remember. I did have a number of my things go to the annual art show again. Once again, I won some ribbons.

The others then worked on their talents and skills until we got into junior high. That's when my true colors came shining through. I loved my art teacher. She introduced me to so many new and wonderful artforms. I got my first set of oil paints when I was in junior high. My art teacher paid for me to go to a workshop on finger painting in oils. I really liked that. I did a silhouette of a succulent with a golden backdrop. It hung in the school office until a Britannica rep saw it and offered to buy it.

I entered a lot of poster contests in junior high and won one two years in a row. I worked with acrylics, tempera, pastels and ceramics. I even tried a little more advanced watercolor but didn't quite get the hang of it. I was in seventh heaven. I blossomed. Each of those two years, I had at least a half dozen pieces selected for the art show. At least half came back with ribbons. I also got a lot of recognition at the semester award ceremonies that were held.

I continued to dominate on into high school. Art became the main thrust of our studies. We only participated in the other classes so we could have the art classes. I lived for art class. My work early in high school was centered around more disciplined art study and not so much the craftsy stuff that I did in junior high. I learned about the human anatomy and had life drawing classes. I was encouraged to be a bit more creative and not so refined. My tendency is toward realism and my teacher wanted me to try to be a little more expressive. I surprised myself.

In high school I was introduced to the dreaded sketchbook. I know I am a damn good artist but I hate for someone to tell me what to draw and when. I would wait till the last day or two when the book was due and then madly hunt for things to sketch. I certainly got creative. I loved to do things that required dimensional shading. I let Bonnie help me out from time to time by drawing buildings.

My freshman year, I did my first portrait for hire. My science teacher from junior high wanted me to do a pastel portrait of his little girl. I had problems getting it just right, but when I finished it I was very pleased with it. He and his wife were both pleased, also. I got $25 for it.

I further developed my technique with oils. I did three paintings that were later framed. The War in Vietnam and Southeast Asia were growing in prominence when I was in high school. There were a lot of magazine pictures around the subject. I did a painting of a mother and her baby. My teacher liked it so well that it was one of the paintings I had framed then donated to the school. I haven't been back to the school hallways since 1984, but when I was there, it was still hanging in the hall. So I know it was on display for at least twelve years.

When we moved to Billings, I continued with my art. I did more painting. I did my first life portrait in oils. It looked the most like the girl that posed than any of the other paintings by the class. I did some playing around, too. We were assigned to do some mood paintings around the way we felt. I was still feeling lost for my father, so did one in black and greens that had a tear-drop and an interpretive portrait of my father. I did another painting that year that was probably the first indication that I was multiple. I had a woman's head nailed to a desert floor with little muscular beings hammering away at my skull and picking up the pieces that had fallen away. It reflected the way I felt. It also had pairs of lips floating around in the air. This represented the voices that were tormenting me and that my mind was slowly falling apart. I was really lost after my father passed away.

In Billings, I was introduced to the silk screen process. I did some rather creative things with designs I created on my class folder covers. I remember one day in the class when I was doing some silk screening the teacher was playing a radio. One of the big hits of the day was Don McLean's American Pie. The radio station was going to move to pop and played that song over and over all that day.

When my mom married Roy and we moved to Denver, I still continued with art. Two pieces of work that I still have to this day from that class are a coat of arms I designed for myself and some interpretive words that were turned into art. It was when I did that piece that I felt I wanted to be a commercial artist. Both of these items are in my portfolio today. I'm very proud of the way they turned out.

I got my first real paying art job in high school. I was hired by a production company to do some blocking for a TV commercial. It was an animated commercial about toilet paper focused around the theme of the Princess and the Pea. I would go to work after school and paint the individual drawing cels on acetate. You had to understand paints and layers with this job. You painted the small detail stuff first then the big background colors. Since the paint was opaque and had a latex base to it, the top colors could be painted right over the other colors and not mess up the art.

About a month into the project, the company moved its offices to a big warehouse where they could have their production studio onsite. Shortly after the move the project artist had a disagree-ment with the owner and quit. We had completed the first set of drawings and had it filmed. The animation was real jumpy and unprofessional looking. They realized they were going to have to almost double the number of drawings. They had a lot of money wrapped up in this project and a contract to complete it. By this time, there was one other high school senior and myself working on the project. We were asked if we thought we could do the drawings. We both agreed that we could.

I ended up doing most of the new drawings. I was able to imitate what had been done already with a few changes. I decided the little angels would look cuter if they had noses. So, I put little pug noses on them. I ended up drawing almost 200 more drawings to bring it up to 500 individual drawings for a thirty second commercial. I worked nights after school until about 10 p.m. and all weekend. It was hard work but I was very proud of my accomplishment. The big disappointment was when my last paycheck for five hundred and some dollars bounced. The company went out of business.

The commercial went out as a pilot in the California market but I never saw it on TV. I did notice, however, after graduating from college that they were still using the angels on the packaging for the toilet paper. And yes, that angel still had the nose I put on him.

I was able to talk everybody into letting me have the major in college. I was going to major in Commercial Art or advertising. Something like that. I was excited about going away to college and going to someplace sunny like Arizona. I couldn't wait for school to start.

I had three art classes my first semester. I had a studio art class, advertising design class and art history class. I found art history to be really fascinating. It developed my appreciation for the market and to have a different perspective on the different styles and periods of art. My studio art class was mainly drawing in pencil, charcoal and ink. It had the dreaded sketchbook assignments. I really liked advertising design. It involved a lot of work focused around lettering and advertising.

My studio art class second semester was frustrating. I would work real hard on a drawing and get it to where I felt I had done enough, then the instructor was not pleased with it. One drawing in particular...involved an aerial photo. We were to create a drawing that camouflaged the photo. I spent two weeks on that drawing. The teacher said he wanted me to work on it a little longer before he would give me a grade on it. Even after trying to do something more to it for a week, I still got a B on it.

That particular incident is what made me decide I didn't want to be that kind of artist. I liked ASU, but did not care for the arbitrary system the art department had for grades. If the teacher did not like your style or technique you wouldn't get a good grade. Grades weren't based on talent, skill or effort, but rather on personal taste of the instructor. No thank you. That's when I bowed out and turned things over to Bonnie and Elizabeth.

I did help Bonnie out with her graphic art classes our junior and senior year. It was pretty structured though and more than I wanted too much to do with. Elizabeth helped her more here than I did.

Since college, I have made cameo appearances from time to time. I come out for art therapy when we ended up in the hospital. I helped to take everyone's mind off of how badly we felt. Art seemed to cheer us up.

Occasionally I would get a wild hair and decide I would help contribute to our income. I would get into an artsy-craftsy mood and make things for Christmas craft fairs. At other times the wild hair was to crochet an afghan...a king size afghan. So far, I have made two of these monsters. They could pass as bedspreads for king size beds.

My greatest accomplishment though was in 1985. A year before then I went to the Women's Bank across the street from our office building and checked on whether they would be interested in seeing some of my work for a possible art exhibit in their lobby. The woman who organizes the exhibits said she would be interested in seeing samples of my work. It was a conservative bank, so I pulled my conservative art pieces together and took them in to her. She was clearly impressed and scheduled me for the month of October 1985.

My assignment was to do several oil paintings that would fill the lobby. I didn't have to do everything though. Elizabeth was going to help out. The exhibit would be a combination of photography and oil paintings. It ended up being more photography than oils. I think I only got a total of about six paintings done plus ones I had done in my earlier years. Two of them were quite elaborate and big. I had a family portrait of my sister, Larry, Daniel and their two dogs. I also did a very large painting of some flamingos. That one was framed when it was still wet.

I think the exhibit went well. I didn't sell anything or get any inquiries for doing other work. I was still very proud of this accomplishment, though. Some extremely talented artists and well known artists have exhibited in the bank lobby. As a token of my appreciation for his stick-to-itness, I gave Dr. Wilets my pride and joy – the flamingo painting. My only resentment is that I never got a photo of the painting. He did buy one of my other paintings later on for his new office.

Since then, I haven't made a major showing until we got the job that put us in the art department at U S WEST. When I worked that job, I was given the opportunity to combine my talents and skills through utilizing the computer. I amazed myself with some of the work I produced. I was a happy camper. Somehow, the others convinced me to pass up that to meet their needs. I reluctantly obliged. I don't know why, because with our new career came new alters. As if it weren't crowded enough in this body.

I still do some things from time to time for my church. I do the monthly singles newsletter. I told the Group that I wanted to design the cover for this book. I went out and bought some new oils and canvas and started the painting. I got as far as getting Whispering Owl painted. Since then I have had a change in plans. I plan to do the cover design on the computer. Don't ask me when. We are so busy trying to make ends meet that this body is absolutely exhausted at night. We even had to get a part time job on weekends. At least it affords us the opportunity to get this book finished.

We are back on a search for a new job. I think many have become disenchanted with retail. We still have hopes and desires for our own store but things look a little dim at present. I have convinced the others that our next job will be back doing what I do so well, graphics and desktop publishing. Katherine is hoping we can land a job as an editor, but I don't think we have as great a chance at that. Shelley and Nicole are looking for office manager type jobs. We will make the best of whatever comes along. I sure hope it swings my way. I have so much to contribute to the Group. I'm sure there is some job out there that will make several of us happy.

That's my story. Not as long-winded as Bonnie. She is one of the dominators, but if you haven't guessed, she is losing out to many of the rest of us. She has served us well and will continue to, I'm sure. It's just time for the rest of us to have some prime time to contribute to the Group effort that we are a part of.

Bobbie

DIANE

There isn't much to me. I am fairly new to the Group. I came along when we were in college. Bonnie wanted to do the mapping but wasn't much interested in all the other classes that went along with it, so voila! I entered the picture. I really dig this geography and geology stuff. It is so cool. I don't care so much for the economics of the science but the physical stuff is so neat.

If we weren't on our third major when we took up geography I might have been able to persuade the Group to change to geology for a major. I'm sure I could have talked Shelley or someone into taking the chemistry and physics classes. But alas, no go. If Bonnie weren't so dominant, I might have even been able to become a meteorologist, and who knows...a TV weather person.

Geomorphology is really intriguing. It is the study of what shaped the earth's features. It deals with climatic influences, glaciers, deposition and all that stuff. I really learned to enjoy the flights to and from school between breaks. I was glued to the window trying to identify all the surface features I had learned about in class. It made those lectures take on a new meaning by actually visualizing what was said.

Because the decision was made to stick it out with geography, I decided that when we got into the Air Force, I would go into intelligence and reconnaissance. Boy, was I ever disappointed when we didn't pass the physical to go on into officer training.

I really enjoyed the air photo interp class I took. We got to view aerial photos through stereoscopic glasses. With the overlap of the photos and the use of the glasses, you could see the photographed image in 3D. It took awhile to adjust and look through the glasses correctly, but when I did I took off. I couldn't get enough of it.

Between my junior and senior year, I had a field methods class that was required. It was a six hour course that utilized field research and mapping. The class went out into the desert and took a survey. We then came back and mapped the terrain. The class then took a week and went out to California to map the avocado groves. We walked the fields and mapped the features making notations on topo maps. Part of the class was to map out the cultural features of lower downtown San Diego and the Red Light district.

My senior year I took a class on Arizona geology. This class took a field trip to the Grand Canyon. What a sight to behold! The second day out, the class hiked down to the Colorado River. We went down the Bright Angel Trail. We were to look for rock formation changes and fossils along the trail. Too bad it was illegal to take any of the fossils. I found some real neat outcrops with excellent specimens. That evening after dinner the whole class went over to the rim to watch the sunset. It was gorgeous. This land is so beautiful!!

I really helped Bonnie out a lot when we got our job with the oil company. I helped her with the interpretation of the notes and sketches of the geologists that brought work into the department. It was so fascinating to learn about the oil industry. I picked up on the technology right away. I would come home and talk for hours with my dad when I lived with them. Roy didn't know that much about geology but he knew about the places that we were working. I was in a different world.

I really think Bonnie would have been lost without my help and support. I would tell her what to draw and how to draw it. She had a way with lines. She could really make a map shine.

Whenever the Group takes a driving trip, I always watch the roadside. I look at the outcrops and trend of the land. The same goes for whenever we fly anywhere. The oil business is in my blood and will always be there whether it is in our career or not. I will always have a fondness for it and do whatever I can to not lose touch with the industry. I feel it has gotten a bum rap from all the environmentalists. You take away all the by-products of oil and they would be lost without their rubber and plastic.

That's about all there is to me. I haven't led a very exciting life but it has been most interesting. I nudge my way back into the scenery from time to time so that I am not forgotten. Besides, without me, there wouldn't have been as prosperous a short life after college. Money is in oil if you can get on board now, but it is real tough. I get a chance every now and then to ponder in the wonders of this beautiful earth. Who's next?

Diane

CAROL

I'm the virtue which lies within this Group. You see, I am the one who holds patience. Early on I wasn't given much responsibility. Later in high school when I helped out as a Girl Scout leader, the Group realized what a great gift I had. They called me out more often. I don't mind being "on call." By not being as prominant as some of the others, I don't get as exhausted. I really worry about some of my sisters. They try to do way too much and too quickly. They need to set back and reflect more often. Instead they get caught up in a whirlwind.

As I mentioned, my birth was around the latter years in high school. Many had been along years before me. They couldn't stand to be around chattering little girls. They wanted to be helpful, but lacked the patience required working with others. That's where I come in. I have all the patience in the world. I can work with someone over and over until they say they've got it. For some people it almost seems to take forever.

I can have patience but I have little tolerance for disrespect. I gave up being a Girl Scout leader when the girls in the troop had very little respect for what belonged to others and the value of another's possessions. I also have patience when there is a desire to learn. When someone displays the attitude that they could care less or are the least bit interested, then I don't tend to waste my time on them. I have encountered people like that. I butt heads with them for awhile then come to my senses and realize that it just ain't gonna work.

I realize that people learn at different paces and I can go with that flow. It takes real skill to know when they have resisted or reached a point when they refuse to learn any more. This seems to be the case more than I would like to acknowledge.

I think I would have made a good trainer. We all have gotten into the world of computers in one way or another. I have watched the others while they do their work and have come to know and understand the software programs extremely well. I think I would make an exceptional software instructor. With the talents and skills that the others have coupled with my patience, we would make a great team.

I have been a tremendous help to the Group to get some of them to slow down and smell the roses. They get such grand ideas from time to time and become overly obsessed with them. I help them take their ideas and sort them out to something that is more realistic and easier to manage.

I am pretty much a background person. I don't like to dominate or be exposed to the daily rituals of life. I help out where I can and step in when the need is there. I like where I am at. Yeh, from time to time I wish a played a bigger role in this life, but I am for the most part, content with what I have and where I have positioned myself. Just knowing that I meet some of the needs of Michele is plenty satisfaction for me. I'm pretty laid back. That's it. There isn't any more to me. Besides, I tend to be a person of few words. I like to sit back and listen to what others have to say.

Carol

SUSAN

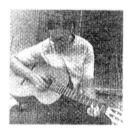

My gift is my voice. It has been a release for how we have felt inside. My singing is a point of some of our therapy and a way to experience some relief from the stressors of everyday life.

I sang a lot when we were young. It helped us maintain some sanity amidst all the turmoil around us.

My first experience with singing was in school, Sunday School and Brownie scouts. It is amazing as to how uplifting it is to utilize your vocal cords in such a way that you are not arguing with others. After a bout of singing, I feel energized and ready to tackle anything that comes along.

Because of the good feeling we got after I would sing, we started to participate in as many singing opportunities as possible. Somehow, it was hard to be depressed after singing a jubilant song.

I got extra singing practice at church when I was old enough for the youth choir. We had practice every other week and would sing every four to six weeks in church. Our church was a small church but we had some good voices in the youth choir. I especially enjoyed Christmas. The songs for that season are real beautiful. When I outgrew the choir I would go to church with my mom just so I could sing. I could care less about the sermon.

Girl Scouts really brought out my love for music. They sing such neat ballads and folk songs. Some of their songs are fun, too. I enjoyed singing around campfires but would get very solemn afterward. In a sense they were depressing, but somehow still made me feel good.

When my mom's parents moved behind us on Fifth Street, my grandmother brought her piano. I could sit for hours and listen to her play Christian music. She would even teach me some simple tunes that I could play. As long as I didn't bang on the keys, she would let me play the piano. Most of the time I just made things up.

When we moved up on Thurmond my third grade year, two instruments came with the house. We got our own piano and a xylophone. My parents caught me playing them and making up music as I went along. They took this for a sign that I wanted to LEARN to play. I guess I did in a way. My parents found a piano teacher who lived a few blocks away from us and signed me up for lessons. I was pretty good at practicing, but once I got the tune, I would turn away from the music. I would memorize the keys and play by ear. This brought tears to my eyes after one lesson. My music teacher yelled at me for not turning the page as I was playing from the songbook. Piano lessons lasted six months. Just long enough to play in the Christmas recital which my parents never attended.

When I got into the fourth grade, the music teacher solicited students for the orchestra. Since my dad had a violin I could use, I signed up. I don't know how I lasted for two years playing that instrument. I practiced just enough so that I didn't embarrass myself. Once again, I would play by ear. I really do not read music very well at all. I could fake my way through a piece if I listened to it a couple times. I didn't want to quit because the music was so beautiful.

I was always looking for ways to get attention. Between fifth and sixth grade I played in the summer orchestra and got to play in a couple concerts on stage. I soon became bored with the violin. I was looking for new ways to express myself and get attention. At the beginning of my sixth grade year, the band teacher was looking for new students. It was announced at an assembly that band students playing the trumpet would get to play at the morning flag raising. That was my cue. I convinced my parents into letting me try playing the trumpet.

I had six months to decide if it was something I wanted to stick with before my parents would have to buy the instrument. I made a real effort this time to learn this instrument. I even caught myself actually practicing a couple hours a week. My parents were not as impressed with the noise that the trumpet made over the violin, but they wanted to keep me happy.

I worked real hard to get to the point where I could play revelry for the flag raising. Finally in November I got my big chance. I was selected to play for two weeks for the flag raising and pledge of allegiance. I was not accustomed to playing outside in the cold. My first attempt was a piddly showing. My horn squeeled and blurted in the cold. Afterward, another student suggested that I keep my mouthpiece in my pocket with my hands on the way to school. It would keep the mouthpiece warm and my trumpet would play much better. I tried it and it worked. I attained my goal of getting that attention and recognition by students and teachers.

When the six months of rental time was up at the end of the semester, I had to make a choice. I went to the music store with my dad. They were having a sale on guitars. My mom was not with us. I had heard some Cadette scouts come and play their guitars at some of our meetings and decided I would like to learn to play the guitar. I told my dad that I really wasn't interested in keeping the trumpet. I had accomplished the goal I set out for and was ready to move onto something else. I begged him to buy me a guitar instead. He gave in and bought me a six string folk guitar. He asked me how I was going to learn and I said I would teach myself and have some of the other scouts teach me the songs we played.

Finally I had an instrument that I could pace myself with. I could go to my room and be by myself and strum away. I got some self teaching books and a few books that showed you the cords when you needed to play them. I learned to play a couple Monkees' songs and about a dozen campfire songs. I couldn't wait for summer to come so I could play with the other girls around the campfire.

I kept that guitar until 1982 when I finally sold it to someone I worked with. We were no longer affiliated with scouts. Carol, of all people, lost her patience with the kids of today and called it quits. We had other activities in our life and if I didn't have anyone other than myself to play with, I wouldn't play.

In addition to teaching myself the guitar, I took singing classes in junior high. In eighth grade I joined an all-girl ensemble. The group consisted of eleven girls. I sang soprano. I did my best to read the music. I picture the notes in my mind as to what I should be singing. I had some trouble with the flats and sharps. When I did learn them, then I tended to sing flat or sharp. There were three other sopranos, so it was important that I sing on key. We rehearsed the first semester for Christmas and sang in at least a dozen concerts around town. In the spring we practiced for springtime performances.

After junior high my only real outlet for music was Girl Scouts and church and we weren't going to church all that regularly. My senior year in high school Karen tried out for the school musical, and got a small cameo part. In addition to the small part we were a part of the chorus, so I got another chance to sing on stage.

When in college, we were a Girl Scout leader but we didn't seem to do as much singing then. I caught myself playing and singing more in my dorm than with the scouts.

My latest big appearance came after our hospitalization in 1989. A group of us decided we needed to get out and be more sociable. We felt the best place to do that was in a singles program at a church. That's when we started going to Trinity United Methodist Church downtown. We felt welcomed right away. We went to church religiously for two solid years missing only a couple Sundays. The church has a fantastic Chancel Choir. I heard you had to try out solo for the choir so was too shy to try. Besides, like I said, I don't read music too well and they do some pretty complex pieces. Because we got real active in the church, Phyllis, the choir director kept trying to get me to join. I always found an excuse.

My excuse was that I couldn't come regularly on Wednesdays for rehearsal. Soon she came back at me and said that I should join the Early Morning Singers. They sang at the early service twice a month and practiced the morning that they sang. She had me there. I thought about it for about a month then decided to give it a try. There were no tryouts for this choir.

As it turned out singing in the choir was a tryout. We regularly had only six to ten people sing at the services. Fortunately most of the time there was one other strong soprano that came to sing. The songs we sang were not overly complicated so I picked them up rather quickly. I did my best to read the music and slowly caught on. I still can't tell you where an "A" or an "E" are. I just know where my voice needs to go with the position of the notes on the music. I soon gained confidence and allowed myself to belt out the music. The group couldn't afford to be shy here, or the people would not be able to hear the music in the sanctuary, because it was a big sanctuary.

I sang in this choir for about a year and a half until we got the part time job delivering newspapers. We usually didn't get done in time to shower and get to the church for rehearsal. Our attendance dropped way low when we got that job. I went once about every six weeks. When we got the job at the computer store, we all but stopped going to church. I had to work every Sunday and could not even get to the early church service.

My attendance started picking up again when we became Supervisor and got every other week off. The only bad thing was that one of my Sundays off was the day we had the store meeting. Couldn't go to church that day. Earlier this year when we became Receiving Supervisor, we had every Saturday and Sunday off, so was real regular at going to church. I even started singing in the choir again.

That all ended about a month and a half ago when we were forced to get a weekend job. Our bonus had dropped from about $200 in December to as low as nothing last month. We can't make it with the new bonus structure and had to get a part time job.

I guess I will have to settle on coming out once a year for the Christmas Eve service and do my year's worth of singing then. I don't mind it so much since we have renewed our faith in Christ. You see, in addition to the musician in the Group, I am the devout Christian. I have helped Carol teach some Sunday School classes even. I have my daily words and meditation with God and am happy with that. Sure I would like to be going to church regularly but we need to eat and pay the bills. Another time will come when we won't have to work seven days a week and I will once again be able to exercise my voice and be nearer to God.

Well, that's the scope of me. I am an old timer that hasn't worn out her welcome. In fact, I feel more alive now than I have in a long time and I am happy with that.

Susan

KAREN

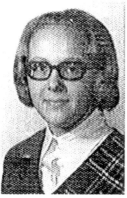

To be or not to be...that's not the question, because I am. I guess you might say I could be the outspoken person in the Group. I never have enough to say. I am always trying to find different ways to say what I feel inside.

I came around when we were in the fifth grade or thereabouts. The Group needed a leader and I stepped forward or outward. I guess I am because of Girl Scouts. They needed girls with leadership tendencies and I felt that would be the ideal opportunity for Michele to get some attention that was long overdue. In my experience with people in leadership roles, they usually get the attention of their audience whether it be in good ways or not. At least the attention was there. Michele was starved for it. She certainly didn't get much at home.

A number of us positioned ourselves in junior high to obtain attention. I really stood out and shined when I got into high school. During orientation, the speech coach got up and gave a speel about public speaking and trips and trophies. That caught my attention. Here was a way to speak out, be heard and have fun doing it. I might even win some recognition, too. I signed up right away.

My freshman and sophomore years speech team was an extracurricular activity. You received no school credit for participating. Later on in my junior and senior years, it was actually a class that I attended twice a week.

I was still quite shy and reserved at this age, so I didn't think I would do very well at debate. I needed something that didn't put me into confrontation and make me think on my feet. What it kind of boiled down to was that I was lazy. I didn't want to have to read all kinds of magazines and newspapers. I wanted to project and not absorb at the moment. As a result, I selected oral interpretation as my event of choice.

Because my life was so dramatic at the time, I chose dramatic interp. My first cutting came from "Gone With the Wind." I selected the excerpt where Melanie was going to give birth and Prissy was acting as a midwife. I was very reserved and had trouble really getting into the part. To me interp was just that...interpretive reading. It was not acting. That was not the way that other students saw it, though. They did everything short of acting, but a few of them actually went all the way. I play by the rules but that is not what the judges were eating up at the time. Needless to say, I did not fair very well that year in competition.

I did go to just about every speech meet that the team went to though. It got us away from the drama of the fighting and arguing at home. Finally I was doing something with kids my own age. I wasn't weird. I was accepted as part of the team.

That year, I also tried a little bit of humor. I was not a funny person. I could not get a rhythm going with the cutting. It did not flow at all. I guess I thought that if I did something funny and got into rounds where there were humorous cuttings, it might take me out of the dread and despair my life had turned into. I needed uplifting. Because I couldn't go it in humor, I would at least go to the final rounds for humor since I usually didn't make it beyond semi's in drama.

Between my freshman and sophomore year, I spent more time than usual at the library looking for cuttings for next season. I don't know what made me find it or what I was looking for when I came across it, but I found the cutting I had been looking for. It had all kinds of horror and drama to it. I hadn't heard it at any of the meets I'd been in. It was free verse reliving the drama and despair of the Nazi concentration camps during World War II. It was a documentary on the trials of Auschwitz. I decided this would be my next cutting. I found what I felt was one of the more dramatic excerpts from the piece and began working with it. I went with it in dramatic interp. What just occurred to me was that I may have been more successful with it in poetry. After all, it was written in verse.

I did much better with this cutting than the one the previous year. I actually got into some final rounds with it. I never did better than fourth place, but helped to gather the necessary points for my school to win top honors at some of the meets. Deep in my heart I would have loved to have won a trophy, but seeing my team win was satisfaction in itself. I got a little more dramatic with every performance when I could get into it. Some days, though, I was empty. I couldn't feel anything. Usually it was a meet that came the next day after a big fight at home. That fight drained me to the point that I had nothing to put into my cutting. When I came around it was usually too little too late.

Nowadays when I go back to relive those cuttings I did, I feel I would have done them so much differently. I am more experienced with life. My life has been a real stage in many respects. Sometimes when I am in denial over this illness we have, I say it was all a big act. There are a lot of professionals out there that would have the public believe that MPD is a big act for attention. Well, I would like to tell you right now, I should be so good. Some of the things we have done, said and whatever could not have been an act for forty years. I am thoroughly exhausted just trying to relive some of the dramatizations of our behavior. I want to believe I am good, but not that good. I tend to be organized. I need to know what comes next. Our life has been a mish mash of this and that with abrupt changes and the key here — unpredictability. I have no clue to the story line. I don't know what comes next. It just comes.

Okay, I'll get off my soapbox. Really, a lot of what has happened has made no sense whatsoever. I am not irrational. I want to believe I am very sane and rational. One thing, though. If they were ever to make a movie about my life, I could be the director. I would at least want to be the technical advisor. I have been around through it all. There is no one better to give direction than someone who has lived it. I would never play the part of me, though.

I stuck with that cutting around those trials for three years. I would do another one for a short time just to have a little different scenery. I stuck with it because it portrayed the doom and gloom I felt I was living. I was stuck in a rut and found no escape from the horror of my life. It was all a bad dream like it must have been for the Jews.

I tried something different my senior year. I tried out for the school musical. That year it was "Carousel." I was one of the side show performers. I was in the magic act. A string of weiners was pulled from my sleeve. I think I had two whole lines and a lot of ad lib. Susan actually got more out of the play than me because she got to sing three or four songs.

My senior year, I tried writing some speeches. I actually wrote two oratories. One for a scholarship contest and one to use in a couple meets. In the scholarship competition I placed third in the city, but didn't manage to get anything but a certificate, my name in the paper and a letter saying how great it was for me to compete.

Right now my role is that of moral support. To give the Group direction and encouragement to not give up. To fight for our rightful place in society. Sure, I think I could do a great job as an actress with what we have been through. I like to watch movies with a critic's eye. To evaluate the actor's performance and then think how I would have acted in that role.

When the Group has to make a business presentation or lead a meeting, I'm there on the scene. It is not as often now as it was two to three years ago. I did have one great feat about a year ago, though. With Carol and Connie's help, I did the all day sales training for associates at the store. I did a damn good job of it if I don't say so myself. To top it off, I had to take a five hour training course and make it last only two hours as we got nearer to the time the store opened.

That's my plain and simple story. Not as vibrant as some of the others' but I know my place within this system and I do what is asked and needed from me. Nothing more, nothing less. Just in case you're wondering, like many of the others, I do have an issue with control. I find I need to have the upper hand on the situation when I am present.

Karen

CORY

I am the shadow for the Group. No one knows much about me. I don't even know much about me for that matter. I am ageless but feel very young. What I am is the shadow that holds all the pain for the Group. I have to be cushioned by a thick pillow of air because it will hurt too much if I am not. Some of the pain is going away now that members are finding forgiveness and resolution to some of our life's issues. I don't think all the pain could ever go away, though.

Life hurts. There are so many bumps and bruises that I am black and blue from head to toe. I can't stand to have people too close to me. It hurts too much to feel the warmth from their bodies. My little body is cold. Another person touching me makes me feel like I am being burned or going to be punished for something I did.

I feel safe when I keep a big distance from me and others. I like it when Michele and the others isolate themselves from other people. They are protecting me from the shouting, hatred and anger of everyone around us. People are too cruel to one another. God did not put us here to be hurtful, but that's the way things are.

Someday, I think the Group may outgrow me. I see signs of it because of the drugs they are taking. It makes them not care about anything. Nothing seems to hate them or anger them. At least much anyway. I'm kinda glad about that because I don't think I could handle any more. I am battered enough as it is. I am ready to heal, but slowly. It is going to take a lot of tender loving care for my little body to become whole and healthy again. I would like to be able to go out and play like a kid for once without the fear of getting hurt.

The others have promised me that even though I may get well, I will still be loved and have a place within this system. Right now, Carol and Susan are nurturing me and nursing me back to health with their patience and goodness. I'm too fragile to be caught up in the rest of the others' lives. It's much too rough for me....But someday....someday I know I will be strong and well. Just don't ask me when. Healing takes time. That's all.

Cory

SHELLEY

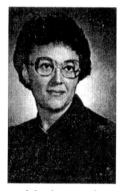

As everyone says, I guess I am the brains of the Group. I really think that Peggy is the brains of the Group, but I am the one that seems to come up with the wild ideas for some of this person's activities. Peggy is rational. I'm wild and a risk taker. To be a keen businessperson, you have to be willing to take risks.

I did get the Group through math class and science when we were in school. It wasn't because I had any brains. It was because I wouldn't give up until I found some kind of sensible solution. It didn't matter whether it was right or not, just so long as it looked right. That approach seemed to work rather well.

I like technical things. I find them intriguing. The more complicated they are, the more inquisitive I become about them. I see them as a challenge. I enjoy a good challenge. Work is a challenge. I don't like a job where you know exactly what is going to happen the minute you walk in. I guess that is what I like about retail. It's kinda unpredictable and what we do now has a routine set of tasks to it, I never know from day to day what is going to happen. There is enough suspense to the day to make me want to come to work to just see what unfolds.

I'm not into computers like Nicole. I do find them very handy and I am not intimidated by them. In fact, when they accomplish the task I set out to do, they are handy gems. All I care about is that they do the job and do it efficiently.

I guess I came around when my mom introduced us to manners and what is "proper." I see that what this system does, does not put my mom to absolute shame. I slip up now and again, but I am one against many. I see that we are dressed appropriately when it counts. When it doesn't I let the others do as they like. I see that we maintain good posture no matter how fat we get. I try to get us to eat the right things and not excessively. I don't know what has happened to our metabolism such that we are unable to lose any of this weight.

I am the one who was always present around my mother's friends. Didn't want to do anything that would embarrass her. I am able to carry on very fitting and proper conversations. I often find myself at a loss for words on many occasions, though. I am still convinced that this is a lingering effect of the ECT treatment we had twelve years ago. Any doctor you talk to will deny it, but I know I didn't fight for words before the treatment like I do now. I am thankful that not all of us had that nasty treatment or our memories would surely be lost. All I know is it wasn't me who signed the papers for the treatments.

I am the businesswoman in the system. I understand business tactics and what is needed to run a smooth operation. Don't ask me to deal with people, because I don't have the talent to talk as a superior to a subordinate. I don't have any problem talking upward or to an equal. That is when I shine. I have excellent communications skills with these people. I work extremely well with clients. I easily make them feel like the superior person.

My dream is to someday have a successful business of my own. I really feel strongly about the Apple computer store but only Nicole and Connie share the same excitement about it. As long as there is enough artwork and marketing to do, I think I can get Bobbie a bit excited about the concept. It will never fly if some are resentful or unwilling. They have the capability to become saboteurs.

I do too much too fast. It isn't that I don't think things through thoroughly. It is just the opposite. Yeh, I'm sure that because of the pace I sometimes move, I may not consider all the sides, but it is close enough for government work. That gives me more leeway than I actually take. I feel dreamers are born. It takes skill, training and hard work for someone to realize their dreams. However, I sometimes think that some people are just born into the luck that allows them to realize their dreams. In all sincerity I think it takes a little of both. I think a large number of the successes in the business world are clearly attributed to luck and good timing.

I'm not one to fly off the handle. I like to set back and observe what is going on around me. I listen to what is being said. I chew it up and use what I think will work for me and go on to the next thing. I am sincere and very serious. Many think I am too serious. I don't think anyone can be too serious when it comes to money and their livelihood.

Many of my sisters would not listen to my caution when we were making all kinds of money at the oil company. All they knew was there was plenty of money to do the things they wanted to do. Never did they dream that it would dry up. Nothing is more humbling than having gone through a bankruptcy. You are stripped of all your possessions and dignity. No one is willing to trust you any more. It takes many years of hard work, fighting and determination to come back on the upside of this. I am still struggling, but am close to peaking out.

I have tried to set a budget for us to work with. I have taught the others how we need to value what we have and not take anything for granted. Every now and then someone will take a leap and get something that is not quite necessary. I have taught them to carefully evaluate the usefulness of whatever we do buy now. If it is not absolutely necessary, does it hold value for the whole?

This store of mine can really fly. It scares me with how much money it will cost, but after having worked in a superstore where thousands and millions of dollars come up in daily conversations, it is not an impossible dream. I have studied the market. After listening carefully to what some seasoned retailers are talking about, it doesn't make sense to try to sell the computers. Too many companies and stores are already doing that. What we need to do is add value to what the consumer has with the support, software and accessories. Let the big guys fight over the skimpy margins they get by selling computers. I will make my money on the higher gross margin products. I can sell a lot of my items at the MSRP because no one locally has it available. It's all based on the principle of supply and demand and selection. My store will have the selection that will continue to bring people back. Mac users are hungry for a place that will cater to their technology. All I need to do is sell someone on it as much as I am sold on it.

As you can tell, I am focused on one key objective at this point. I don't feel I am looking through rose colored glasses either. It will be pure luck if this thing takes off. I know there has got to be somebody out there that will share the thoughts that this can be very prosperous. It would be a niche that no one else in Denver has gone into. That says a lot there.

I'm not totally avoiding the idea that we need to get a better "real" job with a regular paycheck and benefits. If I had my way, it would be an administrator's job. I pull a proportionate number out of the paper to answer along with Bobbie and Katherine. I don't want to get pushy but I know I can play an active role for this system. I would like more time; however, I must admit I have a tendency to get hypomanic with ideas from time to time and can become a real workaholic. Everyone tells me that's not healthy. Granted, I agree we are running on fumes right now because of the ideas I have, but when the right opportunity comes along and everyone is in agreement, I will be accepting of it. I know we will eventually come across the right opportunity that will let us settle down once and for all. Until then, though, I've got to give it all I've got.

We've got to keep on truckin'. Opportunities happen, but I believe they are really made to happen. You have to do the preparatory work for them to happen.

Yes, I have a soapbox, too. Every system needs a few shakers and movers. I am one of these people. I find it very hard to set still. My mind is always one step ahead of the rest. They have to work hard to keep up with me. I don't particularly try to torture them, it's just my nature to keep on the go. Someday I'm sure I will tell myself it is okay to stop and smell the roses.

I guess I haven't told you so much what I have done for the Group as I have told you what I believe. I have given you a little personality orientation and not so much an autobiography. Take that and chew it up awhile.

Shelley

NICOLE

I'm the nerdy person in the Group. I love gadgets, but most of all I live for the computer. The computer is my life. If the others gave me the chance, I'd be on it eighteen hours a day. But, alas, I am not that lucky. Even when the others get on the computer, I am right by their side trying to nudge some time away from them. I'm the one that got the others excited about this technology.

I had my beginning back in college. Bonnie and Diane had a class that required creating a map on the computer. I tried taking a computer science class but ended up dropping it. The technology back then was too complex for me to understand. More than that, I think the teachers themselves didn't quite understand the technology. Anyway, I couldn't quite get the hang of it even though I found it very interesting.

I laid low for awhile after our first orientation to the technology. I would listen to others talk about it and read some of the articles that were written. Back in those days, the technology was mainframes and key punch. I slowly moved from the background as my knowledge and understanding of computers grew. The others were very slow to acquire a taste for this gem of machinery and brains. I think they were more scared of it than anything. The computer is very powerful.

I surfaced when our employer was thinking about getting a computer aided drafting system. I volunteered to research the technology and be on the team that recommended the system to buy. This task force lasted about nine months. I was convinced that the Intergraph system was the better system for doing mapping. Not knowing company politics, I soon found out that the company knew what system it was going to buy all along. It went with an Autotrol system which was geared more for mechanical and architectural drafting. Of course no one would listen to me. I was suppose to be supervisor of the CAD department. Because of our health problems, the others felt that it would be better for all of us if I did not take the position. I was a bit disappointed to say the least. But it was difficult to get excited about something I didn't believe could do what we wanted it to. The disappointment soon wavered.

Other opportunities became available to utilize the computer in the department. Our computer department designed a program that we used to track and chart our department work. I was shown how to use it and was responsible for doing the weekly reports. I enjoyed this menial task. Bonnie and Diane were glad about that.

I was watching a home shopping channel on TV one weekend and they had a computer for sale. I figured I had enough credit left on one of my charge cards and decided to order it. I couldn't wait for it to come. I set it up right away. I am not much for written directions. I learn better by being shown how to do things or by trial and error. Because I refused to read the instructions (actually I tried but didn't understand them), I became frustrated when I couldn't get the computer to do anything but beep at me. It ran on DOS and was an old IBM XT compatible.

The computer sat idle for long periods of time. When the others weren't too preoccupied with their stuff, I would sit down and try to make some progress with the computer. I could never get beyond a certain point. I was hopeful that I could break this jinx with the computer. I was intimidated and afraid that I might mess something up and too scared to experiment with it.

After we left the oil company, the company set up a sort of outplacement department when the layoffs started in early 1986. I was told that any former employee could come into that office and get training on a Macintosh or Wang word processor. I had heard and read a little about the Apple computer about how easy it was to learn and decided I'd take them up on their offer. I made an appointment to go in and was given a half hour of instruction. I was up and running right after that. I came in to use the computer once or twice a week. I did my resume on the computer and wrote my cover letters. I taught Katherine how to use the computer. She began writing a drafting manual and the first attempt at this autobiography.

Soon many of the others in the system realized how easy the Macintosh was and thought of things they could do on it. The excitement became so great that we all agreed it was time to get one of our own. We had sold the IBM compatible when we were selling off most of our other things from the bankruptcy. We got a Mac 512KE and dot matrix printer. It set us back about $1600. That was money we really couldn't afford. Had to wait until money came in from a big drafting project.

Shelley began typing up her invoices on the computer. Our printer was not quite as nice as the laser printer that we used at the company. We would go back over to their office with a disk to print out stuff we wanted a good copy of.

We didn't have much money to buy any equipment and software. We were finalizing our bankruptcy. I just started buying the Macintosh magazines and fantasizing what I would like to buy from mail order catalogs. We just used the software that came preloaded on the computer.

Katherine was introduced to desktop publishing from a woman in the Women Business Owners group we belonged to. Shortly afterward, she was asked to be editor of that organization's monthly newsletter. For the first couple months, she did the typesetting on the other woman's computer. She had a laser printer. Katherine just had to get our own copy of the software. We went to an Apple computer store and forked out $300 for PageMaker. We then had to buy a second floppy drive because we didn't have enough room to run the program on one floppy drive. It seemed that any extra money that came in went toward stuff for the computer. That was fine with me but made things tight. We had to pay cash for everything because we had no charge cards any longer.

Things eventually settled down a bit until Bonnie got the job with Battelle in the fall of 1987. Suddenly money was coming in. I grabbed my share of it and bought a 20MB hard drive first thing. This was sheer luxury. Later came some software to do graphics with. Bonnie and Bobbie were glad about that. There was a little of something for all the main players.

After we moved into our office downtown, it was decided that we would start to offer desktop publishing as a service of ours. We still didn't have a laser printer of our own. The outplacment office was closed. A copy shop across the street from our office had some Macs available for rental time and a laser printer. We started going over there to print out the work we got.

All along, I have been the computer advisor. I help the others as they need it. I recommend what to buy with the money we have. Of course by the time it is paid for it is obsolete. You can't keep up with the technology. You have to use it for what you want to do. As long as it continues to do the job for you it is worth the price. At least that is what I keep telling myself and the others. Who am I fooling, right?! My computer is two years old and already a dinosaur.

I enjoyed working at US WEST in the graphics department. I was able to do the trouble shooting on the hardware and software that ran in the department. I troubleshoot our hardware and software while the others do their thing. On a rare occasion I get to play a game. I'm the only one that likes to play games on the computer. Everyone else is so practical on their usage. Loosen up. Have a little fun once in awhile!

I enjoyed working the sales floor at the store. Once my inhibitions diminished toward IBM compatibles, I picked up on that technology quite quickly. I can sell an IBM just as easily as a Mac. I still feel they are the inferior machine, but there is a hell of a lot of them out there. I will be kind of sorry if the Group decides to quit working at the store. I sure wish our own computer store could get funded. This retail market is real cut-throat and I can see the possibility of the risks with it.

I get such a high from helping people with their computer questions. I know I have developed a wealth of knowledge but had no real clue as to the depth of it until we started working at the store. Lo, what a waste though. There is no money in retail for the peons. The others are constantly razzin' me about the money that we left by going into store management. We could be working forty hours a week and still make more money than we do now at 55 hours. I must admit, though, that it does have its gratification. I'm certain that something will come our way that is akin to everyone's wishes and desires.

No matter what the future does hold, I am bound and determined that something additional will come from my talents and skills. It's no fun having the knowledge that I have chompin at the bit and no place to use it. It is an expensive market, so I will just have to be patient and go with the flow. I don't want to force us into the poor farm again. I'll make the best of whatever opportunity comes along.

I work close at hand with Connie when at the store. She is so good with people. I wish people didn't intimidate me as much as they do. I prefer non-blooded objects, thank you very much. They aren't as cruel and inhumane to someone's feelings.

Well, that's what makes me tick. I'm here for the long haul, but more or less just along for the ride. On to my next sister.

Nicole

CONNIE

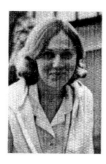

I love to be around people. More than that, I love to watch people. I think we are an interesting bunch of animals. We do some of the screwiest things, especially when we don't think anyone is watching.

I used to love to go to the airport when my dad traveled. My sister and I would sit at the gate my dad was going out on and watch the people hurrying to and from their planes. It would not take long for us to be giggling hysterically. People come in all sizes and shapes and watching their behavior makes things just that much funnier.

I like to go to different places. Just a trip across town puts you in a different cultural environment. It is amazing to see how only 20 miles distance is the breeding ground for different behaviors and attitudes.

I am not shy around people. I have no problem approaching someone and striking up a conversation. The big problem is that I don't get a whole lot of opportunity to do this. The others are so much more domineering with our time and are so very introverted. They would walk in the opposite direction if they thought you might speak to them. They are such home bodies, too. BORING! It is hard to be anybody when you coup yourself up inside of four walls. Experience life! Don't waste it away. Do you guys hear what I am saying? Probably not.

I got my start when we were in high school. We took a job at a local department store in the domestics department as a clerk. The others were too inhibited to approach people and the boss said we needed to see if customers needed help. I broke the ice and got things rolling. It was fun. The others still didn't like being around people that much. When a position opened up in the shipping department, they jumped at the opportunity. I got to do my thing on weekends.

The next summer, I got a job at a local restaurant that was buffet style. I served food and helped prepare it. I also worked the register. People are creatures of habit. They find something they like and become regulars at doing it. Some of the same people would come back religiously and eat at the restaurant. I worked in the German food part of the restaurant. There was this one overweight lady that ate there two or three times a week. She always had to have a kosher pickle. Not just any pickle. She had me fish around in the pan to find the perfect pickle. It had to be not only the biggest, but the best shaped pickle. One other guy ate there at least once a week and always had the Hungarian Goulash.

It seemed that I was the one who put us through college. The only jobs we could find were people oriented jobs. Between my junior and senior year, we took a sales job. It was door to door sales of books. We had to travel halfway across the country to get to my selling location. This was when I was introduced to hard-core selling. The "get your foot in the door and don't leave without the sale" kind of selling. I learned real quickly this was not my style. I do not like to make people do anything their heart is not set on doing. I go for the soft-sell.

Needless to say, I did not do well selling Bibles and sex-education books in the heart of the Bible Belt. After awhile, I got tired of having doors slammed in my face. I took a different approach. I became the peoples' friend. I would stop and visit with people as they were outside. I would talk about everything but selling. I would get to know the people. Then, in passing, I would mention what I was doing out on the street. A few now and then would buy. Others would say they weren't interested and turn away. I didn't push them. I would go on down the road. Needless to say, this approach was not much for making a living. I made just enough to pay the rent and buy food.

The summer as a door to door salesman was short-lived. Two of my roommates came down with mono. It left just one other girl and myself to pay the rent. I didn't sell enough to be able to pay for half the rent. I called my folks. They offered me a plane ticket to come back to Denver for the rest of the summer. I gladly accepted.

It was mid-summer when I returned to Denver. Not enough time to really get into another job. My mom said they had a cook up at church camp back out and her church was looking for someone to take her place. She asked if I was interested. I said, sure, why not? Camp lasted for two weeks. I helped with the cooking. Susan took her guitar and helped with the singing. Carol helped the kids with their crafts. I just enjoyed being in a warm, friendly atmosphere.

We went back to Arizona two weeks before school started to see if we couldn't find a part time job for our junior year. First on the agenda was to find a new place to live, because our roommate from the previous year got married. I located a new complex about a mile from campus. They had just opened and happened to be looking for a rental agent/secretary. I asked if I could apply. I did and got the job. It lasted till just before Christmas, because the managers I worked for were not model citizens and packed up and left one day. The complex was a mess. The owners took over and brought in a professional to run and manage the place.

I waited until the next spring to look for another job. I landed a job in Mesa at the Globe department store in April. It was a part time job that I worked about 28 hours a week at. I started as a cashier, then got a move back into the layaway department. I ran the register back there, set up people's layaway purchases and watched the dressing rooms. I had a lot of people contact. Here, too, I got to recognize the regulars. I had a good time with this job. I worked it through the summer and all the next year. I had to take time off so Diane could go on her field methods excursion to California. I worked right up until a couple days before Christmas since it was the busiest time of the year. I then took a week off for Christmas back in Denver with family.

I kind of took a back seat after college until the opportunity opened up at the computer store. Nicole and I pushed ourselves to the front. If we had to work a second job, why not do something that several of us could enjoy? Nicole loved computers and I loved people. Francie got into the act, too. We made a great trio. We couldn't wait to leave Bonnie and Bobbie behind at US WEST and get to the store. We rarely ever took breaks when we worked evenings.

I started out being very helpful in the software department because that was what Nicole felt most comfortable with. She didn't feel as intimidated there as on the main sales floor. After a couple months, though, they were in need of help in the Apple aisle. A lot of people were in the market for Apple computers for Christmas. I approached the people and provided the liaison between Nicole and the people. I would provide the humanness and friendliness of a helpful sales associate, while her expertise would come out in the words and conversation. Francie is the one that put the fun into the work. She was very uplifting, because even though I am friendly, I tend to be pretty serious about things. She was the lighter side to the trio.

We have since been pulled away from the sales floor to other responsibilities at the store. I make the others walk across the floor every now and then looking for someone who needs some help. The job has become an endeavor amongst many. So much so that we are getting worn to a frazzle with all the switching that goes on throughout the day. That is why we are absolutely exhausted when we get home from work and don't want to do anything but sleep. No matter how much I enjoy the people contact, we are reaching a state of burnout with the job. Some of us keep prodding the others to keep at it awhile longer.

We promise that if we get our own store, things will be different. My suspicions here, though, are I am not thinking too clearly with these thoughts. Something tells me that things would become even more chaotic and exhausting. I think we should go with what reason and our gut says. Granted, our own store would have a lot to offer many of us, but can we really handle the wear and tear that it would pose on us? I think not. I'm sure we would go into overload.

If this is the case, something tells me my days are numbered and it may be time to fade back into the background again. I don't have to go away completely. If we keep the security job we now have on a part time basis, I'll have opportunity to be around people. They still need me to help with people relationships should Bobbie get a job in a graphics department. Whatever we chose to do for work, I will need to be close at hand to give encouragement and help out with the people skills. My selling days may be numbered, but at least I know I will still have something else to offer the Group.

Our survival is, was, and will always be a joint effort of the several. That's something I don't have to worry about. I am glad that we have decided not to integrate. I much rather prefer working together as a harmonious team...and that's my story.

Connie

FRANCIE

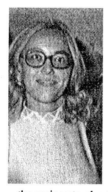

Footloose and fancy free – that's who I am, and why I have the name I have. I love a good time, and I think you have to be around other people to have the best of times. In other words, I love to party.

College was a blast. I had the best time of my life there. If I had my way, we would have become a professional student, but the others were eager to get on with life and make something of ourselves.

I never remembered studying. Of course, I wasn't the one who went to class. That was something for the others to do. I spent most of my time at the AFROTC Detachment with the guys...and other gals. What there were of them.

My freshman year, we took a trip to visit the Air Force base in Las Vegas. I got to meet some pilots and have a good time on the Vegas strip. I wasn't legal, but dressed like an adult and had no problem getting into the casinos to play the slots and drink. I got bored with the slots and turned to watching the other people gamble. I spent my two nights there going to lounge shows. One night, I saw Paul Revere and the Raiders perform for just the cost of two drinks. Food was great in the casinos, too. You could get a full meal for under five bucks. Breakfast was all you could eat for 89¢.

I would go out nights, mainly Friday and Saturday with the guys from the detachment to go dancing. That started mainly second semester of school. First semester, Mike was bent on joining Silver Wing and spent his time studying and going through the pledge program. I could dance my life away. It was great. I had all the partners a girl could want. When one got tired, I would just grab the next likely candidate and pull him out to the dance floor. Disco was hot when I was in school. I remember having a blast doing the bump.

I got invited to a lot of parties with the guys. One of the Silver Wingers was getting married. He was infatuated with me or something. Mainly I think he was drunk. The guys were having his stag party and he kept asking when I was coming. He became obsessed with the idea of me being at his party. So much so, the other guys called me and invited me over. I remember drinking straight shots of Tequila that night and watching stag movies.

I wasn't treated like one of the guys like when Mike was around. They really saw me for the woman that I was. I was fun to be around. They would hang on me and I would party all night with the guys; sometimes sleeping on the floor at someone's apartment.

Finally one of the guys got serious and latched onto me. His name was Bryan. He was a blast. His dad owned an airplane and we went on some interesting dates. The only thing I didn't like about him was that he was never on time when he did set a date. He just kind of expected me to be ready anytime the urge struck him. That was fine for me, but the others did not care for this approach too well.

Bryan was a cartoonist by hobby and made me laugh. That first summer, he would write me almost daily. His letters always had a cartoon in them pertaining to what he had done or was doing at the time he wrote the letter. We had a pretty carefree relationship until it got serious enough that he became sexually attracted to me. For me, that was when the fun stopped. I took off my dancing slippers and let Sally run the show when he got that funny way. I could sleep next to him and cuddle okay, but when the kissing and petting got to be more than I cared for, I split. I did that with all the guys I ever dated. That isn't my kind of fun.

When Mike didn't make it into the officer program. I decided to join Angel Flight. It was the only way I could still hang around the guys and not feel like I was intruding. Bryan eventually became more interested in someone else over Christmas of my sophomore year. That was fine with me because I was feeling a little too strapped tagged as one guy's gal.

My junior year, I turned my attention to older, more mature guys. I would go out to the training base with some of the other Angels. Most of the guys out there in the Officer's Club were pilots, or jet jockies as they were called then. One night when I was out there, I got the feeling that one particular guy had his eye on me. When it is a stranger in a setting like this, I tend to be a bit more reserved. I just kept watching him. Finally, he made a move and came over and asked me to dance. He was great. One of the better dancers I had met. His name was Ken.

We spent most of the night dancing. I guess I left the club around 1 a.m. Before I left, he asked for my phone number and if he could call me later. I was charmed and said, sure. This guy was an absolute doll. He was the best looking man that had ever taken me seriously as a man to a woman. I felt good in his presence. I kept hoping that he would call me again. Later that week he did and made a date to go to a show and dinner. I didn't want this one to get away, so I tried to refrain and be a little conservative on the date. We seemed to really hit it off. We started to become a regular item.

I enjoyed being around Ken. He was lots of fun yet was more mature than the guys at the detachment. We dated regularly until he finished pilot training. At the end of his flight training, he was assigned to a base in Oklahoma for specialized training on the aircraft he would be flying. I hated to see him go. We kept in touch, though. He would send me postcards from some of the trips he took. His folks lived in Scottsdale, so when he came back to Phoenix, he would visit and we would do things for a few days. I don't remember falling in love with the guy. I guess I didn't quite feel I was good enough to have someone as wonderful as him. He was more like a boy doll to play with.

Ken and I remained good friends throughout my last two years in college. Since we were not a steady thing, I didn't feel like it was a problem going out with other guys once he left. I did go visit him in California after Christmas my senior year. That was where he was stationed after his specialized training. We had a good three or four days together. We were still in touch after I graduated.

Ken was planning on coming up to Colorado on vacation to go skiing. He was going to stay with me for a week. Throughout our relationship, I knew he was dating other girls. How could someone as good looking as him not be at his age?

Ken suggested after I moved back to Denver to get out and learn to ski so we could run the slopes together when he came out. I took his advice. Right after Christmas, I bought skis and signed up for a ski trip with a local singles group. I was one of the first ones on the bus. The trip was full, so I knew I would be setting next to someone on the trip. Who would have guessed it would be a guy that would ask to sit next to me? A guy who introduced himself as Gene asked to share the seat next to me. I said sure.

We talked the whole way up to the mountains. We had a lot in common. All my sisters took a strong liking to him from the start because he shared so many of their interests. When I told him I was a real novice skier, he volunteered to give me lessons for the day. I was a real clutz, but he stuck with me through thick and thin. He was an okay guy. We went with the ski club to have dinner when we returned to Denver. He continued to stick by me. When I got ready to go, he asked if he could call. I said I'd love to have him call me and gave him my phone number.

We all became obsessed with this guy. He was a real charmer. Had a little of something for most of us. We couldn't let this one get away. I impatiently awaited his call. He didn't call back until the next Thursday. He asked if he could take me out on Saturday. We went to a movie. He even had the same taste in movies that we did at the time. What a catch!

Needless to say, the relationship took off and got serious very quickly. Soon it was time to make a decision. I talked to Gene about Ken and his pending trip. Do I stick with the guy who is in the same town and very serious about me, or do I lose him for the long distance romance? It was a tough decision. I wasn't sure what was the right thing to do. Finally I decided that my relationship with Ken could never amount to anything serious, whereas, Gene and I had potential. I wasn't looking at getting married right away, but I did like the idea of someone being there for me that I could do things with regularly. Sally and Monique had votes for Gene. I guess if it was going to be a sexual relationship, it had better be with someone that could meet the needs of my sisters. Gene was the man for the job.

As I said earlier, I didn't care for the sexual activities that went along with man and woman relationships, but I did like Gene and he satisfied me in other ways. We did a lot of different and interesting things. We did do a lot of skiing that year and I got much better at it. Almost became a regular snow bunny. We would go to shows, out for dinner, trips to the mountains in the summer and the theater. We even went out dancing and to concerts. He introduced me to a lot of his friends at work. We would go to happy hour every Friday night and have the finger food for dinner.

This relationship got very serious. So serious that I decided to move in with him after dating for a year and a half. We went on trips together. Took a week long trip to San Francisco and one up to Seattle. I was having the time of my life. It was almost as good as being back in college. No better. I had someone all to myself.

This relationship lasted for just about three years. I was pushing him for a commitment because Bonnie and the others were wanting to know what to do with our career. Actually, it wasn't so much that which caused the relationship to topple. It all started falling apart when Gene's mom was killed in a car accident one year the day before my birthday. It shook him up pretty badly. He was an only child and his father had passed away a few years before he came to Denver. He held a lot of anger and resentment toward the boys who were driving the other car. He was bent on seeing justice done, but the boys were under age. He got to a point where he would not share his feelings with me any longer. There was no communication. I had to give him an ultimatum to try and snap him out of it. It didn't work out.

I moved back home with my parents around Easter time in 1979. That really put a crimp in our relationship. My parents knew we had been sleeping together but would not allow me to spend the night with him as long as I was living under their roof. Sally and Monique got creative with where they got their pleasures met. By summer Gene had me talked into buying a condo. He even offered to use part of his inheritance as a down payment. We would be co-signers on the note. Things started to get back to normal for a brief period.

Things really got shot to hell when we had our nervous breakdown that fall. He couldn't handle having his girlfriend in a crazy ward at some psychiatric hospital. He tried to cope but I saw him distancing himself further from us. The amount of time we spent together after we got out of the hospital became less and less. When I asked if he would spend Christmas with my folks, he said he was going with his stock broker to Michigan or thereabouts. He said he would be back New Year's Eve to spend the night with me. It sounded kind of fishy to me.

When he did come back, I noticed most of the spark we had was gone. His mind was someplace else. It quickly occurred to me that he had someone else that he was seeing and must have gone to her place to spend Christmas. I hit the nail on the head. We saw very little of one another after that. I continued to communicate with and see some of our mutual friends but that soon drew to an end, also. He changed jobs. He went to work for a bank.

Six months later, I learned from one of our friends that he was getting married. My heart sunk. How could he be making a commitment to someone so quickly after we broke up and when he couldn't make a commitment to me? I was shattered. I couldn't get him off my mind. I saw him on the Mall one day and congratulated him and told him that I hoped he was happy. He said he was. The next thing I heard was that he was selling his house and he and his wife were moving to Oregon to buy a bed and breakfast place. I just couldn't seem to shake the guy from my thoughts. Three years of hospitalizations and depressions later, I finally resolved that we were through and put him in the back of my mind. Oh I thought about how he was doing now and then, but the fire in my heart was gone for him. I was ready to get on with my life.

After Gene, I could never really find a place for a guy again. I was too afraid of having another hurt like I had with him. We centered our life around Gene. He became our life. Love was too cruel that I swore off it. From time to time I got a little spark under me and would go out to a bar. I even joined a private singles club. I just couldn't get into the scene again. I still like people but I am very cautious with who I become close to. Relationships stay platonic.

I am not the socialite I used to be anymore. I push the others to go out and be around people as much as I can, but they are a little stronger than me. They had a lot riding on the relationship with Gene, too. They were deeply crushed when it ended. I have more or less resorted to being the group historian. I am the communicator within the system. Everyone tells me their wishes and desires and I relay it to those who might not choose to talk or listen to some of the others.

I have since re-established some old relationships. One is with a mutual friend of Gene's and mine. I have shared our secret with her. She has agreed to read this book when it is finished. She has been the one that has kept me posted on Gene's whereabouts over the years. In fact, you will never guess it, but I got a letter from Gene about a month ago. He is back in Denver. He got a divorce but has a son. I also understand that he contracted multiple sclerosis and has become bitter about it. I think that is partly why he got his divorce. If he wants to connect and use my ear, I am here to listen, but I know there will never be what we used to have. And that is my story.

Francie

SALLY

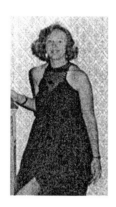

I enjoy men. I enjoy flirting with men. Flirting is a real turn on for me. It excites me to get a man excited about being with me. That sounds plain and simple but my life is by no means that plain and simple. In fact I have lead a rather complicated life.

I was Michele's first sexual alter to be aroused from the depths of this system. I got my start early on. I guess it must have been when we were in the first grade. Mike was playing with Johnny and Rusty one day when they suggested we move our play over to Johnny's basement. Mike thought nothing of it.

Little did he know what plans they had. They suggested playing cops and robbers. Mike would be the cop. Mike got caught sneaking up on their hideout. They proceeded to tie Mike to a chair. They made Mike strip down to his underwear before they tied him up. In steps me.

They decided they couldn't have any witnesses. They were going to torture me then leave me at their hideout. They took my clothes so I would not be inclined to escape. That basement was cold and dark. They tied my hands very tight. They then started exploring my body. They rubbed their hands over my chest then down my front. They then tied a handkerchief over my mouth so I couldn't scream. I tried to tell them that I did not want to play the game any more. They would not listen to me. Next they ran their hands into my underpants and began rubbing me. They rubbed me kind of hard and made me spread my legs apart. I was trying to talk with the gag in my mouth and struggled. Suddenly I felt a tingling between my legs. What they were doing started to feel good to me. I struggled more and the sensation got greater. It was becoming a real turn on for me. I didn't want them to stop. Rusty and Johnny told me not to tell anyone about our secret game.

The others didn't like what happened. They told me it wasn't right. I should not have let them do that kind of thing to me. They wouldn't let me play with Rusty and Johnny any more.

What happened that day caused me to discover something new about my body. I was driven to recreate that sensation that I experienced in the cold, damp basement. One day when we were playing on the monkey bars, we had a rope tied to the top bar that I would try to climb. As I climbed and struggled my way up the rope something began to happen. That tingling sort of thing that happened in the basement that day was happening on the monkey bars climbing the rope.

Soon I couldn't get enough of this activity. I even learned to recreate that sensation by hanging from the top bar and just pretending to climb a rope. Little beknownst to me did I understand that what was happening was that I was masturbating to an orgasm. All I knew was that it felt great.

When we moved off Fifth Street, we did not take the monkey bars with us. I was lost. I didn't know what I could do to satisfy that craving. I tried rubbing my genitals but that didn't quite seem to accomplish the same sensation.

About a year after moving, between fourth and fifth grade, my parents started going out a lot at night. If it wasn't for the business it was with friends out for dinner and drinks. My brother was going into junior high school and starting to go through puberty. He was finding that he wanted to try new things and explore his own sexuality. He had been getting Playboy magazines for a little while and hiding them under his mattress. I found them when I had to change his bed. I got curious and started to look at them.

One night when my parents were gone and the house was dark, I was in my bedroom about ready to go to sleep. I was awoken to a hand coming underneath the covers of my bed. It was reaching for me and touching me. The hand went up underneath my nightgown. I woke alarmed. It was my brother. He said to be quiet so I didn't wake my sister in the next bedroom. I asked him what he was doing. He said he liked my body and how it was maturing. (My breasts were already big enough that I was wearing a training bra.) He knew of a way that he could touch me and make me feel good.

This sounded interesting. I decided to play along with his game. Soon he crawled up into bed with me and took his undershorts off. He rubbed my genitals then suddenly stuck his finger up my vagina. I didn't know I had a hole there until then. What a discovery! He also rubbed and pinched what little breasts I had. I asked him where he learned about this. He said from some of the guys at school and guys he hung around with at my dad's station. He asked if it made me feel good. I said it did. He asked me to rub his penis. He got chills just from me touching it.

The next thing I knew, he had crawled on top of me and was rubbing his penis against my body. I asked him if we should be doing this. He said that mom and dad were not home and nobody needed to know about it other than us. It would be our secret.

From then on, this little game became a ritual on nights that Roger knew my parents would be gone for a long time. I would go to bed early on these nights. I would lie in bed anticipating the sound of my brother sneaking into my bedroom. The secrecy of it all was almost as exciting as what he did in my bed. For once, here was someone that was not afraid to touch and cuddle with me and do things to make me feel good and liked...or loved. I was starved for this kind of attention. I was not going to spoil a good thing by telling him to stop.

For the first couple months my visits were pretty much the same, then one night my brother said he could really make me feel good if I would just let him stick his penis in the hole between my legs. He made me feel good when he stuck his finger in there, why couldn't this be just as good? He was very careful and gentle with me. He said he would stop if it hurt me. I let him on top of me. He made me spread my legs. I had rubbed his penis so it had gotten hard. He then slowly worked it into my vagina. It was scary what would happen next, but it excited me just the same. He then began moving up and down over me pulling his penis in and out. He was very slow and careful about what he was doing. Soon we were building up a sweat. I was moving with his body. Suddenly I started panting and telling him to move faster. Before I knew it a tingling sensation came over me. The one that I experienced in Johnny's basement and on the monkey bars. This was great! I now had a new way to make my body feel good like that.

Roger kind of groaned, then backed out from inside of me. I was all wet between my legs. I thought maybe I was bleeding or something because it felt warm. He said it was him that caused it and I was okay and not bleeding.

This ritual continued regularly for a little over a year and a half. One day in sixth grade, I noticed some red blood in my underpants. Instinct told me to get one of the cotton-like pads that my mom had placed under the bathroom sink. This was the day I became a woman. I had started my monthly periods. I told my mom what had happened. She set me down and gave me the 10 minute version of the birds and the bees. We didn't have sex education in grade school back in those days, but something told me that what Roger and I were doing could not continue. What he was doing to me could make me have a baby. The next time he came to my room, I told him what had happened. He said he could still make me feel good with just his finger. He asked if I would continue to let him come to my room to just lay together and me rub his penis. I said I guessed it would be okay if he promised he wouldn't stick it inside me anymore. He agreed.

This revised play went on for another year or two. Until I had sex education in school and learned that this activity was something we should not be doing. It was wrong and only for grown-ups. It wasn't really my decision to quit, but rather the others in the Group. Some of them have pretty strong moral beliefs and when someone says something is wrong, they refuse to have anything to do with it.

From that point on my means of masturbation and reaching orgasm consisted of finding my brother's dirty magazines, going in the den, laying on my stomach and riding a pillow between my legs while looking at the pictures. A lot of it was fantasizing. Whatever, it got me satisfied when I had the urge.

It wasn't until college that I let a man touch me again. Even at that, I was at school for a whole semester before any intimate contact occurred. At first the activity just amounted to heavy petting with all my clothes on. It wasn't until my sophomore year when Bryan and I were a thing that it went beyond that. First, it started with him putting his hands down my pants. Then we would strip down to our underwear and pretend having sex by rubbing up against one another. Before I knew it, and kind of unexpectedly, we were having intercourse.

I was not using any means of protection when this happened. I had heard about the Pill but was not taking it. I thought there was no need until then. I panicked. The last thing I needed was to get pregnant. I talked to my roommate, Carol, about what had happened. She said she had heard something about a "morning after" pill. I went to a local Planned Parenthood clinic and asked if they had such a thing. There was and I took the pills for the next three days.

Now that the ice had been broken, I knew I would want more of this activity. It made me feel good before and then. I found a local gynecologist and made an appointment for an exam and to see about getting a prescription for the Pill. Bryan and I abstained from intercourse for a month. Just long enough for my exam and to become protected by the Pill.

My sexual activity rose considerably after that. I was a one man woman as long as I dated Bryan. When Bryan and I broke up, I needed to have my needs fulfilled. I began sleeping around. It was mainly with Air Force ROTC guys or pilots. I didn't go in for any kinky stuff. Just clean sex. Monique is the one who plays the games with the guys. Back then there was no worry about getting AIDS like there is today.

Things kind of settled down when I met Ken. He was a real gentleman. He knew how to make me feel good. He is the only man that could get me to have simultaneous orgasms. He held off for himself until I had reached my state of ecstacy.

Ken and I took a trip to the mountains one weekend. He had a convertible and we were riding with the top down. It was such a gorgeous day. We had packed a picnic lunch. We found a nice shady, grassy, wooded area off the side of the road to have our picnic. We went far enough away from the road not to be bothered by cars. We had wine, cheese and chicken. By the time we had finished lunch and the bottle of wine we were feeling sleepy so cleared off the blanket and laid next to one another. One thing led to another and before we knew it, we were undressing one another. I had never had sex outside before. It was great! Back to nature and all. The only thing I didn't like about the whole experience was the big mosquito bite I got on my butt!

After Ken, my next great romantic encounter was with Gene back in Denver. We got into heavy petting and kissing right off, but I didn't want to come across as easy prey, so I made him wait to get the real thing. We dated a month before we partook of intercourse. The wait was worth it, though. Gene was great in bed. Because of some of Gene's pleasures, I shared him with Monique. Gene liked oral sex and that isn't my forté so I'd let her take him on for that.

I spent almost all my weekends over at Gene's place. We would have sexual marathons; a little sex, a little pinball, more sex, some food and wine. We did other things, too. I shared him with several of my sisters. They learned to play racquetball and played tennis with him. They went to the theater and concerts and good restaurants. Sex was a big part of our relationship but everyone got a little something from it. We were one big happy family.

Our relationship changed after I moved in with him in his old Victorian house. We went from having sex almost every night to three or four times a week. I was having difficulty reaching orgasm. It must have been the stress Bonnie was under at work. To keep our relationship from deteriorating, I found myself often faking an orgasm. I didn't want Gene to think he couldn't satisfy me any more.

Soon, I learned to enjoy frolicking in bed almost as much as reaching a climax, though it definitely was not the same. Just being close and hugging one another showed me that someone cared about me and that was what I would look forward to.

One of our last crazy flings was when we christened my new condo before I moved in. We had sex and cuddling for an hour straight on the floor in the living room. The last time Gene and I did it was on New Year's in 1980. That was when we found out that he was definitely involved with another woman. I just couldn't feel the same about him any more after that. I don't remember doing it again after that. We stayed friends for awhile longer, but quickly drew apart.

Since then, I have had one night with Bryan and one night with Ken. They happened to be passing through Denver on two separate occasions and spent the night with me in my house. It was fun while it lasted but nothing like it was before. Nothing could equate to what Gene and I had.

With so little sexual activity in our life, I kind of faded off into la la land. The others didn't have much need for me. I did need to blow off some pressure every now and then and would surface. I learned a new way to masturbate that was almost as great as climbing the rope. I had one of those shower massaging shower heads in the house where I could adjust the stream of water. When it was adjusted just so, I found that I could massage my clitoris enough with the pressured water to reach orgasm. It was wonderful! I thought I had forgotten what an orgasm felt like. I soon became addicted and took showers for Michele regularly.

After the one nighters with Bryan and Ken, I wasn't with another man until about 1985. I developed a thing for my next door neighbor, Mike. We were good friends and he had a liking for me, or a need for fulfillment just like me. We came to a mutual understanding and started engaging in casual sex. Our relationship was strictly platonic and not romantic at all. It was a plain case of two people with needs that needed to be met who were ready and willing. The others didn't care much for it. Mike knew Michele was multiple and some people we talked to thought he was taking advantage of us. I don't think that at all. I had needs that weren't being met. I was all for the little arrangement we had.

He knew how to get me to come out. He would play an arousing sexual movie. The others would begin watching it until they got turned off. I would peek out and really get into the movie. Then that was all she wrote. The only thing I didn't like about the thing with Mike was he talked about having his needs met but would not let himself go completely. He knew I was no longer on the pill and he would abstain from ejaculating. I don't see how he could have been enjoying himself, unless it was a turn-on for him to see me aroused. I always wondered but just couldn't quite find the right way to ask him.

Mike has since gotten married and seems very happy. I am very happy for him. We remain good friends and I have become a good friend of his wife. I talk to him from time to time on the phone but that is about all. I have gone to their place on a couple occasions but just as a friend.

It's been a couple years now since I have seen any action. I think this body is starting to approach menopause, because the desires that once used to be there aren't any more. I just can't get enthusiastic about masturbating. I have a stash of Playboy magazines that I sometimes will pull out to look at and read but that is about all. I have had some erotic dreams, but that has been the only real turn on for about a year now. I still prefer to look at beautiful women's bodies, but don't pass up the opportunity to stare at a good piece of man's ass from time to time as we walk around out in public.

I guess to sum it up, I enjoy good, clean sex, but more than anything, I love the feeling of being needed and wanted when you are intimate with another person. Last but not least, you will hear from Monique, my darker half. I don't know that there was any real planning to save the juiciest for last. I guess she is the outcast of the group if we have one. I like sex, but not her kind. Let her tell you herself.

Sally

MONIQUE

I have a great little treasure with my body and I am not afraid to share it as long as it is done my way. I think I am sexy and voluptuous and what every man dreams of. I wasn't always this way, though. We have been in and out of various skins all our life, but this picture is the way I saw myself in college and continue to see myself. I don't care how many layers of fat Michele chooses to wrap around me. She is just screwing herself over.

I love sex...hard core sex. I think forced sex is a real turn on. I constantly fantasize about being raped. That's why I get to walk the streets late at night. I'm the only one not afraid of meeting someone on the street. I would turn on the guy and rape him. Ha!

The one thing with me and sex is – I have to be in control. When with a guy, I have to be on top. If not, I control how much muscle power he is going to get on his prick.

Sally is okay, but she is too delicate. I like it rough and tough. I need it that way to get off. When she had trouble reaching an orgasm during masturbation I would take over. I would ram anything and everything I could find up my vagina. Things like multiple tampons, brushy hair curlers, candles, Ping-Pong balls. You gotta be careful about those ping pong balls. They are liable to get stuck up there. Have to go fishin' for them. When they get lubricated with all my secretions, they become slippery little devils and hard to grab a hold of. I freaked the others out a number of times.

When that didn't seem to satisfy me, I decided to bring our dog into the act. I would force her to lick my clitoris and vagina. At first she resisted, but soon she learned to like it and then couldn't get enough of it. She would start licking, then would reach for whatever secretions she could get. She would try to bite me and ram her tongue deep into my vagina. What a gas! I did this with Sheri and Toshi. For some reason, Nikki was too cute and tiny to get on to.

When I first got started, I convinced our sister, Karla, to experiment with me. We would explore one another's body. We would see what it was like to suck a nipple till it was black and blue. I could only get her to do this about half a dozen times. I guess I was too rough on her. The rest of the time it was myself, dog and/or brother.

I learned how to control my muscles with my brother. He would tell me what felt good to him, then I would work at it each time we had a fling. I really built up my butt and vaginal muscles. Later on when I was in college, I put my technique to good use. I could drive the guys crazy with my muscle control.

Speaking of college, what a great time that was! I had a real blast. Especially when we started going to parties. I'd pick out a guy and coerce him into the bedroom. All along making him think he was getting me into the sack. I would act semi-frigid and real nervous and tell him that I really didn't do this sort of thing. I'd say that I never went all the way with a guy before – just heavy petting and kissing. Oh, I'm a great French kisser, too. More about that later. Eventually, I'd let him into my pants. I would stroke his penis rigorously and get him real hot and turned on, all the while trying to hold him off. Finally, he would get so burning hot, that I'd almost let him rip my clothes off and fuck his brains out. As he was thrusting himself inside of me, I would use my strict muscle control to excite him further. His orgasm would become my orgasm. Once he had a chance to come up for air, I would start stroking his penis more and get him turned on all over again. I would make this go on and on for two to three hours. I fucked those guys' brains out, when they thought they were fucking me. I probably did this a couple dozen times in between Sally's boyfriends.

Now about my kissing. I do the deep throat kind of kissing. I ram my tongue deep inside the guy's mouth, circling his tongue. I then prod his tongue into my mouth. I would then lightly grasp his tongue with my teeth and lips and begin sucking on it using my lips to mimic my vaginal muscles on his penis. This would drive the guys wild. He couldn't wait to get into my pants after I started kissing him this way. Of course I would try to push him away making him even more hot and hungry to want to fuck me.

There was a Mike in college, too. He was an Air Force Cadet. He is the one who taught me to go down on a guy and suck his cock. Guys were like putty in my hands when I would do this. It excited them even more when I would let them come in my mouth. Instead of spitting out the semen, I would swallow it. I put my kissing deep throat technique to work on their cock. I would tease them with my mouth action until they were about to scream. Then I would go down deep and hard sucking with all my might.

I was not overly orgasmic when I got it on with guys. In fact I probably faked more orgasms than I had. I wasn't in it so much for the physical orgasm as the emotional orgasm that the power I had over someone else brought me. I lived to manipulate the men I encountered.

I liked Bryan. He was different. He was kind of boyish in nature and kind of rough. Like he didn't know how to handle a woman. When we finally got it on, I think I surprised him with my abilities and kept bringing him back for more.

As Sally said, Ken was a real gentleman. I know he got enjoyment from what I did for him, but I found him routine and not much of a challenge.

There was this one guy in college. We had a thing my senior year. He was a year behind me and real short...But what a boner. He had the biggest damn prick I have ever encountered. Now that guy excited me. He had more than I could fit in my mouth. I nearly choked on him on several occasions. We were a wild couple that would experiment with all kinds of kinky positions and techniques.

Then there was Gene. The love of my life. We all loved him for various reasons. But I was able to live out some wild fantasies with him. I regularly went down on him while he was driving down the highway. We took this one trip to California and drove through the Napa Valley. We took in a lot of the winery tours and tastings. I love that Burgundy wine. It is dry like a man's semen. It was a real aphrodisiac for me. I couldn't wait to get him to turn down a side road for a quicky. I would stick my hands down his pants and get his cock nice and hard so it burst out of his pants. I would then relieve the tension by unzipping his pants. To relieve the tension further that I had created, I would suck him to orgasm, then zip him back up. He had to go and spoil it all by telling me some story about how a man had hit a tree and killed him and his wife or girl. When they pulled them from the wreckage, the woman was still in the man's lap with his penis in her mouth.

Gene and I would often take showers together and fuck in the shower or bath tub. That was a turn-on. He always let me on top. That was a turn-on for him. He liked to have the woman in control. We would sometimes fuck all night into the wee hours of the morning. The others didn't mind quite so much as long as they didn't have to be present. This activity was a real stress reducer for us all.

When Sally would masturbate in the shower, I would make things exciting by turning up the hot water until we could barely stand it or came close to burning us. That spoiled her fun, but made it feel great for me. A little water torture. I torture myself in other ways, too. I got into this hot wax thing for awhile. I would drip hot wax on my nipples and genitals. It hurt at first, but the torturous pain excited me. Once again I was roll playing.

I really get hot and turned on watching triple X-rated movies. The only thing I thought was a turn off in the movie was that none of the women would let the guy ejaculate in their mouth. I really liked it when two men were working over a woman. One has his cock in her mouth and the other is fucking her brains out. I would put myself in her place and pretend to be controlling the guy's prick in my cunt and driving the guy with his cock in my mouth crazy. Real power over man. Who said the woman was the innocent weakling? They just think they have control. I dare any man to take me on. I would welcome a gang bang any day.

Now my life is boring. I haven't had a good fuck in ages it seems. Mike, our neighbor was okay, but I didn't have as much fun with him, because he controlled how much he put into the sex. Sally liked it, so I let her have him. They got along great. I tired quickly of him.

Of late, all I have had to work with is a vibrator and some other prosthetic devices. Real crude at best, but I guess more real than hair curlers and the such. If he was up to it, I would get our Mike to come out and pretend he was raping me. This added to the use of my toys was a real turn-on. My orgasms have not been much to write home about lately. They are tiny little bubbles that pop so quickly and don't last. A real bummer. So much so that I don't masturbate much any more. It is too much work for so little pleasure.

What I miss most is the hospital struggles. That has been my best feat since Gene. I would help Kim do something dumb that got the staff in the psych ward concerned and then resist that con-cerned behavior...and voila! the struggle. I first learned about this at Mt. Airy during our first hos-pitalization. It was great struggling and squirmming with guy's hands all over me trying to hold me down or get me to the seclusion room. I also loved the restraints. Especially the full four-point restraints. I once got 5-point restraints. I was flying high. I felt like I was in a medieval torture chamber, or even like back in Johnny's basement. Even when I am being tortured, I have the feeling of being in control of the situation and that gets me going. That is the game of all games as far as I am concerned. Too bad we haven't been in the hospital for several years, let alone re-straints. Being healthy is okay, but sure takes a lot of fun out of my life.

I think I have painted a fairly colorful picture of just who I am for you. Talking to Michele, you would never guess that she had someone as wild as me inside her and capable of the things I am. In fact every time she thinks about having me around, she gets grossed out and sick to her stomach. Isn't life wonderful? Well, this has been our story. Hope we have informed, amused and educated you about the life of someone with MPD. This kind of life is not so bad. I have found it to be real challenging and exciting. Like, when I can get Michele into an awkward situation...or when I can really make others take a second look at Michele. Really, I am not that bad, am I? That's all folks!!!!!

Monique

Epilogue

A lot has evolved in my life in just the short year since this manuscript was completed. My life is moving forward in a more sane and rational manner. I'll briefly bring you up to date.

I quit my job with the computer store in April 1996. Personnel morale had dropped to an all time low with most of the associates and many were leaving. Since I filed discrimination charges against them with the EEOC in October 1995, the store manager was fired and regional manager took and early retirement sabbatical. Charges were for sexual discrimination and discrimination based on an established disability (MPD). Personality conflicts existed with management and subordinates because of alter defense mechanisms. I can't afford legal representation to take them to court, so am having to wait out the 2-year government backlog before the case even gets assigned to an investigator.

I had no job lined up when I quit. I knew the day was coming, but promised myself to stick it out until I did get a new job, but could not accept further humiliation and intimidation when they wanted to reassign me to clerical duties after being a manager. That was the "final straw."

I still had my weekend security job as an income source. I fought to get unemployment due to quitting under duress, but lost my case in the hearing. I immediately registered with several temp agencies and added additional floating shifts with the security company during the week. In May, I got a weeknight, part time position working in the warehouse for a local national gift and nutritional book distributor.

I had one or two job interviews a week, but nothing seemed to materialize. I sincerely believe this was due in great part to my weight problem/appearance, and that my intelligence and experience threatened many of those who interviewed me. I received a letter from one company following an interview stating that the job was offered to someone whose experience better matched their needs. Funny, though, for at least the next three weeks, the very same ad for that job appeared in the paper.

Financial resources became tight. I tried to start an Internet marketing company, but received minimal response and shoved that idea aside. I was still hoping to get my computer distribution business funded, but was unsuccessful. I closed both businesses the end of last year.

I became an Amway distributor just before leaving the computer store. I signed up initially for the dreams and promises of financial freedom it promised were possible. I'm sure that may come some day down the road, but have decided to redirect the other values of the business. I have received something almost as rich as great wealth this past year from that business. I have become very close with my sponsors and receive the kind of encouragement I lacked growing up. They listen to me, and are sincerely interested in my growth and progress whether business related or not.

When I left the computer store, I lost my health benefits. I was forced to cut back drastically on my therapy program. My therapy quickly became the motivational tapes available through my distributorship. They included life stories of the struggles, hard times and successes of other distributors. These changed my perspective on life and gave me a more hopeful outlook. It wasn't long before I didn't miss my weekly therapy sessions.

My relationship with my mother also changed directions. We are now closer and more open and understanding of one another than I ever remember. I'm so excited with life, that the one night a week I visit her, I don't assume the role of her sounding board. I control much of the conversation with enthusiasm behind who I am, my accomplishments and goals.

Last spring, Katherine spent many weekends at the PowerBook keyboard pumping out one manuscript after another. She completed a second book based on the discrimination experience with the computer store in less than four months. Concurrently, she took a complimentary screenplay software program received from a vendor we had contacted with our computer business, and began turning our story into a movie screenplay. She didn't stop with that. She finished another screenplay and almost a third by the end of August.

By fall, I had a long-term, full time temp position with U S WEST. I was still working my other two part time jobs at the same time. All total, I was working over 80 hours a week. The project was suspended in early October.

I wasn't getting enough temp assignments to remain busy with the agencies I was registered with and enlisted with a couple new ones. Most of my assignments seemed to be of an administrative nature instead of graphics; however, I did develop and expand my knowledge and skills on the IBM compatible PC. The first assignment with one of the new agencies landed me a new full time permanent job and career. Since December 9, 1996, I became employed as a secretary in the managed care department of a major national life and health insurance company headquartered in Englewood, Colorado. It was difficult at first to accept a position as a secretary with all my experience, knowledge and skills, but quickly realized it was my foot in the door and only temporary. This company has a tremendous employee training and development program. I see this new career opportunity presenting me with unlimited growth and potential. The company has the typical problems of a large, major corporation experiencing fast growth. Though sometimes difficult to understand or accept, I try to look beyond the individual problems toward the big picture. I find myself excited about what I am doing and learning, but most of all, excited about the people I work with.

Never, in my entire 20-year professional career, have I worked for people who actually acknowledge what I have to contribute to the team, *and* express it to me daily. Despite the typical corporate shortcomings, this company is truly people-oriented and interested in growing and advancing its people resources.

This may all sound exciting and uplifting based on the past I carry with me, but doesn't say everything. I still need to work three jobs for over 80 hours a week to pay off debts from the past few years. I have no social life but feel I am vibrant and alive! I promised friends and family it is only temporary, but find myself faced with a real dilemma when the time comes that I can afford to quit one or both of my part time jobs. Each job has attributes that would be very difficult to walk away from. My security job is not strenuous and gives me a chance to earn wages while being around people and have the opportunity to write, read, catch up on my personal matters, or just drop my pace into a lower gear. I love the warehouse job because of the people I work with. It gives me the exercise I wouldn't otherwise get. I have variety with the tasks I can do and get more computer time. I acknowledge the fact I have become a computer geek.

The changes this past year have not all been work related, though. I experienced some major personal breakthroughs not already mentioned. Mentally, I reached an impasse and decided to do something about my weight problem. Sure, my mom's constant prodding and nagging, and my acceptance that it could be contributing to my not getting a permanent job influenced my decision; however, I do believe it had a lot to do with just finding myself with the right mental aptitude regarding the problem, and ready to make a change. The nutritional resources available through Amway and my warehouse employer influenced my change in the kinds of food and way I ate. It has been a slow, but steady process. I have been able to lose and "keep off" 40 pounds and several inches since March 1996, solely through my own efforts. I hope to continue this gradual process and lose another 60 pounds.

Last year, Gene came back into my life. Not as a lover, but someone I could share my new awareness of hope and encouragement with. I learned at Thanksgiving, from mutual friends, that Gene had some major setbacks after I last spoke with him at the beginning of last year. Sometime in the summer, he suffered a stroke and then a heart attack in addition to suffering from Multiple Sclerosis – and he's not even 50. He was alone in Denver with no other friends or support except that of our mutual friends, and he was deteriorating quickly.

I remembered back to my first hospitalization for depression my freshman year in college. All my close friends from AFROTC came to visit and cheer me up. I was embarrassed for them to see me in a weakened condition, but they made me feel cared about and gave me the encouragement to get through what I was dealing with at the time. Gene is pretty much confined to a wheelchair and the rehab hospital. The stroke partially paralyzed his right side and had a major affect on his speech system.

Since December, I have gone to visit him a few times a month. Weekends, after work, are the only possible times for me to go visit. My mom's not excited that I visit him and places demands on me that cause me to juggle the time they both get. I don't find my visits easy. It is very difficult to understand what he is saying when we do converse. I often don't know what to talk about. My visits only last 10-20 minutes, but are hopefully long enough and interpreted as coming from a concerned friend who cares. I have this interest in giving back some of what others gave me when I needed it.

All of these changes have evolved rather matter-of-factly, but I see them as major events leading to a new me. However, none have affected me more than the discovery I made last fall. During one of my weekend security shifts, I found myself experiencing difficulty organizing my thoughts and generating the desire to do anything. I couldn't understand why Katherine's third screenplay hadn't been finished, let alone touched, for at least three months. This went on for at least two weeks in a row. I soon became troubled by this awareness and looked deeper within myself for the answer. To my surprise, I got no response and soon recognized that sometime during my hectic schedule of the preceding months, I had lost that constant "chatter" I always seemed to have inside my head. Things were now quiet. I even concluded that despite the hectic pace I was keeping, I no longer felt chaos, confusion or being tugged in many directions as in the past. There was a sense of peace to my persona. At first I just thought my sorority of alters had gone on a hiatus. My awareness of this strange phenomena heightened. I began to think I had been abandoned and was alone, but, somehow, didn't really feel alone. I could also recall most of my days and activities with almost no gaps. That's when it hit me...

I hadn't talked to anyone about what it was like when someone with MPD integrates or fuses with their alters, because my system decided long ago against integration. (Okay, I decided against it.) I did remember something that Faith with Justus told my support group. She said alters evolve as protective defense mechanisms when someone is threatened or faced with traumatic issues or events. When a person takes control of their situational environment and come to terms with past traumas, their alters know they have accomplished their task and the independent identity (shield) is no longer needed to protect the host. When the time is right, alters mesh themselves back into the whole being of the core or dominant personality. Another thing Faith said is that this process often seems to just "happen" when you least expect it. The alters don't often ask your permission to integrate or fuse. They decide when the time is right.

This past year I accepted what happened in the past and was ready to "let go;" the big issue surrounding the deep, inner grief I held for my real dad, finally got fully processed, and I allowed myself to let go and move on with my life. I'll never be able to change my mom and her behavior and personality because she is who she feels comfortable with. I have come to accept it and acknowledge that who she is was not completely her choice, but due to her childhood environment and own protective mechanisms. I have allowed myself to forgive her and remove any blame I may have imposed.

Expressing normal love in my birth family was nearly nonexistent. Because of my illnesses and dark past, outside support mechanisms have demonstrated new ways to learn and accept and give love. Hugs are steadily becoming less painful to give and receive. Seeing the unconditional love that has flowed through Karla's family since Stephanie was born with her difficulties and handicaps, and little hope for life beyond a vegetative state, has opened my eyes and shown me the hope and miracles love creates. This past January, Karla's husband, Larry, unselfishly risked his life and underwent day long surgery to donate part of his liver to Stephanie so she could see her 11th birthday. Her difficult life has opened the hearts of my family and brought us closer together, valuing each other for who we are.

I'm amazed with the progress I have made in the past seven years. I have grown, changed, evolved and matured considerably. Just ten short years ago, I was near defeat and ready to accept a shortened life of turmoil, pain and suffering. Today, I can't get enough of life. This is greatly due to reaffirming my faith in my God and asking Him to share my burdens. I miss my internal family and what they accomplished for me. I'm much stronger now and ready to accept full responsibility for my life and future. Since I feel I have assumed all their talents and skills, I also accept that I will never be quite as good as each was, individually, but am thankful for what I do have. I now have allowed others outside my mind and body to accept and love me as my Group did. I still hold this warmth inside my heart that tells me they are not gone for good – that they're quietly off stage watching my progress, and giving me the sense of security that they will come running should I ever need their help again.

I hope that my story will give others who are sick or troubled that, with the proper attitude, faith and support, their situation is temporary and can improve. I don't think anyone who lives on this earth has a perfect life; even those with great wealth and material possessions. Life can never be perfect. There will always be imperfections, but life is what we chose it to be. We chose to be happy or miserable. Life is good and worth living fully if *you* give yourself permission to love, forgive and hold the faith that you will receive the means for happiness once you open your heart and drop the excess baggage you carry. We can't travel back in time to change the past nor right the wrongs done to us. We can chose to make the lives of our perpetrators miserable or "do unto them", but that behavior would lower us to their level. We need to come to terms with those issues, turn the other cheek and forgive them.

Good luck in your personal search and journey for the answers which will provide you with a brighter, happier, and more loving life for you and those you touch.

Michele

APPENDIX

NOTE: This is the published report of the study which I participated in at the National Institutes of Health in the fall of 1986. I am the Patient number 2 that they refer to in their report. Since this hospitalization, my seizures have all but disappeared. Their findings made me more aware of what was happening to me and allowed me to have more control over my episodes. I still suffer from occasional episodes as reported in the study but they are infrequent and don't last as long as earlier in my illness.

* * * *

Dissociative States and Epilepsy

O. Devinsky, MD; F. Putnam, MD; J. Grafman, PhD;
E. Bromfield, MD; W.H. Theodore, MD

Article abstract — Since symptoms of chronic dissociative disorders such as multiple personality disorder (MPD) may be shared by patients with seizure disorders, we investigated the possible relationship between dissociative state and epilepsy. We monitored 6 MPD patients with intensive video-EEG recordings to determine whether epileptic phenomena have any correlation to the dissociative symptoms experienced by these patients. Previously, physicians had diagnosed epilepsy in all 6 patients; however, none proved to have epilepsy. In addition, we studied dissociative symptoms in 71 epileptic patients with the aid of a standardized questionnaire, the Dissociative Experiences Scale, and compared them with age-matched controls. While the group median score of cases with complex partial seizures was higher than that of normal controls, it was significantly lower than that of the psychiatric patients with MPD. Partial seizure patients with dominant hemisphere foci had higher depersonalization subscale scores than those with nondominant foci. Our data suggest that epilepsy is not a primary pathophysiologic mechanism for developing dissociative symptoms.

NEUROLOGY 1989, 39:835-840
Vol. 39, No. 6 pp.835-840, June 1989
Copyright 1989 by Edgell Communications, Inc.

Multiple personality disorder (MPD) is a psychiatric condition in which 2 or more distinct personality states (alters), each with its own relatively enduring pattern of perceiving, relating to, and thinking about the environment and self, exchange control over the behavior of the individual.[1] MPD belongs to a larger category of psychiatric conditions, the dissociative disorders, characterized by disturbances of a sense of oneself, and of memory. The disturbances of self may be (1) loss of memory for self-referential information (psychogenic amnesia), (2) elaborations of secondary identities (eg, psychogenic fugue, multiple personality), or (3) depersonalization. Memory changes typically consist of amnesia (complete or partial) for recall of events occurring while in a dissociative state. Dissocia-

---

[1] American Psychiatric Association. Diagnostic and statistical manual of mental disorders, 3rd ed, rev. Washington, DC: American Psychiatric Press, 1987.

tive disorders such as psychogenic amnesia may occur as acute responses to overwhelming trauma and are common in combat or disasters.[2] Chronic dissociative conditions such as depersonalization syndrome and MPD may be a response to extended stress and repetitive trauma.[3] MPD in particular is closely linked to severe childhood physical and sexual abuse.[4]

Many symptoms reported in MPD are shared by patients with seizure disorders. These include blackouts, fugues, depersonalization, derealization, déjà vu, jamais vu, dreamy states, hypergraphia, and auditory, visual, and olfactory hallucinations.[5] As early as the 19th century, Charcot and Marie and others linked multiple personality with epilepsy.[6] While no EEG data are available on these early cases, recent reports in both the psychiatric[7] and neurologic[8] literature describe patients having MPD and epilepsy or EEG abnormalities. Furthermore, duality of consciousness is clearly recognized as an ictal symptom in patients with temporal lobe epilepsy.[9] Several authors have suggested a pathophysiologic relationship between MPD and seizures. Mesulam suggested[10] that ictal and interictal behavior disturbances related to chronic temporal lobe epilepsy may, in susceptible individuals, produce dissociative states. Putnam has advanced a kindling model of MPD in which repetitive child abuse is the kindling stimulus for the development of MPD.[11] Most MPD patients, however, have normal EEGs.[12]

---

[2] Putnam, FW. Dissociation as a response to extreme trauma. In: Kluft RP, ed. This childhood antecedents of multiple personality. Washington, DC: American Psychiatric Press, 1985.

[3] See above.

[4] Putnam FW, Guroff JJ, Silberman EK, et al. The clinical phenomenology of multiple personality disorder: review of 100 recent cases. J. Clin Psychiatry 1986; 47:285-293.

[5] See above.

Putnam FW. The scientific investigation of multiple personality disorder. In: Quen JM, ed. Split mind/split brains. New York: New York University Press, 1986.

[6] Charcot JM, Marie P. On hysteroepilepsy. In: Tuke H, ed. A dictionary of psychological medicine, vol 1. London: Churchill Publishers, 1892.

Taylor WS, Martin MF. Multiple personality. J. Abnorm Soc Psychol 1944; 39:281-300.

Sutcliffe JP, Jones J. Personal identity, multiple personality, and hypnosis. Int J Clin Hypnosis 1962; 10:231-269.

[7] Cutler B, Reed J. Multiple personality: a single case with a 15-year follow-up. Psychol Med 1975; 5:18-26.

Brende JO, Rinsley DB. A case of multiple personality with psychological automatism. J Am Acad Psychoanal 1981; 9:129-151.

Schenk L, Bear D. Multiple personality and related dissociative phenomena in patients with temporal lobe epilepsy. Am J Psychiatry 1981; 1311-1316.

[8] Mesulam MM. Dissociative states with abnormal temporal lobe EEG. Arch Neurol 1981; 38:176-181.

Benson DF, Miller BL, Signer SF. Dual personality associated with epilepsy. Arch Neurol 1986; 43:471-474.

[9] Kamiya S, Okamoto S. Double consciousness in epileptics: a clinical picture and minor hemisphere specialization. In: Akimoto H, Kazamaturi M, Seino M, et al, eds. Advances in Epileptology: XIIIth Epilepsy International Symposium. New York: Raven Press, 1982.

[10] See note 8 above.

[11] See note 5 above; Putnam Scientific.

[12] See above.

Coons PM, Milstein V, Marley C. EEG studies of two multiple personalities and a control. Arch Gen Psychiatry 1982; 39:823-825.

Concores JA, Bender AI, McBride E. Multiple personality, seizure disorder, and the electroencephalogram. J Nerv Ment Dis 1984; 172:436-438.

This study investigates the possible relationship between dissociative symptoms and epilepsy from 2 perspectives. The first is the intensive video-EEG monitoring of MPD patients to determine what, if any, relationship epileptic phenomena have to dissociative symptoms experienced by the patients. The second perspective is to investigate dissociative symptoms in epileptic patients with the aid of a standardized questionnaire, the Dissociative Experiences Scale (DES).[13] If there is a primary pathophysiologic relationship between dissociation and epilepsy, we hypothesize that there should be an elevation of DES scores in epileptic patients comparable to those seen in the dissociative disorders.

METHODS. *Diagnosis of MPD.* The diagnosis of MPD was made independently on each patient by 1 investigator (F.P.), and by 1 or more treating psychiatrists. All MPD patients satisfied the Diagnostic and Statistical Manual of Mental Disorders (DSM-IIIR) criteria for MPD.[14]

Dissociative Experiences Scale methodology. The DES is a 28-item, self-administered questionnaire that reliably discriminates patients with MPD from other psychiatric patients.[15] The completed questionnaire yields an overall score, ranging from 0 to 100, and 3 subscale scores (dissociation, depersonalization, absorption). The DES was administered to 71 patients with generalized seizures (n=12) and complex seizures (n=59) who fulfilled the criteria in the 1981 International Classification of Epileptic Seizures.[16] Among those right-handed individuals with complex partial seizures, 17 had dominant hemisphere seizure foci, and 16 had seizure foci in the nondominant hemisphere. The DES was also administered to age-matched comparison groups of 34 normal controls and 42 MPD patients participating in National Institute of Mental Health research protocols. Because dissociative phenomena are not normally distributed within the population, all DES scores are analyzed nonparametrically.[17] Pairwise comparisons between groups were done with the Kruskal-Wallis test.

RESULTS. The first set of data consists of the results of the intensive video-EEG monitoring of 6 patients with MPD who were evaluated at the National Institutes of Health, Clinical Epilepsy Section (NIH/CES), in whom the diagnosis of epilepsy was strongly suspected. The clinical features of these cases are summarized in table 1. Table 2 presents the clinical-EEG correlations of behavioral episodes in these same patients. The 2nd portion of this section presents the results of our administration of the DES in patients with epilepsy or MPD, and normal subjects.

Report of cases. The following 2 case reports are typical of the 6 cases seen between 1981 and 1987 at the NIH/CES for evaluation of possible seizure disorders. All patients were intensely monitored with telemetered video-EEG recordings as previously de-

---

[13] Bernstein EM, Putnam FW. Development, reliability, and validity of a dissociative scale. J Nerv Ment Dis 1986; 174:727-735.

[14] See note 1 above.

[15] See note 13 above.

Ross CA, Norton GR, Anderson G. The Dissociation Experiences Scale: a replication study. Dissociation 1988; 1:21-23.

[16] Commission on Classification and Terminology of the International League Against Epilepsy. Proposal for revised clinical and electroencephalographic classification of epileptic seizures. Epilepsia 1981; 22:489-501.

[17] See note 13 above.

scribed.[18] In 4 of the 6 subjects, sphenoidal electrodes were used during intensive monitoring. The diagnosis of MPD was made in 4 individuals prior to admission, while in 2 it was made afterward. EEG recordings (with the standard 10-20 scalp electrode placement) were performed at the NIH EEG Laboratory. Hyperventilation, photic stimulation, and stage 1-2 sleep recordings were obtained in all patients except no. 6.

Patient 1. A 40-year-old right-handed woman was admitted to the NIH/CES for evaluation of a possible seizure disorder. She had a history of physical and sexual abuse by her father since early childhood. She also had a sister who had been diagnosed as schizophrenic. Initial psychiatric presentation was at age 32, with depression and suicidal ideation. However, the patient admitted to affective symptoms since childhood. Between ages 32 and 37, she had 11 hospitalizations for depression and various suicide attempts (overdosages, wrist slashing, hanging). The diagnosis of MPD was made at age 37. Since then, 28 separate personalities had been identified.

A seizure disorder was first diagnosed at age 14 during a 3-week hospitalization for vertigo. In the hospital she had an episode of loss of consciousness that she now states was due to hyperventilation and "bearing down" (i.e., Valsalva maneuver), but it had been concealed from the doctors. Her EEG was interpreted as "mildly abnormal," and she was started on phenytoin, which she discontinued during college. Since age 32, she had had 2 episodes of nocturnal enuresis that were considered to be possible seizures. In addition, the patient reported "zings," which she characterized as electric shocks moving rapidly up and down her spine, and then passing down through her extremities. These were usually concomitant with changes in personality.

A neurologist diagnosed temporal lobe epilepsy because of depersonalization and fear and 3 previous EEGs that all revealed bursts of temporal theta activity. The patient was started on carbamazepine, and despite serum levels of up to 12 μg/ml, there was no change in episodic or affective symptoms.

On admission to NIH, the general medical and neurologic examinations were entirely normal. Medications included carbamazepine (1,000 mg/day) and alprazolam (2.0 mg/day); they were discontinued within 4 days of admission. A 90-minute EEG recording (including sphenoidal electrodes) was normal; theta activity was recorded only during drowsiness. During 6 days of video-EEG telemetry with sphenoidal electrodes, at least 5 episodes of each of the following behavioral changes were recorded: (1) confusion; (2) personality change; (3) "zings" (see above), and (4) brief paroxysmal feelings of fear or sadness. There was no observable change in the background rhythms during any episodes.

On 18-month follow-up, the treating psychiatrist reported that the patient made significant progress in working through her traumatic memories. However, she has had no change in the frequency of her "spells." There has been increased depression and suicidal ideation associated with the recovery of these memories, and the patient has required 3 psychiatric hospitalizations. Auditory hallucinations, self-mutilation, and headaches are reportedly decreased. There has been no change in the degree of dissociative symptoms.

Patient 2. This 32-year-old right-handed woman with MPD was admitted to the NIH/CES for evaluation of a possible seizure disorder. She had been physically abused by her father, and during childhood had an incestuous relationship with her older brother. Initial psychiatric presentation was at age 26 with depression and attempted suicide. She was subsequently treated with tricyclic antidepressants, monoamine oxidase inhibitors, and electro-

---

[18] Porter RJ, Wolf AA Jr, Penry JK. Human electroencephalographic telemetry. Am J EEG Technol 1971; 11:145-159.

convulsive shock, with limited success. MPD was diagnosed at age 28. Since then, 15 personalities have been identified.

This patient has had several types of paroxysmal episodes that were considered seizures. These included (1) "blackout spells" with initial distortion of sounds, dizziness, and progressive constriction of her visual field over several minutes, which at times progressed to blindness (1 spell in childhood was associated with a loss of consciousness); frequency was once a day, duration was 20 seconds to 5 minutes; (2) confusional episodes, usually preceded by paresthesias in the left or both hands that sometimes spread to the elbow after 2 minutes, followed by a "fading away" feeling and an inability to comprehend speech (frequency was 1 to 20 per day, duration was 20 to 40 seconds); and (3) rare tonic or clonic movements lasting less than 2 minutes. She had 6 EEGs; 3 revealed no abnormalities, 2 had bursts of anterior theta activity, and 1 had rare temporal spikes. Previous video-EEG monitoring included several episodes thought to be potentially epileptic, with no background changes (despite use of sphenoidal electrodes). The patient had been treated with clonazepam, primidone, valporic acid, phenytoin, carbamazepine, and methsuximide. None of these medications was effective treating the paroxysmal episodes.

On admission to NIH, the general medical and neurologic examinations were entirely normal. Medications included clonazepam (4 mg/day) and lorazepam (1.5 mg/day). All medications were discontinued within 4 days of admission. A 90-minute EEG (including sphenoidal electrodes) was normal. During 5* days of video-EEG telemetry with sphenoidal electrodes, 12 confusional episodes (all preceded by paresthesias) and 8 episodes of clonic activity (usually starting in the upper extremities, but spreading to all 4 limbs, with preservation of consciousness) were recorded. There was no change in the EEG background activity during or after any of these events. When informed that the episodes were probably not epileptic, the patient was disappointed, and responded, "My mother will be very upset that I do not have epilepsy."

On 18-month follow-up, the patient's treating psychiatrist reports an almost complete disappearance of psychogenic seizures and a refocusing of therapy on vocational functioning. Concurrently, there has been a decrease in depression, suicidality, conversion symptoms, panic attacks, and depersonalization. No further hospitalizations have been required.

DISCUSSION. The 6 patients with MPD illustrate the clinical profile typically found in MPD patients.[19] They had extensive complicated psychiatric histories beginning an average of 7 years before the diagnosis of MPD. These patients were polysymptomatic with depression, mood swings, anxiety, self-destructive behavior, depersonalization, and conversion reactions. Neurologic symptoms consisted of amnesia, headaches, seizure-like confusional or black-out episodes, and paresthesias; medical complaints were often of abdominal pain and gastrointestinal distress. These individuals were refractory to the standard treatments for these disorders. As with previously reported MPD series,[20] our patients acquired various psychiatric, neurologic, and medical diagnoses over the course of their illnesses. While many met diagnostic criteria for personality disorder diagnosis (DSM-IIR Axis II), the superordinate diagnosis was MPD, and the other symptom clusters can be understood as part of the dissociative disorder.[21] A history of childhood physical

---

[19] See note 4 above.

[20] Coons PM, Bowman ES, Milstein V. Multiple personality disorder: a clinical investigation of 50 cases. J Nerv Ment Dis 1988; 176:519-527.

[21] Putnam FW, Loewenstein RJ, Silberman EK, et al. Multiple personality disorder in a hospital setting. J Clin Psychiatry 1984; 146:81-89.

and sexual abuse was uncovered in each case, and is thought to play an instrumental role in the development of dissociative states.[22]

All 6 patients were referred to the NIH/CES with a diagnosis of definite or probable seizure disorders. Paroxysmal behavioral episodes and equivocal abnormalities demonstrated on EEG suggested epilepsy to the referring physicians. However, additional studies and clinical follow-up did not support seizures as the pathophysiologic mechanism for these events. There was no evidence of epileptiform discharges on video-EEG telemetered recording during prolonged interictal (in all patients) and ictal (patients 1, 2, 4, and 5) periods. Moreover, there was no improvement in "seizure-like" episodes in response to antiepileptic medications with therapeutic serum levels for all patients, but in 2 patients (nos. 2 and 4) there was a reduction in these episodes after the patient was told that laboratory studies did not suggest a diagnosis of epilepsy.

The clinical episodes that were thought to be seizures may be divided into 3 principal types: (1) transient sensory, affective, cognitive phenomena similar to simple partial seizures; (2) dissociative states, including periods of confusion with subsequent amnesia but without automatisms; and (3) convulsive movements. The first type, which includes symptoms such as "electric shocks," paresthesias, and epigastric and olfactory hallucinations, are not diagnostic of seizures. Silberman et al[23] found that affective and seizure patients were similar in terms of the number and frequency reported symptoms in relation to illness. This finding may be relevant, since depression was present in 5 of the 6 patients in this study (4 had attempted suicide).

Dissociative states have been reported in patients with seizure disorders and may occur during prodromal,[24] ictal,[25] postictal, or interictal[26] periods. Amnesia, depersonalization, and bizarre feelings are common to both seizure-related and functional dissociative episodes, and differentiation between these entities may be difficult. The pathophysiologic role of epilepsy in the development of dissociative states is supported by definite epileptiform discharges on EEG, a clear temporal relation between seizures and behavioral episodes, and improvement following antiepileptic therapy.

The referring physicians used EEG data to support the diagnosis of seizures in 5 of the 6 patients. Of the 29 EEGs obtained in these patients (11 at the NIH), 14 were normal (8 at the NIH), 11 revealed nonspecific abnormalities (2 at the NIH), and 4 demonstrated potentially epileptiform discharges (1 at the NIH). Intermittent theta activity or "slowing" over the temporal region during drowsiness was the most prominent EEG "abnormality" in 2 patients; however, this may be a normal occurrance during the drowsy state.[27] Fourteen- and 6-Hz positive spike discharges were present in the outside EEGs obtained in patient 3; however, these are not considered epileptiform, and are rarely the only findings in patients with proven seizures.[28] The 4 EEG studies with epileptiform discharges were obtained from 3 patients (nos. 2, 4, and 5) Patient 2 had rare temporal spikes in 1 of 7 EEGs; however, the EEG with such temporal spikes was unavailable for our review. The importance of this finding is questionable, since 1 or more epileptiform transients, usually spikes, were

[22] See note 2 above.

[23] Silberman EK, Post RM, Nurnberger J, et al. Transient sensory, cognitive and affective phenomena in affective illness: a comparison with complex partial epilepsy. Br J Psychiatry 1085; 146:81-89.

[24] See note 8 above; Benson.

[25] Daly D. Ictal affect. Am J Psychiatry 1958; 115:97-108.

[26] See notes 7 & 8 above; Schenck & Mesulam.

[27] Niedermeyer E, Lopes de Silva F. Electroencephalography. Baltimore: Urban and Schwarzenberg, 1987:193.

[28] See above.

present in 24% of normal subjects who were sleep-deprived for 24 hours.[29] In patient 5, there were sharp waves over the right temporal area in 1 recording, but this was during drug withdrawal. Patient 3 had 3 normal EEGs and 2 with occasional temporal sharp transients. Since the interictal EEG contains epileptiform discharges in more than 90% of patients with complex partial seizures,[30] the EEG findings in our patients do not clearly support the diagnosis of seizure disorder. However, the high incidence of nonepileptiform abnormalities in our patients suggests that a neurophysiologic abnormality may contribute to the pathogenesis of MPD.

The temporal relationship between dissociative episodes and seizures is critical, but most significant is the recognition that not all episodes of impaired consciousness or tonic and clonic movements represent seizures. In 5 patients (nos. 1, 2, 4, 5, and 6), behavioral episodes (including 13 with confusion and subsequent amnesia; 24 with clonic shaking movements) previously considered to be seizures were recorded with telemetered video-EEG (table 2). These events were atypical for seizures (see below) and were not associated with EEG changes during the prodromal, ictal, or postictal periods. Although the incidence of EEG changes using scalp electrodes during nonmotor simple partial seizures is less than 25%,[31] the incidence during complex partial seizures is approximately 90%.[32] We recorded 57 personality changes in 2 patients (nos. 1 & 4), but found no epileptiform EEG changes. The description of behavioral episodes by nonmedical personnel strongly suggested epilepsy, but the results of simultaneous video-EEG recordings discount this diagnosis.

There is difficulty differentiating between complex partial seizures and dissociative states with confusion and subsequent amnesia. Although all 6 patients had periods of altered consciousness and amnesia, we identified atypical features. Complex partial seizures usually last less than 5 minutes and include automatisms in approximately 90% of the cases.[33] In contrast, all our patients had episodes of impaired consciousness for more than 10 minutes, and none had automatisms reported during these episodes. Another important aspect of complex partial seizures is the postictal period, which begins when the patient first responds to a command or questions, and ends when responses are complete and accurate.[34] A postictal period is present in 80% of complex partial seizures, and lasts approximately 90 seconds.[35] We did not observe distinct postictal periods in our 6 patients. Also atypical for true seizures is the modification of clonic movements by suggestion as seen in patient 2. The failure of epileptic drugs to alter paroxysmal behavioral episodes is another indication that seizures are not the relevant mechanism. Although 16 anticonvulsants were administered to the 6 patients, there was no definite improvement in any subject. However, 2 patients had fewer "seizures" after we discussed the nonepileptic nature of the events with each of them.

---

[29] White JC, Langston JW, Pedley TA. Benign epileptiform transients of sleep. Neurology 1977; 27:1061-1068.

[30] Escueta AVD, Basca FE, Treiman DM. Complex partial seizures on closed-circuit television and EEG: a study of 691 attacks in 79 patients. Ann Neurol 1982; 11:292-300.

Theodore WH, Porter RJ, Penry JK. Complex partial seizures: clinical characteristics and differential diagnosis. Neurology 1983; 33:1115-1121.

[31] See above.

[32] See above.

Ajimone-Marsan C, Ralston BL. The Epileptic Seizure. Springfield, IL: Charles C Thomas, 1957.

[33] See above.

Devinsky O, Kelley K, Theodore WH, et al. Clinical and electroencephalographic features of simple partial pressures. Neurology 1988, 38:1347-1352.

[34] See note 30 above; Theodore.

[35] See above.

As a 2nd perspective on the relationship between epilepsy and dissociative states, we compared the number and types of dissociative experiences in complex partial seizure patients with those from MPD patients and normal controls. Although the DES scores of the seizure patients were moderately elevated as compared with those of normal individuals, these patients' scores were similar in range to those previously reported for psychiatric patients with anxiety or phobic disorders.[36] However, we found a 20% overlap between the DES scores of seizure disorder and MPD patients, demonstrating that about 1/5 of patients with epilepsy have significant dissociative experiences.

Our data do not support the hypothesis that epilepsy is a primary pathophysiologic mechanism for developing dissociative symptoms. Six MPD patients who suffered from a chronic dissociative disorder did not prove to have epilepsy although all had been diagnosed and treated for a seizure disorder at some point during their illness. If epilepsy plays a primary role in the development of dissociative symptoms, we might have expected to see higher levels of dissociative symptoms as indicated on the DES in our seizure patients. When we reviewed the clinical records of the 5 epileptic patients with the highest DES scores, we found no evidence of psychiatric disorders. While some dissociative patients have epilepsy,[37] the etiologic role of seizures is uncertain. Coons et al[38] found a 14% incidence of psychogenic seizures and a 10% incidence of epilepsy (40% of whom had post-traumatic seizures) in 50 patients with MPD. These authors concluded that the dissociation in MPD is not due to ictal or interictal limbic system epileptic discharges.[39] However, in selected individuals, seizures may play an important role in the manifestation of dissociative states.[40]

Note: "Sorority" author's records indicate this testing lasted 11 days.

---

[36] See note 13 above.

[37] See note 20 above.

[38] See above.

[39] See above.

[40] See notes 7 & 8 above; Schenk, Mesulam & Benson.

Table 1. Clinical features

Pt. No.	Age, Sex	Seizure pattern	Diagnostic studies	Anticonvulsant treatment & type of response	IQ score	DES score
1	40 F	(1) Nocturnal enuresia; (2) electric shocks moving up and down spine and extremities	EEGs mildly abnormal in 1 episode, bursts of theta in 3 episodes; normal in 1 episode	Carbamazepine and phenytoin: no response	V-96 P-100 FS-98	63.4
2	32 F	*(1) Distortion of sounds, dizziness, progressive constriction of visual field; (2) confusion preceded by parethesias in left or both hands; (3) tonic and/or clonic jerking movements*	*EEGs had rare temporal spike in 1 episode, bursts of anterior theta activity in 2 episodes; and normal activity in 4 episodes*	*Clonazepam, mysoline valporic acid, phenytoin, and methsuximide: no response*	*V-107 F-104 FS-105*	43.2
3	38 F	(1) Dissociative episodes; (2) Blank stare with "glassy eyes"	CT normal; 6- and 14-Hz positive spike or sharp activity in 4 episodes	Carbamazepine: no response	V-99 P-104 FS-105	19.0

Table 1 (Continued)

4	26 F	(1) Forced staring without alteration of consciousness; (2) Feelings of "darkness, scrunched up" with impaired responsiveness	CT normal; EEGs showed left temporal transients in 2 episodes, and were normal in 4 episodes	Pheytoin, carbamazepine, primidone, and valporic acid, equivocal improvement	V-102 F-98 FS-100	51.1
5	40 M	(1) Syncopal episodes with confusion; (2) Agitated behavior	24-hour Holter monitor was normal; normal CT; EEG showed sharp waves over right temporal area during nticonvulsant withdrawal in 1 episode; nonspecific abnormalities in 1; and normal in 1	Phenytoin, primidone, and methsuximide: no repsonse	Not Available	70.9
6	26 F	(1) "Foggy feeling" with impaired memory	EEG was normal in 5 episodes	Carbamazepine: mood improvement	V-122 P-102	Not Available